CARCIOVASCULAR GENETICS FOR CLINICIANS

Developments in Cardiovascular Medicine

VOLUME 239

The titles published in this series are listed at the end of this volume.

Cardiovascular Genetics for Clinicians

edited by

P.A. Doevendans
Academic Hospital Maastricht,
Maastricht, The Netherlands

and

A.A.M. Wilde
Academic Medical Center,
Amsterdam, The Netherlands

SPRINGER-SCIENCE+BUSINESS MEDIA, B.V.

A C.I.P. Catalogue record for this book is available from the Library of Congress.

ISBN 978-94-010-3888-1 ISBN 978-94-010-1019-1 (eBook)
DOI 10.1007/978-94-010-1019-1

Table of Contents

List of Contributors

W.R.P. Agema
Department of Cardiology, LUMC, P.O. Box 9600, 2300 RC LEIDEN, The Netherlands
Co-authors: J.W. Jukema

C. Basso
Department of Biology, University of Padua, Via U Bassi 58/B, 35131 PADOVA, Italy.
Co-authors: G.A. Danieli, A. Rampazzo, G. Thiene, A. Nava

H.J. Blom
Department of Internal Medicine, Academic Hospital St. Radbout, P.O. Box 6500, 6500 HB NIJMEGEN, The Netherlands
Co-authors: F.F. Willems, G.H.J. Boers

R. Brugada
Section of Cardiology, Department of Medicine, Baylor College of Medicine, Houston,Texas 77030, USA
Co-author: R. Roberts

G.H.J. Boers
Department of Internal Medicine, Academic Hospital St. Radbout, P.O. Box 6500, 6500 HB NIJMEGEN, The Netherlands
Co-authors: H.J. Blom, F.F. Willems

G. Bonne
INSERM UR523, Institut de Myologie, Batiment Babinski, Groupe Hospitalier Pitie-Salpetriere 47, bd de l'Hopital, PARIS, France
Co-authors: P.A. Doevendans, C. Marcelis

B.J.C. van den Bosch
Department of Molecular Genetics, Academic Hospital Maasticht, P.O. Box 5800 AZ MAASTRICHT, The Netherlands
Co-authors: H.J.M. Smeets, R.J.E Jongbloed, I.F.M. de Coo

L. Carrier
INSERM UR523, Institut de Myologie, Batiment Babinski, Groupe Hospitalier Pitie-Salpetriere 47, bd de l'Hopital, PARIS, France
Co-authors: R.J.E. Jongbloed, H.J.M. Smeets, P.A. Doevendans

I.F.M. de Coo
Department of Neurology, AZR Sophia, P.O. Box 2060, 3000 CB ROTTERDAM, The Netherlands
Co-authors: B.J.C. van den Bosch, H.J.M. Smeets, R.J.E Jongbloed

R. Corrocher
Department of Clinical and Experimental Medicine
Policlinic GB Rossi, 37134 VERONA, Italy
Co-authors: D. Girelli, O. Olivieri

G.A. Danieli
Department of Biology, University of Padua, Via U Bassi 58/B, 35131 PADOVA, Italy.
Co-authors: A. Rampazzo, G. Thiene, A. Nava, C. Basso

J.C. Defesche
Vascular Medicine, Academic Medical Center, Meibergdreef 15, 1105 AZ AMSTERDAM, The Netherlands
Co-author: J.J.P. Kastelein

P.A. Doevendans
Department of Cardiology, Academic Hospital Maastricht, P.O. Box 5800, 6202 AZ MAASTRICHT, The Netherlands
Co-authors: L. Carrier, R.J.E. Jongbloed, H.J.M. Smeets

D. Girelli
Department of Clinical and Experimental Medicine
Policlinic GB Rossi, 37134 VERONA, Italy
Co-authors: O. Olivieri, R. Corrocher

P. Grossfeld
UCSD medical Center, Division of Pediatric Cardiology, University of California, 200 West Arbor Drive, SAN DIEGO, CA 92103-8445, USA

R.J.E Jongbloed
Department of Molecular Genetics, Academic Hospital Maastricht, P.O. Box 5800, 6202 AZ MAASTRICHT, The Netherlands
Co-authors: B.J.C. van den Bosch, I.F.M. de Coo, H.J.M. Smeets

J.W. Jukema
Department of Cardiology, CS-P, LUMC, P.O. Box 9600, 2300 RC LEIDEN, The Netherlands
Co-authors: W.R.P. Agema

J.J.P. Kastelein
Vascular Medicine, Academic Medical Center, Meibergdreef 15, 1105 AZ AMSTERDAM, The Netherlands
Co-author: J.C. Defesche

A.A. Kroon
Department of Internal Medicine, Academic Hospital Maastricht, P.O. Box 5800 6202 AZ Maastricht, The Netherlands
Co-authors: W. Spiering, P.W. de Leeuw

I.M. van Langen
Department of Cardio Genetics, Academisch Medical Center, Meibergdreef 15, 1105 AZ AMSTERDAM, The Netherlands
Co-authors: C. Marcelis, Wilde A.A, J.P. van Tintelen

P.W. de Leeuw
Department of Internal Medicine, Academic Hospital Maastricht, P.O. Box 5800 6202 AZ Maastricht, The Netherlands
Co-authors: A.A. Kroon, W. Spiering

M.M.A.M. Mannens
Department of Clinical Genetics, Academic Medical Center, Meibergdreef 15, 1105 AZ AMSTERDAM, The Netherlands
Co-authors: H.J.M. Smeets

C. Marcelis
Department of Clinical Genetics, Academic Hospital Maastricht, P.O. Box 5800, 6202 AZ MAASTRICHT, The Netherlands
Co-authors: P.A. Doevendans, G. Bonne

A. Nava
Department of Biology, University of Padua, Via U Bassi 58/B, 35131 PADOVA, Italy.
Co-authors: C. Basso, G.A. Danieli, A. Rampazzo, G. Thiene

O. Olivieri
Department of Clinical and Experimental Medicine
Policlinic GB Rossi, 37134 VERONA, Italy
Co-authors: R. Corrocher, D. Girelli

G.B. van Ommen
Department of Human Genetics, Leiden University Medical Center, Wasenaarseweg 72, 2333 AL LEIDEN, The Netherlands

L. Pérez Jurado
Department of Experimental and Health Sciences,University Pompeu Fabra, Dr. Aiguader 80, 08003 BARCELONA, Spain

A. Rampazzo
Department of Biology, University of Padua, Via U Bassi 58/B, 35131 PADOVA, Italy.
Co-authors: G. Thiene, C. Basso, A. Nava, G.A. Danieli

R. Roberts
Section of Cardiology, Department of Medicine, Baylor College of Medicine, Houston,Texas 77030, USA
Co-author: R. Brugada

P.N. Robinson
Institute for Medical Genetics, University Clinic Charité, Schumannstr. 20/21, 10098 BERLIN, Germany

H.J.M. Smeets
Department of Molecular Genetics, Academic Hospital Maastricht, P.O. Box 5800, 6202 AZ MAASTRICHT, The Netherlands
Co-authors: L. Carrier, R.J.E. Jongbloed, P.A. Doevendans

W. Spiering
Department of Internal Medicine, Academic Hospital Maastricht, P.O. Box 5800 6202 AZ Maastricht, The Netherlands
Co-authors: P.W. de Leeuw, A.A. Kroon

G. Thiene
Department of Biology, University of Padua, Via U Bassi 58/B, 35131 PADOVA, Italy.
Co-authors: C. Basso, A. Nava, G.A. Danieli, A. Rampazzo

J.P. van Tintelen
Department of Clinical Genetics-AZG, Academisch Hospital Groningen, P.O. Box 30001, 9700 RB GRONINGEN, The Netherlands
Co-authors: C. Marcelis, I.M. van Langen, Wilde A.A

M.A. Vos
Department of Cardiology, Academic Hospital Maastricht, P.O. Box 5800, 6202 AZ MAASTRICHT, The Netherlands
Co-authors: X.H.T. Wehrens, A.A. Wilde

Wilde A.A
Department of Cardiology, Academisch Medical Center, Meibergdreef 15, 1105 AZ AMSTERDAM, The Netherlands
Co-authors: C. Marcelis, J.P. van Tintelen, I.M. van Langen

F.F. Willems
Department of Internal Medicine, Rijnstate Hospital, P.O. Box 9555, 6800 TA ARNHEM, The Netherlands
Co-authors: G.H.J. Boers, H.J. Blom

X.H.T. Wehrens
Department of Cardiology, Academic Hospital Maastricht, P.O. Box 5800, 6202 AZ MAASTRICHT, The Netherlands.
Co-authors: M.A. Vos, A.A. Wilde

PREFACE

All physicians practicing medicine encounter patients suffering from cardiovascular disease. This book has been outlined in such a way that vascular surgeons, general internists, neurologists and cardiologists should be able to use it. The book covers the complete scope of cardiac diseases in addition to chapters on hypertension and atherosclerosis. In many patients there is a family history of cerebrovascular accidents, myocardial infarction or peripheral arterial disease. Also in patients reporting collaps, palpitations and arrhythmias the family is crucial and can provide clues to a genetic cause of the disease. This book is published to guide physicians in the process of determining whether a genetic component is likely to be present. Furthermore, information is provided what the possibilities and limitations of DNA diagnostic techniques are. Finally, the importance of newly identified categories of potential patients, i.e. gene carriers without symptoms or any inducible sign of disease, is highlighted. For some patients a genetic diagnosis is essential to determine appropriate therapy and for counseling? In some other diseases DNA diagnostic tools are available but the relevant for the patients may be less clear. In other families the search for a disease causing gene is ongoing and the possibilities to find genes and to unravel the pathophysiology of the disease is limited by the lack of patients. To give insight into the current state of genetic diagnostics, the authors have classified the cardiovascular diseases. Category A indicates a disease state for which the molecular diagnosis is crucial for the pharmacological treatment. In category F diseases are included that have a positive family history, but in whom we have no clue where the disease gene is positioned in the genome. The classification should provide the handlebars to select and inform patients. Molecular diagnosis is a very active field and we realize that the moment the book is published the possibilities will have changed for some diseases. Furthermore, new drug development could have genotype dependent effects, which would be another reason to consider re-evaluation of the information in this book. Where possible we included internet references and hint to where you can look for up to date genetic analysis available. We hope you enjoy reading the book and that it gives you true support in making clinical decisions.
P.A. Doevendans, A.A. Wilde

* Acknowledgement
We are indebted to Nicolle van Geleen and Xander Wehrens for their help in preparing the manuscript.

PA Doevendans and AA Wilde (eds.), Cardiovascular genetics.

INTRODUCTION TO GENETICS

P.A. Doevendans

Introduction

Molecular Cardiology is changing our concepts of cardiovascular development, disease etiology, pathophysiology and therapy at a rapid pace. The power of the biological approach for cardiovascular pathology and therapy, is based on the strict relation between DNA (carrying the genetic code), RNA (the messenger between the nucleus and the cytoplasm, containing a copy of the genetic code) and proteins (the final gene product with a specific function). Every gene (DNA) contains the code for one or more related proteins. In addition to the coding DNA, every gene has a regulatory DNA sequence, controlling the expression level of the gene. It is this regulatory part, that has to be activated to start RNA production (transcription) A scheme is presented in figure 1. For additional cartoons look at www.translational-med.nl) [1]. Which genes are active in different cell types depends on the interaction of the regulatory DNA of various genes with nuclear proteins. These nuclear proteins, the so-called transcription factors, can recognize regulatory DNA sequences and modulate the level of transcription. Once a gene is activated and transcribed mRNA is produced. mRNA subsequently migrates from the nucleus to the cytoplasm, where the genetic code is translated into amino acids (appendix I and II). The chemical binding of adjacent amino acids leads to peptide and protein formation. The function of the protein determines eventually the impact of changes at the DNA level.

Molecular genetics

Single nucleotide polymorphism

Several tools have been developed in molecular biology to identify genetic differences between individuals [2]. It is estimated that there is a single nucleotide polymorphism (SNP) in every 1000 basepairs (bp) of DNA. As 95% of the genomic DNA seems to be without function and does not contain genes, most SNPs (2.6 million) are positioned outside genes [3]. Therefore, only a minority of the SNPs has been detected within genes. SNP can be indicated by base and position in the gene like G346A. This means that the Guanine base at position 346 from the start site of transcription, has been substituted by the base Adenine. SNPs in coding DNA (exons) can have consequences if the genetic code is altered leading to an amino acid substitution.

PA Doevendans and AA Wilde (eds.), Cardiovascular genetics.

This is often indicate by A1490D or Ala1490Asp. This implies an amino acid switch at position 1490 form Alanine to Aspartic acid. Due to redundancy in the genetic code some SNPs will have no effect (Appendix II). SNPs positioned in either the regulatory sequences or introns can effect transcription regulation. Some polymorphisms will increase transcription, where others will block it. This has been shown for instance for the cholesterol ester transferase protein (CETP). CETP is responsible for cholesterol ester transport from HDL to LDL. A SNP in the first intron is associated with increased CETP levels and decreased high density lipoprotein (HDL) levels [4].

Mutations

The terms polymorphism and mutation can be confusing. The most frequently used definition is based on population studies, where genetic variation is considered to be a polymorphism when it is found in at least 1% of the population. Some variations are very rare, only present in a few % of the studied individuals. This could indicate a short history for the genetic change or an unfavorable genetic makeup. Other variations are found in almost 50% of the people and for these changes it remains unclear what should be considered normal and what is the variant.
The other definition considers every variation a polymorphism and the term mutation is reserved for variations with measurable effects on gene activity or protein composition. It is not clear by which mechanism the SNP in intron 1 of the CETP gene influences transcription. The identified change may not even be the real cause of the difference in circulating CETP levels. Possibly this altered base is just a genetic marker for another base substitution elsewhere in the gene. Therefore the base alteration is considered a polymorphism, a genetic variant which is associated with -but not necessarily causally related to- a certain parameter, here the CETP level. Genetic changes that are causally related to disease are termed mutation.

Mutations have been identified as the cause of monogenic diseases that can cause congenital cardiac defects (chapter 3), atherosclerosis (chapter 4-8) connective tissue disorders (chapter 9-10) cardiomyopathy (chapter 11-13), and arrhythmias (chapter 14-17). In these monogenic diseases the mutations appear to be positioned in exons leading to an amino acid substitution (missense mutations). Other mutations introduce a stop codon (triplet codon that does not match with any amino acid), leading to a premature termination of translation and a truncated protein. When one base is missing a shift in the reading frame occurs leading to a new (often nonsense) protein (figure 2). In addition, the processing of RNA involves steps to remove introns from the precursor RNA (splicing). Some mutations (one or more bases) can interfere with the process of splicing and obstruct the formation of messenger RNA, that is required to bring the genetic code to the ribosome for translation. Several bases can be missing (deletion) or extra (insertion). Insertion of DNA fragments can occur in introns with unpredictable consequences for RNA and protein processing (Angiotensin Converting Enzyme gene) [5].

Classification of monogenetic diseases

To guide clinicians in referring patients for DNA diagnostics we classified the monogenetic diseases into 6 categories form A to F. For category F diseases, no chromosomal locus or gene is known, but from the family history and pedigree analysis a genetic factor appears obvious. In these families and diseases the genetic analysis has still to be initiated. In category E disease a locus has been identified. However as one locus contains many different genes the further elucidation of the disease mechanism awaits the recognition of the affected gene. The solid establishment of the relation between disease and chromosomal locus, is sometimes enough to recognize individuals at risk. As various diseases can be caused by different genes often the gene is identified in some families whereas in other families only the locus is known.
As indicated above the role of polymorphisms is often unclear, as a SNP can be genetic marker of variance instead of the explanation of the disease (category D). In general, a specific polymorphism can be found significantly more often in patients compared to healthy individuals. But the impact can be very limited and the polymorphism if present does not always lead to disease. Therefore the significance is often a matter of debate, related to genetic background, and environmental factors. The importance of DNA analysis is therefore limited and rarely indicated, except for patients included in well defined studies. With category C diseases we indicate the group of monogenic diseases where DNA diagnostics are available, but contribute little to clinical decision making. This in contrast to category B, where diseases are included that could lead to counseling advice. Once a mutation within a family has been identified, DNA diagnostics can be used early in pregnancy, which is only relevant if extensively discussed during counseling. In category A disease, the correct diagnosis guides the actual treatment of the patient, either pharmaceutically or by mechanical intervention. Here DNA diagnostics can also be used to decide upon preventive treatment. Preventive treatment should be considered in any genetic cardiovascular disease.

Preventive treatment

The availability of DNA diagnostic approaches leads to the recognition of predisposed 'healthy' individuals. A good example is the long QT syndrome (category A). We can now distinguish patients, they have symptoms, an abnormal ECG and carry the mutation. However family members may carry the mutation, have a prolonged QTc interval but still be asymptomatic. Should we treat these individuals preventively? What should be done if individuals have a normal ECG, no symptoms but in whom a mutation has been documented? The new genetic tools, allow us to recognize new, disease prone individuals. In the future we will have to monitor closely, what the impact of DNA diagnostics is on well being and social behavior of our customers. In addition, a careful follow-up on the effectiveness of preventive treatment should be warranted.

Multigenic disease

In monogenic disease the relation between the mutation and cardiac disease is straight forward. Most mutations will however have a less pronounced impact. Therefore the importance of one mutation may be hard to prove (category D). In addition, a number of unfavorable mutations in various genes could lead to a summation of subtle effects and to cardiovascular diseases like atherosclerosis and hypertension. When several genes are involved the disease cause is multigenic, which brings us to the next level of complexity in genetic analysis. To compare affected with healthy individuals many genes will have to studied, which is time consuming and expensive. Fortunately the technology to analyze genes faster and more effectively, like micro-arrays and DNA-chip technology is being developed and will soon be available for universal research use [2].

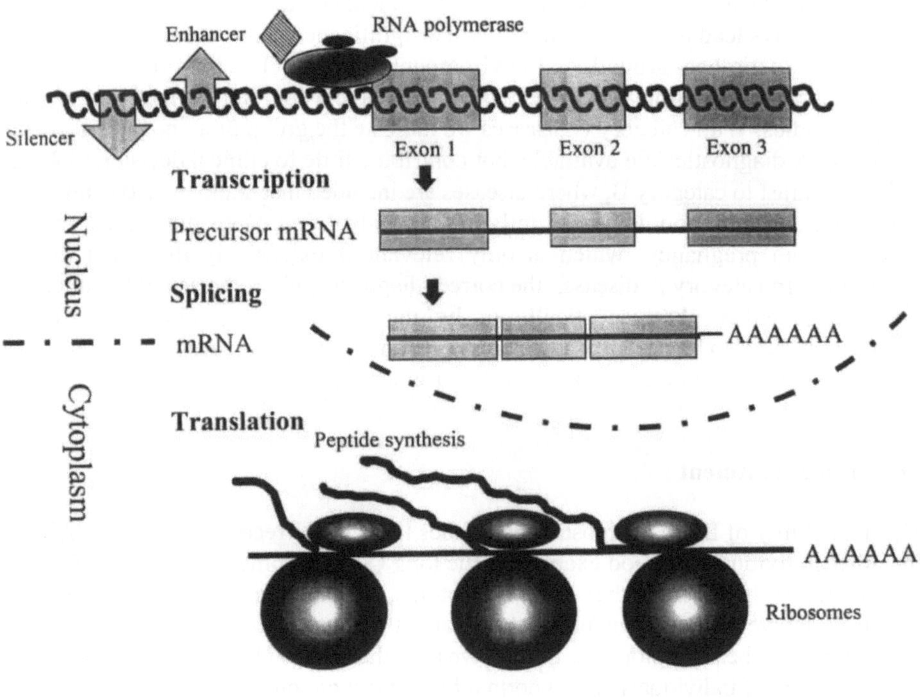

***Figure 1**. A schematic representation of the structure of a gene, transcription and translation.*

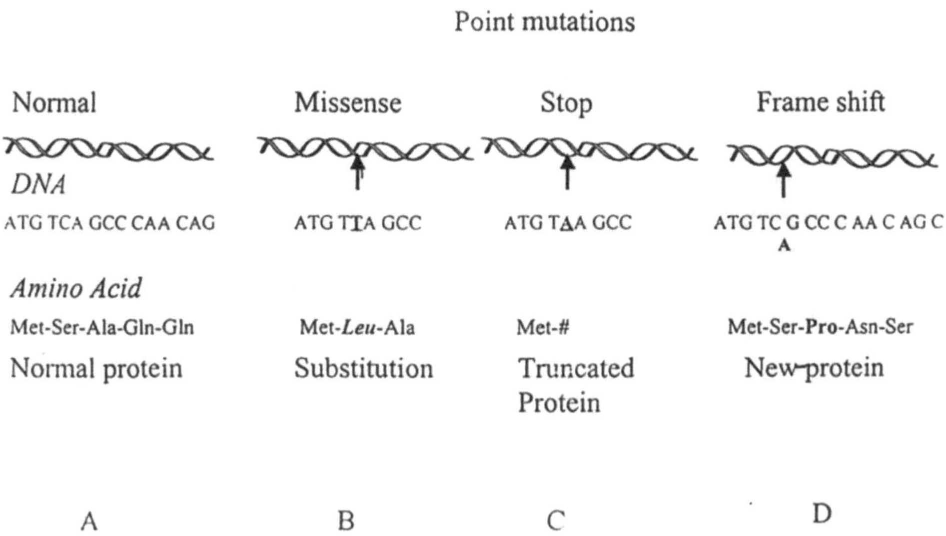

***Figure 2**. Point mutations. The normal situation of transcription and translation is shown in panel A. Panel B missense: the change of one base cytosine (C) at position 5 into thymidine (T) results in one amino-acid replacement (Serine-Leucine). Panel C stop codon: C to A (adenosine) change introduces a stop codon. This base triplet does not code for an amino acid and therefore translations stops. Panel D frame shift: the loss of A at position 6 leads to a shift in triplet codes, and therefore a new protein product.*

References

1. Rosenthal N. Molecular medicine. Recognizing DNA. N Engl J Med 1995; 333:925-927.
2. Collins FS. Shattuck lecture--medical and societal consequences of the Human Genome Project. N Engl J Med 1999; 341:28-37.
3. Doevendans PA, Mummery C. Pluripotent Stem Cells: Biology and Applications. Neth Heart J 2001;9:103-107.
4. de Knijff P, McPherson R, Bruschke AV, Lie KI, Kastelein JJ. The role of a common variant of the cholesteryl ester transfer protein gene in the progression of coronary atherosclerosis. The Regression Growth Evaluation Statin Study Group. N Engl J Med 1998; 338: 86-93.
5. Doevendans PA, van Empel V, Spiering W, van der Zee R. Clinical Perspectives of Molecular Cardiology. Ned Tijdschr Klin Chem 26, 48-51. 2001.

APPENDIX A

THE GENETIC CODE AND AMINO ACID SYMBOLS

A = Ala = Alanine
C = Cys = Cysteine
D = Asp = Aspargine
E = Glu = Glutamine
F = Phe = Phenylalanine
G = Gly = Glycine
H = His = Histidine
I = Ile = Isoleucine
K = Lys = Lysine
L = Leu = Leucine
M = Met = Methionine
N = Asn =Asparagine
P = Pro = Proline
Q = Gln = Glutamine
R = Arg = Arginine
S = Ser = Serine
T = Thr = Threonine
V = Val = Valine
W = Trp = Tryptophan
Y = Tyr = Tyrosine

APPENDIX B

SCHEME TRIPLET CODE

TTT } Phe	TCT	TAT } Tyr	TGT } Cys
TTC }	TCC Ser	TAC }	TGC }
TTA } Leu	TCA	TAA - Stop	TGA - Stop
TTG }	TCG	TAG - Stop	TGG - Trp
CTT	CCT	CAT } His	CGT
CTC Leu	CCC Pro	CAC }	CGC Arg
CTA	CCA	CAA } Gln	CGA
CTG	CCG	CAG }	CGG
ATT	ACT	AAT } Asn	AGT } Ser
ATC Ileu	ACC Thr	AAC }	AGC }
ATA	ACA	AAA } Lys	AGA } Arg
ATG Met	ACG	AAG }	AGG }
GTT	GCT	GAT } Asp	GGT
GTC Val	GCC Ala	GAC }	GGC Gly
GTA	GCA	GAA } Glu	GGA
GTG	GCG	GAG }	GGG

APPENDIX C

All authors tried to implement this classification in their chapters

Classification of genetic disease

A. Molecular diagnostics available and diagnosis is relevant for treatment (TREATMENT)
B. Molecular diagnostics available and relevant for genetic counseling (COUNSELING)
C. Diagnostics available. Molecular diagnosis does not alter treatment, but could be relevant for risk assessment (RISK)
D. Polymorphism with implications for predisposition, but minor phenotypic consequences (RISK)
E. Chromosomal loci have been identified, but no genes are known (RESEARCH)
F. No locus nor gene is known (RESEARCH)

See also introduction pages

1. MOLECULAR GENETICS IN CARDIOLOGY

M.M.A.M Mannens, H.J.M. Smeets

Introduction

Genetics and genomics are being introduced rapidly into clinical practice. Knowledge on genes and gene defects, gene expression and gene products are being gathered as part of the recently completed human genome project at a rapid pace [1,2]. The genetic cause of the vast majority of important monogenic disorders is known, the more rare disorders are being unravelled fast. Technical developments enable molecular geneticists an accelerated and detailed characterization of genetic defects, predisposition or background of individual patients. The introduction of genetic tests for heritable cardiac abnormalities is of a recent nature. Disorders, like the Long QT-syndrome, Brugada syndrome or hypertrophic and dilated cardiomyopathies have only recently been unravelled and research is ongoing to improve DNA-diagnostics [3,4]. Genetic testing offers many opportunities, but also a considerable number of risks and uncertainties, and introduction in the clinic has to be performed with great care. Not every test that can be done, should be done. It is evident that genetic testing must be beneficial for the patient. If he or she is affected, then the test can either be performed to make or confirm a diagnosis or to predict prognosis and adjust treatment. It is clear that a genetic test affects not only the patient involved, but also concerns relatives or future offspring. Even if patients are unaffected, it is possible to determine their genetic status and to predict what the chances will be of developing symptoms in the years to follow. Especially these studies are becoming more and more important in the field of genetic cardiovascular diseases, enabling the discrimination between carriers of a genetic risk and non-carriers. These investigations should be embedded in a multidisciplinary approach of cardiologists, clinical geneticists, laboratory specialists and psychologists. It is obvious that in this area of predictive medicine, ethical and social (health insurance) aspects play a role as well. Society should establish the rules by which genetic testing may be performed, preventing the exclusion of patients because of their genetic burden.

Mendelian and non-Mendelian inheritance

Genetic diseases can be divided in Mendelian and non-Mendelian diseases [5]. The first group is caused by defects in autosomal or X-chromosomal genes that have a dominant

PA Doevendans and AA Wilde (eds.), Cardiovascular genetics, 1-12.

or recessive manifestation. In case of a dominant disorder (figure 1), the disease will become manifest if only one gene is affected, in case of recessive segregation, both homologous genes must be affected to develop symptoms. Dominant and recessive are no absolute terms. Some carriers of dominant mutations remain healthy, which is called non-penetrance [6]. This can be disease, age- and sex-dependent. A penetrance of 90% means that 90% of the carriers of a gene defect will be affected (at that age). Another possibility is that not every case in a family has to have the genetic cause. These patients are called phenocopies and can be a problem in disorders with a common environmentally induced counterpart. It is also possible that the manifestations of genetic diseases vary among gene carriers, which is called heterogeneous expression. Sometimes mutations in the same gene can lead to different disorders, as do mutations in the SCN5A gene involved in Long QT syndrome, Brugada syndrome or isolated conduction defects [7,8,9]. Some specific neuromuscular disorders, like myotonic dystrophy or Friedreich Ataxia, become more severe in following generations. This phenomenon is called anticipation and the molecular basis is unstable DNA, which increases in size from generation to generation [5]. The size of the unstable DNA fragment is in general related to disease severity.

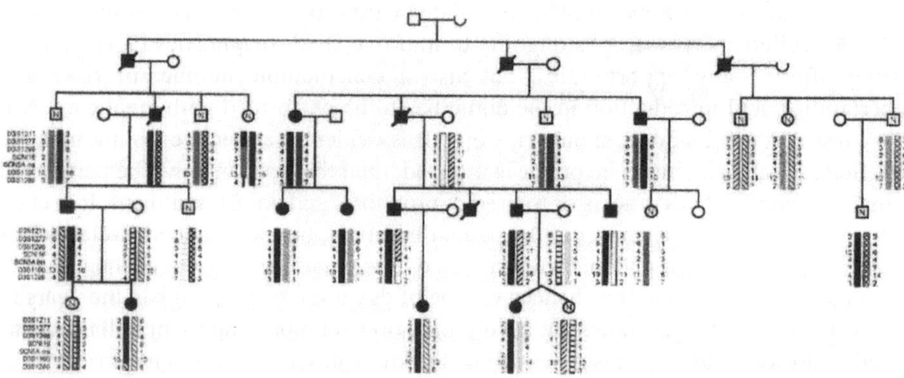

Figure 1. (see color section) *Linkage analyses in a family presenting with "Brugada" syndrome and LQT3. The haplotype indicated with a black bar segregates with the disease. Affected persons are indicated with filled symbols. N = not affected. Deceased persons are indicated with a crossed line. Alleles are numbered for each marker on chromosome 3.*

Carriers of recessive disorders are usually without symptoms. However, in some disorders it is possible to identify them by biochemical defects, reduced enzymatic activity or by expressing only partly the clinical spectrum (as a marginally increased QT-interval in Jervell Lange-Nielsen syndrome). Finally, some disorders, like inherited cancers can be dominant at the family level and recessive at the gene level. One mutation in a gene segregates in the family and a second hit occurs somatically. If the chance of this second hit is high, then a dominant segregation pattern occurs. Therefore, these terms of dominant and recessive segregation should be carefully explained, when used. This is also the case for X-chromosomal diseases, which are predominantly encountered in males, because they only have one X-chromosome and while females have two. Dominant or recessive are terms related to genetic diseases and not to genes. In a specific gene, both dominant and recessive mutations can occur, either leading to the same or a different phenotype. Dominant mutations in the KCNQ1 gene lead to Romano Ward syndrome, whereas recessive mutations in the same gene cause the Jervell Lange-Nielsen syndrome [10]. The latter may also occur in the KCNE1 gene, displaying the genetic heterogeneity of this disorder. Often the nomenclature and classification of genetic disorders are adjusted from the moment when the genes, causing the disorders have been identified.

In addition to Mendelian inheritance other segregation patterns exist for monogenic disorders. Some diseases show a maternal segregation pattern and are caused by defects in the mitochondrial DNA, which is for example the case for a number of isolated or rare syndromic dilated or hypertrophic cardiomyopathies [11]. Other gene defects only become manifest when transmitted by either parent. This phenomenon is called genomic imprinting [12] and indicates that for some genes only the paternal or maternal copy is active. Therefore, a defect in such a gene only has an effect, if it is present in the active copy of the gene. As can be deduced from phenomena like penetrance and heterogeneous expression, it is clear that manifestation of monogenic disorders is not constant and that no clear discrimination between monogenic disorders with one major gene defect and modifying factors, and complex genetic disorders with more minor gene defects and environmental factors, exist. Polygenic diseases are caused by more than one gene, which often contribute in a quantitative manner to the clinical manifestations and are considered risk factors, as the manifestations are often not constant, dependent on the genetic background. Complex genetic disorders are polygenic disorders, which can be influenced by the environment. These disorders are much more frequent than monogenic disorders and the role of the environment is often much stronger, which means that a disease-state does not always have a genetic cause [13].

Genetic heterogeneity of monogenic disorders

Diseases like familial hypertrophic cardiomyopathy or the congenital Long QT syndrome are genetically heterogeneous monogenic disorders (see also chapters 12 and 15). The diseases are caused by single gene defects in patients, but defects in a number of genes can lead to the same disease. Familial hypertrophic cardiomyopathy (chapter 12) is a disease of the cardiac sarcomere and 9 sarcomeric genes have been detected with mutations [4,14]. At this point, a complete screening of all genes is technically not possible in a routine diagnostic setting. It is also not necessary for those families in which hypertrophy can be clearly demonstrated and progression of disease is relatively benign. However, testing is essential for those families in which sudden cardiac death (SCD) occurs, especially in those cases where hypertrophy is mild. It is obvious that with the speed of the technical developments in this field, a more optimal and more complete protocol, covering all possibly involved genes, will become available for diagnostics in the years to come.

When no phenotypic selection criteria for genes exist, the frequency of mutations in the genes can be used to establish a protocol. For familial hypertrophic cardiomyopathy one could start with the beta-MHC gene (35% of the mutations), followed by the Troponin T gene (15%) and the myosin binding protein C-gene (15%). It should be stressed that the chances of identifying rapidly a mutation in a patient, increase, if affected family members are available, and genetic markers can be used to identify the locus involved (in large families) or exclude loci not involved (in smaller families). The latter situation is often present in families with SCD. It should also be noted that careful clinical examination is a prerequisite as any false diagnosis will lead to a wrong conclusion with respect to the gene or genetic locus involved. The combination of clinical and genetic data is also important for extending the knowledge on the disease (frequency of non-penetrant carriers, number of de novo mutations), developing selection criteria for the gene involved, like in the congenital Long QT syndrome, and for establishing a more exact genotype-based prognosis. Genotype-phenotype correlations are important for counseling (but as long as not all contributing factors are known should be used with great care in individual cases) and for therapy. In case of severe mutations, aggressive treatment can be defended. Congenital Long QT syndrome (chapter 15) is caused by mutations in cardiac potassium or sodium channel genes [3,15]. Based on gathered knowledge on genotype-phenotype correlations, it is possible to select the most likely gene involved from the clinical information, like the trigger of cardiac events (physical stress points to the KCNQ1 gene and acoustic stimuli to HERG gene), or the electrocardiographic characteristics [16]. The identification of the causative mutation has to performed however. This is specifically important, because gene-specific prophylactic therapy exist and can save lives, if carriers are identified quickly and early. It can be expected that gene-specific therapy may evolve to mutation specific therapy in the future.

This book deals with disorders, in which genetic testing forms a clear contribution to patient management, either to direct therapy or to give advise concerning life-style. This is most important in asymptomatic carriers, who can only be identified by screening family members at risk for the gene defect. Some chapters are on complex diseases, like hypertension, and cardiovascular risk factors with a miscellaneous contribution to often frequent phenotypes. In case of monogenic disorders, it is possible to perform DNA-diagnostics, if the underlying genetic defect has not yet been elucidated. A prerequisite is that genetic loci are known for the disorder and, in case of genetic heterogeneity, that the size of the family is such that segregation of the disorder with a specific locus can be proven with high likelihood. Finally, disorders are being discussed in which the value or the possibilities of genetic testing are far from clear and have to be considered as research. Thus far, every genetic disease has started this way and developments in research have paved the way for diagnostic applications. The switch point from research to diagnostics is critical. The discovery of genes and pathogenic mutations in a genetic disorder does not solve all diagnostic or prognostic problems. Gene carriers and segregation patterns can be determined with certainty, but in case of unique mutations and small families, it can be quite difficult to give a clear risk estimate for the development of clinical features, nor is it initially evident, whether there is a treatment and how successful it is.

This is of specific concern as the identification of a gene, gene mutations or risk factors, trigger a direct request from clinicians to perform genetic testing, often at a moment at which the real implications of the findings still have to be determined. However, given the often severe nature of the disorders involved, it is usually no option to refrain from testing and the patient should be informed and guided through this process by a multidisciplinary team of experts in this new field of cardiogenetics. Although DNA-diagnostics is becoming available for an increasing number of cardiovascular disorders, this does not mean that in all cases a molecular diagnosis can be achieved. To improve the success rate, a good collaboration between the laboratory and the referring cardiologist and clinical geneticist is necessary. Often, the clinical data such as the patients' history or an ECG can be extremely helpful to identify the most likely causative gene.

DNA-diagnostics - basic strategies

DNA-diagnostics is usually performed on DNA isolated from blood. As only DNA-analysis is concerned specific tissues are not required, except for mitochondrial DNA mutations, which can vary among organs. DNA-isolation is not very critical and EDTA or Heparin blood samples can be kept at room temperature for several days without interfering with the analysis. If RNA-analysis is required or immortalized cell lines need to be prepared for gene expression or protein studies, then the blood needs to be delivered within a single day at the DNA-laboratory. DNA-diagnostics falls apart in strategies, established to identify known mutations and strategies to screen for unknown genes or mutations. The identification of known mutations is straightforward and can be completed within days, which is a big advantage for predictive testing. Dependent on the mutation, either Polymerase Chain Reaction (PCR) or Southern blot technology can be applied [5]. In most cases, the amplification by PCR of the DNA fragment that is to be investigated (genes, exons) is required. For PCR, two synthetic oligonucleotides (small single stranded DNA fragments called primers), are added to single stranded DNA. These primers flank the DNA fragment that has to be analyzed. Each primer hybridizes to one of the DNA strands and serves as a starting point for the synthesis of new DNA by the enzyme Taq DNA-polymerase (Taq stands for Thermus aquaticus, the bacteria from which it was isolated). After the first round of amplification, the DNA is denatured and a second round of amplification follows, followed by a third and so on. After about 20-30 rounds of amplification, the DNA fragment to be analyzed has increased a million folds and can be visualized by gel electrophoresis and ethidium bromide staining. The PCR fragments can be analyzed for the specific mutation by a variety of techniques, such as Allele-specific Oligonucleotides (ASO), Allele-specific Primer Extension (APEX), Oligonucleotide Ligation Assay (OLA) and mutation-specific restriction digestion [17]. For large rearrangements, deletions or duplications in genes, Southern blot analysis is still performed. DNA can be size separated directly on a gel after being cut by restriction enzymes. Numerous enzymes are available that cut at specific places in the DNA, generating DNA fragments of various sizes. These size-separated DNA fragments can be transferred to a membrane to which the DNA is bound. The relevant DNA fragments on this membrane can be visualized by hybridizing the membrane to labelled (radioactive or fluorescent) DNA fragments of the genes/exons that are investigated (see figure 2b). An alternative for some cases can be long range PCR, by which fragments of more than 10 kb can be achieved (figure 2a) [18].

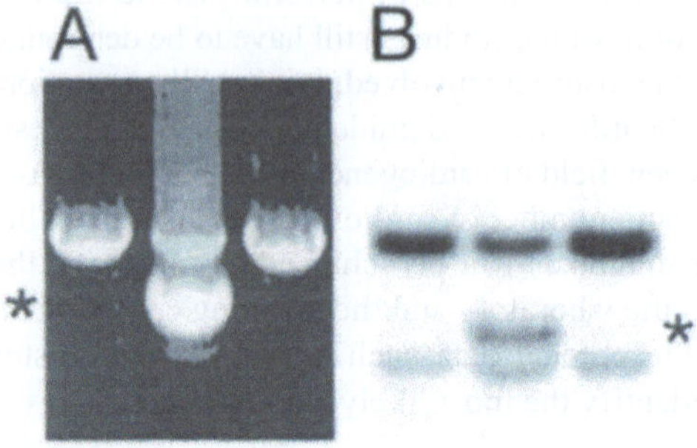

Figure 2a. *Gelelectrophoresis of a long-segment PCR fragment containing exon 6-11 of the LDL gene. In lane 2, a 2.5 kb deletion encompassing exon 7 and 8 is visible (arrow).*
Figure 2b. *Autoradiograph of the same 2.5 kb deletion (lane 2, arrow) as analyzed by Southern blotting and hybridization with a radioactive probe containing exons 2-11.*

In case the genetic defect in an affected family is unknown, then basically two strategies are applied in DNA-diagnostics to identify the causative genetic locus or defect. Wherever families are available with multiple affected persons, linkage analysis is performed. The segregation of an affected allele can be followed by use of closely linked, preferably disease locus flanking, polymorphic DNA markers (microsatellites, Single Nucleotide Polymorphisms) that identify the two homologous chromosomal loci. Without knowing the actual defect (gene mutation), a prediction can be made about the mutation carrier status of an individual. In most cases, the accuracy will be >>95%. If the family is too small, linkage analysis is no option when different genes can give rise to a similar phenotype (as in Long-QT syndrome).
In addition, meiotic crossover events (naturally occurring exchange of DNA between homologous chromosomes during gametogenesis) and lack of informativity of the polymorphic markers used can obstruct a molecular diagnosis. Linkage analysis for known disease loci can usually be rapidly performed, however, in case of unknown disease loci it is quite laborious as a complete genome scan has to be performed. To avoid problems associated with linkage analysis, mutation screening of disease genes can be done, which can be very time-consuming, depending on the size and number of potential candidate genes. The coding and, wherever applicable, regulatory sequences are scanned in patient DNA and compared to the known, unmutated sequence. The technology used is usually PCR-based and involves either sequencing, which can be quite time-consuming and costly if the genes involved are large, or gene scanning, followed by sequencing in case of an aberration. Many methods all with specific advantages and disadvantages to quickly scan through a gene exist. Apart from HPLC and mass spectrometry, most of this scanning technology (Single Strand Conformational Polymorphism, Denaturing Gradient Gel Electrophoresis, PCR or Southern blotting) is based on electrophoresis. DNA fragments are separated on a gel where the mutant fragment shows an aberrant mobility through the gel. To identify large gene rearrangements, duplications or deletions, Southern blot analysis is applied. These mutations can be missed if only PCR-based strategies are used.

In addition to the big advantages, also pitfalls exist in DNA-diagnostics. Identification of a sequence variant does not always mean that this variant is causative for the disease. Apart from obvious mutations such as deletions or full stops, there are many DNA-polymorphisms in the general population that are not pathogenic. In most cases, mutations leading to single amino acid changes need to be further investigated to rule out the possibility of a normal sequence polymorphism. Population studies have to be performed in appropriate controls and functional analyses are desired, but often not possible in a diagnostic setting. Literature and mutation database searches are necessary and the position of a mutation within important domains of a gene or evolutionary conservation of the altered amino acid can provide additional evidence. Finally, it can be helpful to demonstrate segregation of a mutation with the disorder in a family or to demonstrate that the mutation is not present in de parents DNA and thus occurred de novo.

Indirect DNA-diagnostics: Linkage analysis

With polymorphic DNA markers a disease locus can be followed within a family (figure 1) [5,13]. In this way, the carrier status of a patient can be determined indirectly. If a polymorphic marker is close to the disease locus (1-5 cM), it will segregate in the vast majority of cases with the disease locus since the occurrence of chromosomal cross-over events during meiosis is unlikely (< 1-5%). If markers on both sides are available, the chance of double cross-over that could negatively influence the interpretation of the test is even smaller (1-5% X 1-5% = 1/10.000 – 25/10.000). The polymorphic markers are often PCR fragments that, due to the variations in DNA, differ in length or sequence and can be separated with electrophoresis or alternative techniques. In general, linkage analyses can only be used in cases where the disease locus and carrier status of at least two individuals is known and/or the family is large enough to exclude segregation of a marker with the disease locus by chance. Computer analysis are necessary but linkage of a marker with a disease locus is proven if the chance of linkage compared to non-linkage is 1: 1000. Linkage is excluded at chances 1:100. These likelihoods are given in logarithms or LOD scores (log of the odds). A lod score of 3 means a chance of 1:1000 for linkage. Lod scores of 3 are only achievable in large families (roughly over 11 informative meioses i.e. heterozygotes for whom the segregation of the homologous chromosomes in relation to the disease can be determined). This means that the disease status of at least 11 individuals should be known without doubt. Smaller families are often studied to give an indication of the gene involved or exclude genes not involved, but conclusive DNA-diagnosis is not possible. Figure 1 gives an example of a linkage study. Polymorphic markers are numbered according to their length. The "black bar" combination of polymorphic markers (haplotype) is segregating with the disease locus, a combination of LQT3 and "Brugada" syndrome segregating in one family. These markers on chromosome 3 segregate with the disease giving a lod score of 6.5. Analysis of the relevant gene (a sodium channel SCN5A) revealed a 3 nucleotide insertion (TGA) at position 5537, causing the disease.

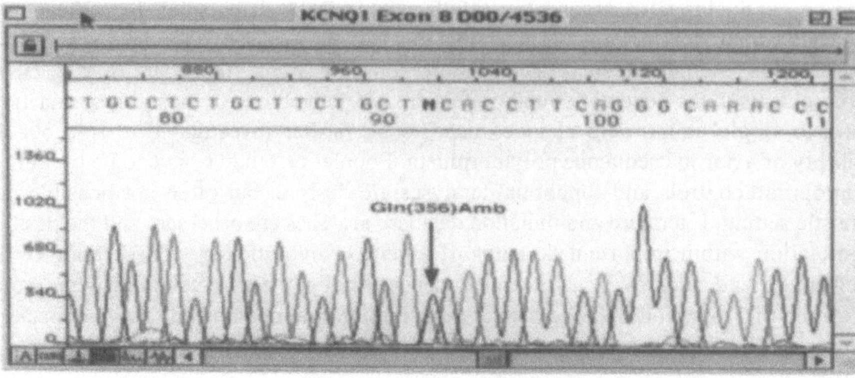

Figure 3. (see color section) Sequence analysis. A DNA mutation was found leading to a change from aminoacid glutamine to a full stop at position 356. The result is an incomplete non-functional ion channel protein (KCNQ1) that causes the long QT syndrome type 1 (Romano-Ward syndrome) in this patient.

Direct DNA-diagnostics – screening for small mutations

Sequencing

The sequence of a particular DNA fragment can be determined by using a primer sequence (short oligonucleotide complementary to a small DNA fragment adjacent to the DNA fragment to be sequenced) [5]. Using this primer as a starting point, the sequence of a single stranded DNA fragment can be artificially copied by an enzyme called DNA-polymerase and the addition of the chemical components of DNA (the nucleotides adenine, cytosine, thymine, guanine). The newly synthesized strands are chemically modified by the addition of small amounts of dideoxynucleotides that are labeled with fluorochromes or radioactive isotopes. The dideoxynucleotides represent all four existing nucleotides (A,T,C or G) that are added in 4 distinct reactions or are labeled differently so they can be recognized as such. Incorporation of a dideoxynucleotide stops the synthesis of DNA. This occurs randomly. Addition of modified adenine for instance reveals the position of all adenines in the genetic code by creating partially synthesized DNA fragments that stop at all positions of adenine. By doing so with all 4 modified nucleotides and by separating fragments with a resolution of one nucleotide by high voltage electrophoresis, the genetic code can be read simply by determining the length of the fragments. The nucleotide present in a particular fragment comes before that of a longer fragment. Figure 3 shows an example of such a sequence reaction. The procedure is nowadays fully automated and in most cases the dideoxynucleotides are labelled with fluorochromes of 4 different colors. The separated fragments are detected with laser technology (colored peaks). By comparing the known sequence with the sequence in patients, a mutation can be found. In the case shown, a DNA mutation was found leading to a change from amino acid glutamine to a stop at position 356. The result is an incomplete non-functional ion channel protein (KCNQ1) that causes the long QT syndrome type 1 (Romano-Ward syndrome) in this patient.

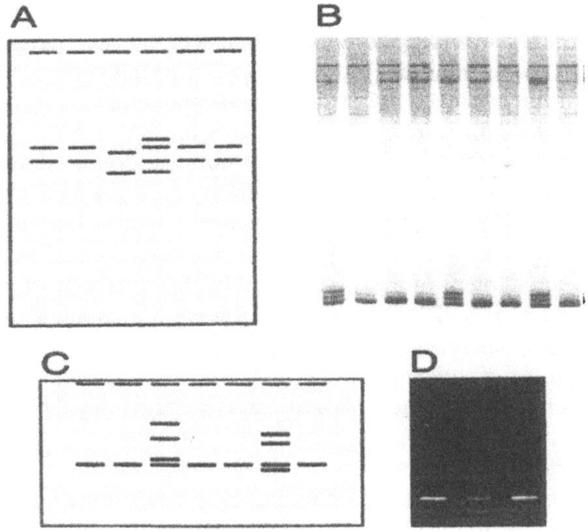

Figure 4. (see color section) *SSCP-analysis. The theoretical change in mobility is shown (figure 4a). Normally 2 bands are visible, the sense and antisense strand of the DNA (controls in lanes 1,2,5 and 6). If a DNA fragment is homozygously mutated, theoretically 2 new bands might appear since both sense and antisense DNA changes for both alleles (lane 3). In case of a heterozygote (one normal and one mutated gene, lane 4), a total of four bands can be seen. Figure 4b shows a base deletion at position 754 in the HERG gene of a Long-QT2 patient. Affected family members are shown in lanes 1,5 and 8. Figure 4c shows a theoretical DGGE analysis. Mutants are seen in lane 3 and 6, revealing homo and heteroduplexes. Figure 4d shows a N543H heterozygous mutation in the LDL receptor gene (lane 2) causing familial hypercholesterolemia compared to control DNA (lane 1 and 3). The aberrant homo and heteroduplexes are clearly visible on this DGGE gel.*

Single-strand conformation polymorphism (SSCP) and denaturing gradient gel electrophoresis (DGGE) analysis

SSCP and DGGE [5] are methods based on altered electrophoresis patterns for DNA fragments due to sequence changes. They are relatively easy to perform but do not detect 100% of mutations (on average between 90-95%). For SSCP, the DNA fragments of at maximum 300 basepairs (bp) are made single stranded by melting and immediate cooling. This single stranded DNA molecule will form intra-molecular interactions leading to a molecule specific structure. This tertiary structure is dependent on the sequence of the entire fragment. If a mutation exists in a given fragment, the conformation will usually be altered. This alteration often results in a change of mobility during electrophoresis, under conditions where these weak tertiary structures are not disturbed (non-denaturing). In figure 4a the theoretical change in mobility is shown. Normally 2 bands are visible, the sense and antisense strand of the DNA. If a DNA fragment is mutated, 2 new different bands will appear since both sense and antisense DNA strands are different. In case of a heterozygote (one normal and one mutated gene), a total of four bands can be seen. In practice, bands might co-migrate and can thus not be visible or extra bands can be seen due to additional conformations or the formation of double stranded DNA, or just artificial PCR reactions. An example is given in figure 4b where a base deletion at position 754 in the HERG gene of a Long-QT2 patient leads to a frameshift and premature stop.

Affected family members are shown in lanes 1, 5 and 8.
DGGE is a technique in which the DNA strands of the two alleles are also separated but these 4 strands are re-annealed afterwards. In case of mutations, DNA molecules existing of homo or heteroduplexes occur. Two wild type strands may re-anneal, as may two mutated strands to form homo-duplexes. If a mutant and wild-type strand re-anneal, heteroduplexes are formed. These newly formed double-stranded DNA molecules demonstrate changes in electrophoretic mobility on a gel with a gradient of denaturing agents. Because of the mutations, DNA fragments will melt at different positions in the denaturing gel and thus get stuck at different positions due to the formation of "Y" structures. Heteroduplexes are easiest to identify, but also homoduplexes of mutations can often be detected, thus making detection of homozygous mutations possible. Figure 4d shows a N543H heterozygous mutation in the LDL receptor gene causing familial hypercholesterolemia compared to control DNA. The aberrant homo- and heteroduplexes are clearly visible. DGGE allows fragments to be larger than SSCP-fragments.

DHPLC-analysis
One of the most promising new technologies in DNA mutation detection is denaturing high-performance liquid chromatography (DHPLC) [19]. In contrast to the above mentioned detection methods, DHPLC uses chromatography instead of electrophoresis to detect aberrant DNA fragments such as insertions, deletions but also single base substitutions. The sensitivity of the technology is comparable to sequencing, although a sequence reaction is needed to determine the actual sequence change, but the detection level is higher (1% mutation is detectable [20]). PCR fragments are denatured and reannealed thus forming homo- and heteroduplexes. These newly formed DNA fragments are transferred to a HPLC column and eluted in about 10-20 minutes. Elevated column temperature causes partial denaturation, starting with the less stable heteroduplexes, and consequently heteroduplexes are separated from homoduplexes. Partial denatured molecules are generally less well retained on the column, due to their decreased interaction with the ion pairing reagent (triethylamonium ion). The optimal temperature for a specific DNA fragment can be determined by computation or experimentally. In theory, two homo- and two heteroduplexes can be found. In practice one wild-type and one or two mutant peaks are mostly seen as shown in figure 5. In this figure, a wild type DNA fragment is shown (figure 5a) compared to splice mutations in the same fragment of the LDL receptor causing familial hypercholesterolemia, figure 5 b (the 313+1 G>A mutation in intron 3) and figure 5c (the 191-2 A>G mutation in intron 2).

Alternative technology
Many alternatives techniques are available that fall outside the scope of this book. Some techniques to identify specific mutations are currently being adjusted to screen entire genes. By using micro-array or DNA-microchip approaches the entire sequence of the gene can be rebuild by overlapping oligonucleotides and the hybridization pattern of the DNA of the patient resolves its sequence [21]. Mass spectrometry is another example of new technology, that can be used to quickly screen large numbers of samples for known mutations.
However, in general practice, these techniques are not yet available or applicable.

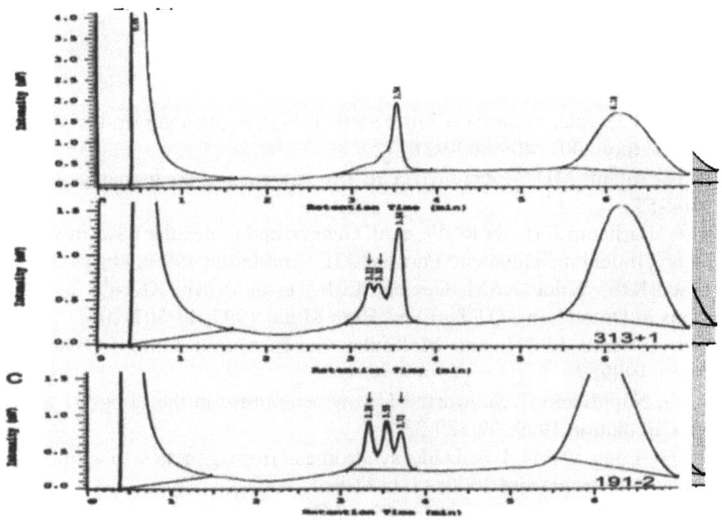

Figure 5. *DHPLC-analysis. A wild type DNA fragment is shown (figure 5a) compared to splice mutations in the same fragment containing exon 3 of the LDL receptor causing familial hypercholesterolemia, figure 5 b (the 313+1 G>A mutation in intron 3) and figure 5c (the 191-2 A>G mutation in intron 2). Aberrant peaks are indicated with arrows.*

In case of quantitative differences, like deletions and duplications, real-time PCR is very valuable since this technique can provide information on gene (or chromosome) copy number within hours. Sometimes, analyses at the RNA or protein level are necessary to predict the result of a DNA change or as alternative in cases where no DNA alteration can be found. A major breakthrough is expected from the micro-array or DNA-microchip approaches mentioned above. This technology can be used to screen the complete sequence of a gene for small mutations or to analyze large numbers of clones (cDNA or genomic clones) for major rearrangements. In a different application oligonucleotides or cDNA clones are attached on the array and the expression level of those genes can be determined in RNA samples from normal or affected tissue [22]. Specific expression profiles may exist for specific gene defects or pathogenic states, allowing a refined characterization of the underlying genetic cause or disease state in the patient. As the micro-array approach can also be used to determine large numbers of risk factors, it is clear that the time where a more complete knowledge of genetic defects and predisposition of patients emerges is nearby. It is, however, also clear that interpreting this information and explaining it to patients will be the major bottleneck in the years to come. It will be important to focus on relevant information and established knowledge in health care. Scientists, clinicians and society will have to collaborate closely to make the genomic revolution a success and of benefit for humans and the human population.

References

1. International Human Genome Consortium. Initial sequencing and analysis of the human genome. Nature 2001; 409:860-921.
2. Venter JC, Adams MD, Myers EM, et al. The sequence of the human genome. Science 2001; 291:1304-51.
3. Priori SG, Barhanin J, Hauer RNW, et al. Genetic and molecular basis of cardiac arrhythmias: impact on clinical management. Part I and II. Circulation 1999; 99:518-28.
4. Jongbloed RJE, Wilde AAM, Geelen JLMC, et al. Novel KCNQ1 and HERG missense mutations in Dutch Long-QT families. Hum Mutat 1999; 13:301-10.
5. Strachan T, Read AP. Human Molecular Genetics; 2nd edition. Oxford: Bios Scientific Publishers 1999.
6. Priori SG, Napolitano C, Schwartz PJ. Low penetrance in the Long-QT syndrome. Clinical impact. Circulation 1999; 99:529-33.
7. Priori SG. Long QT and Brugada syndromes: from genetics to clinical management. J Cardiovasc Electrophysiol 2000; 11:1174-8.
8. Bezzina C, Veldkamp MW, Van den Berg MP, et al. A single Na^+ channel mutation causing both long-QT and Brugada syndromes. Circ Res 1999; 85:1206-13.
9. Bezzina CR, Rook MB, Wilde AAM. Cardiac sodium channel and inherited arrhythmia syndromes. Cardiovasc Res 2001; 49:257-71.
10. Neyroud N, Tesson F, Denjoy I, et al. A novel mutation in the potassium channel gene KVLQT1 causes the Jervell and Lange-Nielsen cardioauditory syndrome. Nat Genet 1997; 15:186-9.
11. Towbin JA, Lipshultz SE. Genetics of neonatal cardiomyopathy. Curr Op Cardiol 1999; 14:250-62.
12. Reik W, Walter J. Genomic imprinting: parental influence on the genome. Nat Rev Genet 2001; 2:21-32.
13. Haines Jl, Pericak-Vance MA,eds. Approaches to gene mapping in complex human diseases. New York: Wiley-Liss 1998.
14. Bonne G, Carrier L, Richard P, Hainque B, Schwartz K. Familial Hypertrophic Cardiomyopathy. From mutations to functional defects. Circ Res 1998; 83:580-93.
15. Nicol RL, Frey N, Olson EN. From the sarcomere to the nucleus: Role of genetics and signaling in structural heart disease. Annu. Rev. Genomics Hum Genet 2000; 01:179-223.
16. Wilde AAM, Roden DM. Predicting the long-QT genotype from clinical data. From sense to science. Circulation 2000; 102:2796-8.
17. Hawkins JR. Finding mutations, the basics. Oxford University Press 1997.
18. DeCoo IFM, Gussinklo T, Arts PJW, Oost van BA, Smeets HJM. A PCR test for progressive external ophthalmoplegia and Kearns-Sayre syndrome on DNA from blood samples. J Neur Sci 1997; 149:37-40.
19. Underhill PA, Jin L, Lin AA, et al, Detection of numerous Y chromosome biallelic polymorphisms by denaturing high-performance liquid chromatography. Genome Res 1997; 10:996-1005.
20. Bosch van den BJC, Coo de RFM, Scholte HR, et al. Mutation analysis of the entire mitochondrial genome using denaturing high performance liquid chromatography. Nucl Acids Res 2000; 28:89-96.
21. Lipshutz RJ, Fodor SPA, Gingeras TR, Lockhart DJ. High density synthetic oligonucleotide arrays. Nature Genet 1999 21 suppl:20-5.
22. Young RA. Biomedical discovery with DNA arrays. Cell 2000; 102:9-15.

2. CLINICAL GENETICS

J.P. van Tintelen, C. Marcelis, I.M. van Langen

Introduction

Clinical genetics is a relatively young specialism in the field of medicine. Recent advances in the knowledge of the clinical and molecular aspects of genetics have led to an increase of diagnostic, prognostic and in some cases even therapeutic possibilities. This progress has also entered cardiology. However, some physicians do not give sufficient information to patients prior to performing a genetic test and not all other physicians have yet the skills or knowledge to interpret results of genetic tests correctly, as was recently shown in a study of patients with a hereditary form of colorectal cancer, familial adenomatous polyposis [1]. Because genetic aspects of health and disease are substantial to an individual, both in a physical and psychological way, it is important for physicians to be aware of these elements. They have to be properly trained to be able to handle both "technical/medical" and "emotional/psychosocial" elements of genetic (aspects of) disease in their patients. Besides it is important that cardiologists and physicians are able to recognise their limitations so that co-operation with clinical geneticists can be established. There is an increasing awareness that cardiological disorders can be familial. This not only holds true for some disorders following an established, so called monogenic or mendelian inheritance pattern like long QT syndrome (LQTS), hypertrophic and dilated cardiomyopathy (HCM, DCM) or arrhythmogenic right ventricular cardiomyopathy (ARVC), but also more common for multifactorial or polygenic inherited diseases in cardiology like coronary heart disease, coagulation disorders, hypertension etc. To be able to handle these elements, knowledge of basic aspects of inheritance patterns and genetic counselling is necessary. In this chapter information on pedigree construction, patterns of inheritance and genetic counselling and testing is given.

Pedigree construction [2,3]

The family history is a compilation of information on the health of a person's family and therefore provides a basis to determine risks, and facilitates diagnostics in familial disease. Collecting and reproducing relevant, accurate and detailed information on disorders in family members of a patient with a certain disease is an important step in

PA Doevendans and AA Wilde (eds.), Cardiovascular genetics, 13-28.

genetic counselling. Drawing a pedigree is a very helpful tool in assessing any familial disorder. It gives a quick, accurate and visual record of the family, and enables assessment of the possible inheritance pattern, which is of course important to determine the risk of recurrence for an individual or its offspring. The symbols commonly used are represented in figure 1.

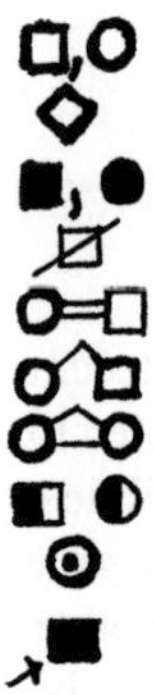

male, female unaffected
sex unknown
male, female affected
deceased
consanguineous marriage
twins
monozygotic twins
heterozygote (carrier) in autosomal recessive disorders
heterozygote (carrier) in an x-linked recessive disorder
propositus/proband: the person through whom the family is ascertained

***Figure 1**. Commonly used symbols in construction of a pedigree*

A few points have to be taken into account to make pedigree construction more reliable and easy:
-additional information can easily be added to a pedigree, underneath the symbol of the person concerned like e.g. his/her QTc time, septal thickness in HCM or other relevant information (convulsions in a LQTS family), cause and age of death etc. (see figure 2)
-numbering: this makes it possible to add more detailed information on an individual as a footnote to the pedigree and makes referral to that person more easy. Generally, a generation is numbered in Roman numerals, with a succeeding number for each person in a generation. E.g. II-3, is the 3rd person from the left in the second generation in the pedigree (see figure 2)
-consanguinity should directly be asked for
-add details about both sides of the family: unexpected results might have consequences for your patient
-note date or year of birth instead of age. Add age at time of death.
-always start drawing a pedigree in the middle of your paper

Inheritance patterns [2,3].

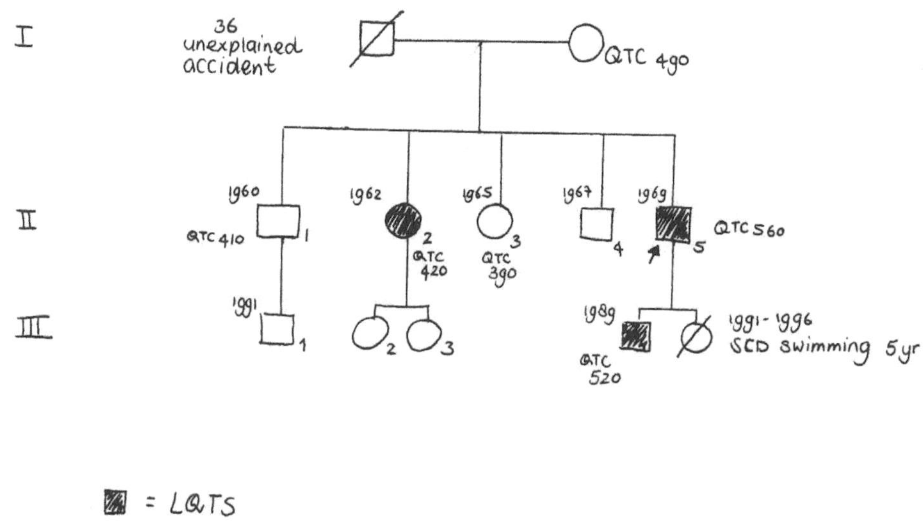

Figure 2. *Example of a pedigree in a medical record taken from a LQTS family*

Sometimes the information gathered in the pedigree can lead to the recognition of a certain **pattern of inheritance** following certain genetic "laws". If a single gene causes a disorder the pattern of inheritance is called mendelian or monogenic. All our cells contain 46 chromosomes, these form 23 pairs of identical chromosomes. So all genetic information (on our chromosomes) is present twice. One chromosome is paternally and the other maternally inherited. During meiosis, when the gametes are formed, identical chromosomes of a pair are separated so that each gamete contains only one chromosome of a pair. Exceptions are the sex chromosomes in males. Because males do have only one X and one Y chromosome genetic information on these chromosomes is singularly present (hemizygous).

The patterns of inheritance can be subdivided depending on the localisation and expression of the gene involved. In an **autosomal** inheritance pattern, the gene is on one of the autosomes –not sex chromosomes-; if the gene concerned is located on the X-chromosome, there is a **X-linked** pattern of inheritance. A **dominant** (mutated) gene is expressed when it is singularly present in a so-called heterozygous form, and a **recessive** gene will cause symptoms (express) only when both genes are mutated (homozygous).

More commonly this recognition is established by knowledge of the diagnosis with a compatible pedigree pattern. Pedigree information itself is not sufficient to make a diagnosis.
When a disorder follows a clear mendelian inheritance pattern, it is usually not difficult to give information on the chances that the disease will occur in family members. The different patterns of inheritance are discussed below.

Autosomal dominant inheritance (see figure 3)
An autosomal dominant disorder can be defined as a disorder that is largely or completely expressed in heterozygotes. The major characteristics are:
- It affects males and females equally.
- 50% of offspring (irrespective of the sex of the affected parent) is affected.
- Male-male (father to son) transmission occurs.
- Vertical transmission (affected persons in succeeding generations).

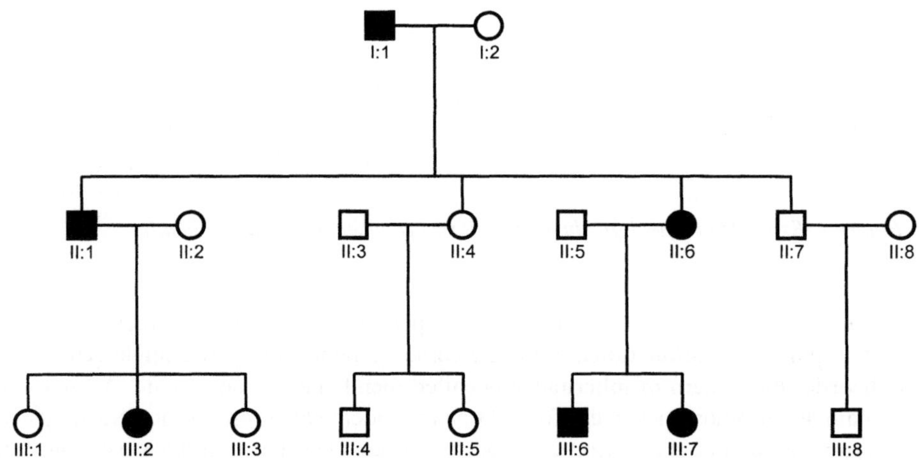

***Figure 3**. Example of an autosomal dominantly inherited disorder. Note male-male transmission*

Some aspects, also clearly present in autosomal dominant cardiac disorders like LQTS, HCM, DCM or ARVC can make it hard to give precise risks on occurrence of the disorder in family members. These are:

1. Reduced penetrance: no evidence of a disorder is found in a person known to possess a certain disease gene (by DNA analysis, or by having an affected parent and an affected child)

2. Late or variable onset /age dependent penetrance: the chance of getting signs of a disorder rises with age

3. Variable expressivity: the variable degree in which a disorder is expressed in different patients. This variable expressivity is present between families, due to a different mutation for example, but also within a family where one single mutation segregates. In this case the influence of other genes or environmental influences might cause the variability of clinical aspects.

Autosomal recessive inheritance

In an autosomal recessively inherited disorder (see figure 4), an affected person is born to healthy parents who are heterozygous for the disease allele (often called "carriers"). The disease only comes to expression when a person has two abnormal alleles. Vertical transmission, one of the characteristics of an autosomal dominant inheritance, is rare. Given the small size of families nowadays, mostly only 1 or 2 persons in one generation or family are affected.

The basic characteristics are:

- It affects males and females equally.
- Carrier parents have a 25% chance of getting a diseased child
- Affected persons are found in one generation. Seldom more distantly related affected family members are identified. Vertical transmission is rare.
- The presence of consanguinity favours, but does not prove, autosomal recessive inheritance.

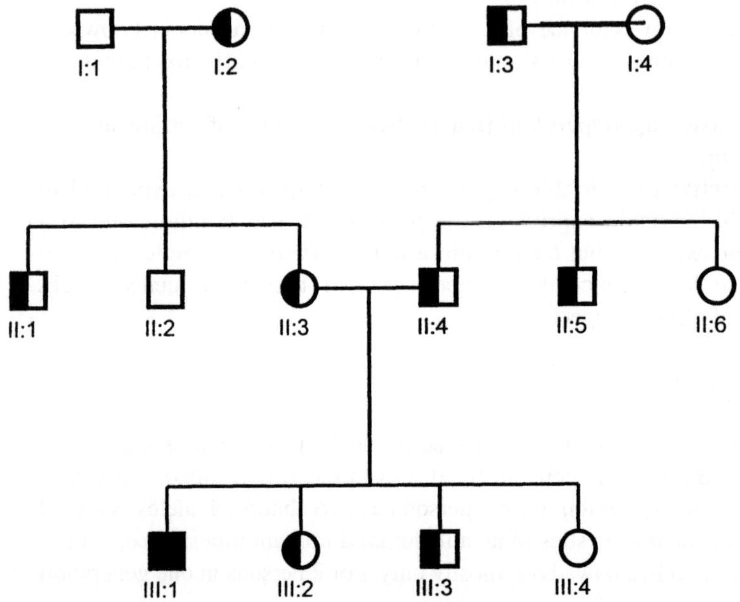

***Figure 4**. Example of an autosomal recessively inherited disorder*

X-linked inheritance

In X-linked disorders (see figure 5), the mutated gene is located on the X chromosome. Depending on the dominant or recessive character of the gene involved certain features can be recognised:

- No male to male transmission (a man passes his Y-chromosome, not his X-chromosome to his son).
- All daughters of an affected male have the gene (which will affect them if it is a dominant gene, or make them all carriers if it is X-linked recessive).
- Unaffected males do not transmit the gene.
- Sons of carrier women (recessive gene) or affected females (dominant gene) have a 50% risk receiving the gene
- 50% of daughters of carrier women will be carriers themselves (if X linked recessive), or patients (if X-linked dominant)

When a disorder is X-linked recessive, carrier women generally do not have signs or symptoms of the disorder. One has to be aware that these X-linked patterns are not always obvious. Carrier women of a mutated dystrophin-gene, causing Duchenne or Becker muscular dystrophy in their family, have an increased risk of developing DCM (see also chapter 13) and slight elevation of CPK values can be ascertained. In this case the mutated gene can neither be considered recessive, because it does express, nor dominant because carrier women do not develop muscular symptoms and not all carrier women develop elevated CPK levels or DCM. This difference is caused by non-random inactivation of the X-chromosome.

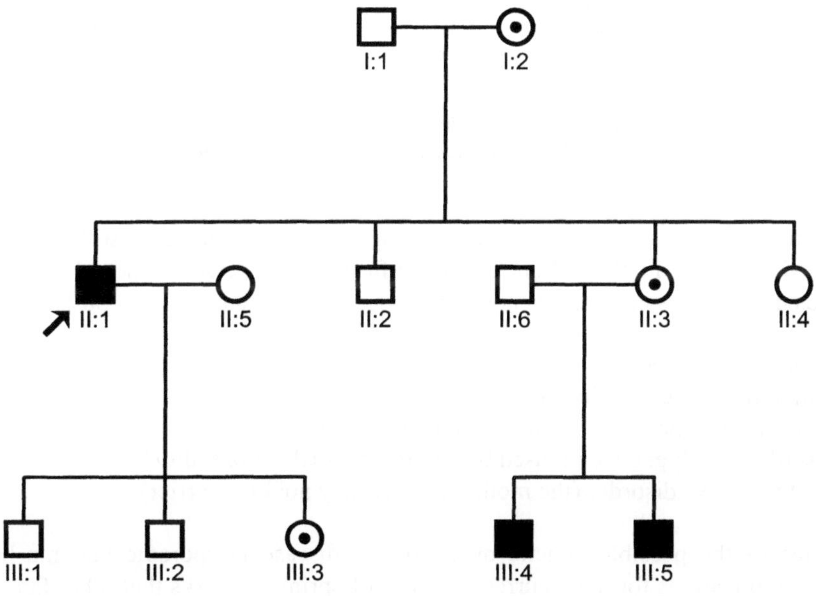

***Figure 5A**. Example of an X-linked recessive disorder (e.g. haemophilia A)*

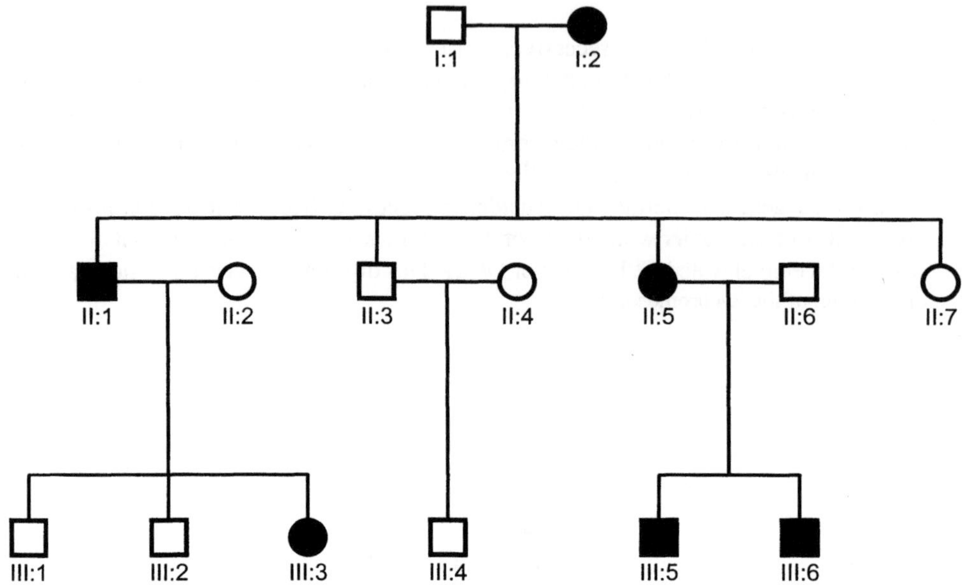

***Figure 5B**. Example of an X-linked dominant disorder. Note similarities to autosomal dominant inheritance, but sons of affected males are always unaffected (no male-to-male transmission), half of the daughters are affected.*

The situation where a heritable disorder is suspected in a sporadic case has to be approached with care. First of all one has to confirm that the person is indeed the only one affected. This does not exclude non-penetrance (see chapter 1). Other possibilities are:

- The disease is non-genetic
- Autosomal recessive inheritance
- Spontaneous autosomal or X-linked dominant mutation
- The disorder is polygenic or caused by a chromosomal abnormality
- X-linked recessive disorder (the mother may or may not be a carrier)

Knowledge of the possible genetic origin of the disease in sporadic patients has important implications for the recurrence risk in offspring and risks that other family members have to develop the disease. This risk can vary between 0 and 50%!

Other (non-mendelian) patterns of inheritance

Mitochondrial inheritance

Mitochondria have their own 16,569 base pair DNA molecule. Every mitochondrion contains 2-10 copies of this molecule. Mitochondrial diseases are inherited maternally because only oocytes transmit their cytoplasm (including the mitochondria) to the zygote. So only mothers will have affected children. This pattern of inheritance and related disorders are described in chapter 11.

Multifactorial/polygenic disease

A large number of diseases or conditions appear to result from a considerable genetic component (in which one ore more genes can be involved) in combination with environmental or unknown influences. So a single genetic factor cannot be held responsible for the condition. Examples of these are numerous in cardiology e.g. hypertension or atherosclerosis.

The estimation of risks in this inheritance pattern is generally based on observed data rather than theoretical predictions. One has to be aware that the data are collected in an unbiased manner and that the population in which the data were collected is comparable to the one the patient or his relative belongs to. The risk increases when one is more closely related to a proband, when multiple family members are affected, when the disease is more severe or more commonly present in a population.

Genetic Counselling

Genetic counselling is considered a communication process, which deals with human problems associated with the (risk of) occurrence of a genetic disorder in a family [4,5]. In this process an appropriately trained professional (physician, genetic counsellor) should help an individual and/or his family to:

- Comprehend medical facts (disorder/diagnosis, course, and management)
- Understand the heredity contribution to the disorder and recurrence risks (in relatives and for future children)
- Understand the options available for dealing with the recurrence risk (like prenatal diagnosis, reproductive alternatives)
- Choose a course of action in view of their risk, compatible with family goals, values, religious beliefs and act in accordance with that decision
- Make the best possible adjustment to the condition in an affected person and/or to the recurrence risk of the disorder.

Common reasons for cardiovascular genetic counselling (see also table 1) or consultation of a clinical geneticist are e.g.

- Parents who have a child with a structural heart defect or (who are suspected of) a disorder or syndrome with cardiac implications, who want to be informed about recurrence risks, discuss prenatal diagnostic methods, or when syndrome evaluation is indicated.
- Individuals with a known (or suspected) cardiovascular disorder or those who are at risk for a specific cardiovascular disease on the basis of their family history.
- Risk assessment and pre-test counselling in individuals prior to genetic testing, interpretation or explanation of results of genetic tests and/or discussion of the implications of the results for family members.

Table 1: Indications for genetic counselling in cardiology:

-Parents of a child with:	-a (suspected) cardiovascular disorder with a known genetic component like e.g. congenital structural heart defect -a cardiovascular disorder associated with other (dysmorphic) features or organ dysfunction e.g. Marfan syndrome, Williams syndrome
-Persons who have a cardiac disorder themselves who want to be informed on the genetic risks for themselves or their offspring	
-Persons at risk for a cardiac disorder on the basis of family history, or proven or suspected familial cardiac disease (risks for themselves or their offspring)	
-Persons seeking risk assessment prior to genetic testing and/or interpretation of genetic tests for cardiovascular disorders	

In order to achieve the objective of genetic counselling, four major components compromise the genetic counselling: diagnosis, informative counselling, decision making /supportive counselling and follow-up.

1. *Diagnosis*:
Collection of necessary information to confirm or establish the diagnosis in the patient or family. Strategies to be utilised are e.g. taking a detailed (family) history and preparation of a pedigree, collection of medical and autopsy records of family members to confirm suspected diagnosis, additional clinical evaluation in the proband or family members, assessment of the counselee.
2. *Informative counselling*:
Impartion of disease facts like diagnosis, natural history, prognosis, treatment and management modalities, genetic implications and possible options. Discussion about this and perception of these facts and risks with the counselee.
3 *Process of decision making and supportive counselling*:
Support and reinforce choices in couples wanting to raise a family or in individuals wanting predictive testing to be informed on their own health status or risks. Helping individuals and families to cope with the discovery of a genetic disorder in the family or in an individual.
4 *Follow-up*:
Send a letter summarising the information given, encourage people to pose questions or to return for follow-up sessions to comprehend the information or to discuss concerns or feelings. At most departments of clinical genetics trained social workers or psychologists are available for supportive care, if needed.

Because genetic counselling fulfilling the above-mentioned criteria requires expertise of both cardiologists and clinical geneticists, in the Netherlands multidisciplinary cardiogenetic outpatient clinics have been initiated. Goal is to offer genetic counselling according to the above mentioned guidelines. In our setting a cardiologist and a clinical geneticist in co-operation with a genetic associate evaluate and confirm the diagnosis, gather information on family members, offer/perform genetic counselling and if required perform additional cardiologic investigation and DNA tests. Results are discussed with the proband and a plan is made to offer investigations to family members if they want to. We offer so-called cascade or step-wise screening in which first-degree relatives (parents, children, siblings) of a patient with a suspected or proven genetic cardiovascular disorder are being screened first. If a further family member turns out to be affected, his or her first-degree relatives will be offered screening as well. If the family history points towards a familial character of the disorder, other family members are offered screening as well, see figure 6.

The advantage of the combined out-patients' clinics is that the counselling procedure can take place in one or two settings and that both specialists know what information is communicated to a patient. Besides immediate plans can be effectuated for additional investigations like directed DNA investigations or echocardiography.

This service is very much appreciated by the patients and referring physicians. The cardiologists and clinical geneticists involved feel it is an efficient way to take care of patients with a genetic cardiovascular disease and their families. GP's and cardiologists refer patients to our outpatient clinics. In case of referral by a cardiologist it's our goal to refer the patients back to their local cardiologist with advises on treatment.

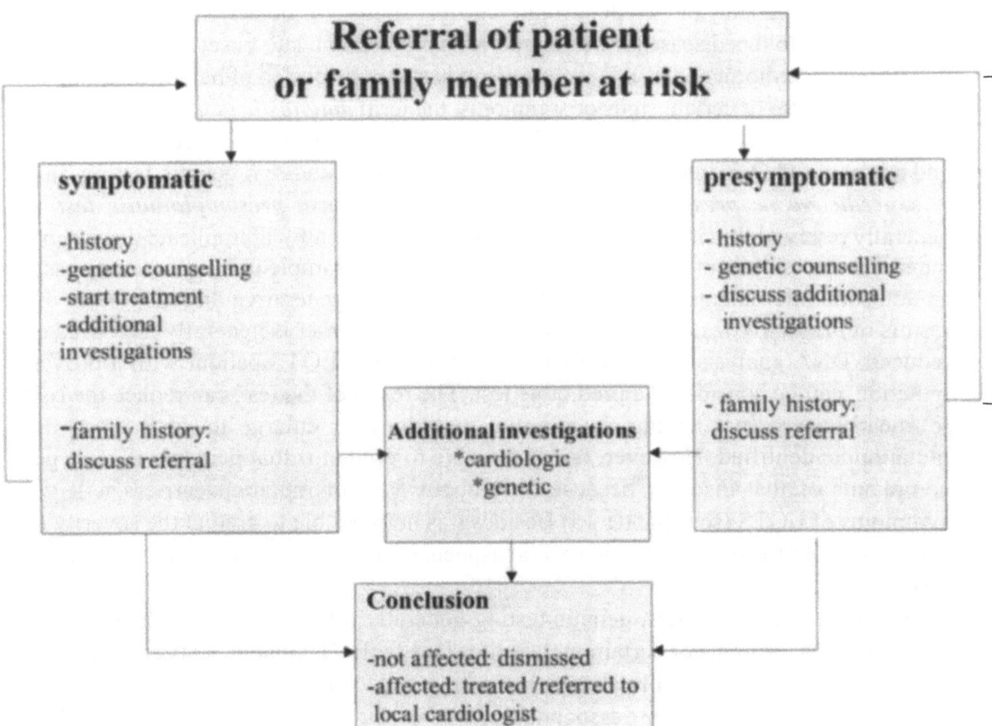

***Figure 6**. Flow chart applied in our combined cardiologic-clinical genetic outpatients'clinic*

In genetic counselling two situations have to be distinguished. First: ***affected*** individuals (or the parents of an affected child) coming for genetic counselling to discuss reproductive aspects of the disorder or to confirm a diagnosis (by cardiologic or physical examination or the use of genetic techniques). Second: ***healthy***, ***asymptomatic*** people who want to be informed about their genetic status and their risk of developing a specific disorder during their life, often after identification of a familial disorder. This is called presymptomatic or predictive genetic counselling (see 1.4). In recent years, clinical geneticists have obtained a lot of experience in presymptomatic testing from dealing with neurodegenerative disorders like Huntington's Disease, Spinocerebellar ataxia (SCA), myotonic dystrophy and hereditary forms of cancer like hereditary breast and ovarian cancer (HBOC), hereditary non-polyposis colorectal cancer (HNPCC) and Familial Adenomatous Polyposis Coli.

Genetic testing/genetic screening/Presymptomatic testing/predictive testing [2,4,6]:

Genetic testing is the use of specific tests for the analysis of a gene, its product or function in individuals who are at increased risk for a genetic disorder because of their family history or symptoms. Genetic testing can be established for diagnosing a specific disease in a patient or to determine carrier status to detect susceptibility or predisposition to this disease (in healthy persons predicting a late-onset disease like e.g. hypertrophic cardiomyopathy). When a person has or is suspected of having a particular disorder, because of certain signs or symptoms, the term ***diagnostic genetic test*** is being used. An example is the use of genetic investigations in a person with recurrent syncope and a prolonged QTc interval. When healthy individuals undergo genetic testing, this is a ***predictive or presymptomatic genetic test***. The term ***presymptomatic test*** is generally reserved for situations where an abnormal test result will implicate the, almost inevitable, development of the disorder later in life. An example is Huntington disease, an autosomal dominantly inherited progressive neurodegenerative disorder. With the results of ***predictive*** *testing*, the risk of developing a disorder is generally increased or reduced. DNA analysis in a healthy person related to a LQTS patient with a proven mutation, can be considered a predictive test. The result of the test, can reduce the risk to –nearly- zero (not having the familial mutation), or enlarge the risk when the mutation is identified. However, one is not able to predict if that person will ever get complaints of that disorder because only about 50% of mutation carriers will get symptoms of LQTS (see chapter 15) Besides it is not possible to predict the severity or age of onset of the disease. Some special aspects of predictive testing are discussed in below.

In (cardiovascular) genetics, genetic testing generally refers to the analysis of DNA, chromosomes, proteins or certain metabolites (see table 2). Genetic tests are available for some "pure" cardiovascular disorders (like e.g. LQTS, HCM, certain types of DCM) or disorders that can be associated with cardiovascular abnormalities (like haemochromatosis, mitochondrial diseases, neuromuscular diseaseor coagulation disorders).

Table 2: specific genetic tests available for cardiovascular disorders

Chromosome analysis: e.g. for Turner syndrome (45,X) or Down syndrome (trisomy 21), Fluorescent In Situ Hybridisation analysis deletion 7. (Williams syndrome), deletion 22q11 (velocardiofacial syndrome)
DNA analysis*: dyslipidemias, homocystinuria, LQTS, HCM, certain forms of DCM, ARVC, catecholamine induced ventricular tachycardia, Brugada syndrome
certain syndromes like e.g.: Holt-Oram syndrome, Marfan syndrome
Protein tests/metabolic investigations: Marfan syndrome (fibrillin), homocystein (homocystinuria), Ehlers Danlos syndromes (collagen), dyslipidemias (cholesterol incl. fractions, triglycerides,chylomicron)

note: mutations are not detected in every patient because not all genes responsible for the disease have been identified (or are offered as diagnostic service) yet, or because the sensitivity of the genetic tests is not 100%.*

It is generally accepted that genetic testing can be performed in the context of treatment, management or implementation of preventive measures in disease to modify the severity of a certain disorder. Other indications are to supply information on reproductive counseling, or to enable prenatal diagnosis in certain disorders.

Before a genetic test will take place a risk assessment should be performed and genetic counselling should take place. This holds particularly true for predictive and presymptomatic genetic counselling because of the possible medical, psychological and social implications. The decision to undergo genetic testing should be an individuals own free choice and there should be no obligation from insurance companies, employers or other persons or authorities. To prevent people from making decisions they might regret later, genetic testing should be provided along with genetic counselling. In the Netherlands special cardiogenetic outpatient clinics provide care and counselling facilities for patients or their relatives with a (suspected) heritable cardiovascular disorder.
Genetic screening differs from genetic testing. The main difference is that in genetic screening a population is searched for certain disorders to identify persons at risk, independent of positive family history or symptom manifestations. Goal of genetic screening is to prevent deleterious effects of the disorder by treatment or life style rules (e.g. dietary measures in PKU, hypercholesterolemia or G6PD).

Special elements of genetic/presymptomatic/predictive testing [4,6].

In predictive testing there are some important issues that have to be considered before the actual testing takes place:

Medical-therapeutical aspects

1. The relevance and consequences of identifying the gene mutation in an individual. The identification of a mutant gene in a person, doesn't necessarily predict the outcome:

some mutation-carriers will only develop symptoms later in life, so-called age-dependent penetrance (like e.g. in DCM or HCM), while other mutation carriers never develop symptoms (non-penetrance; e.g. in LQTS estimated to be about 50%). There can be an enormous clinical variability. In ARVC some family members develop severe episodes of ventricular arrhythmias at young age, while others have only mild abnormalities on cardiac ultrasound at an older age without any complaints. Reduced penetrance and variable expression are typical elements of autosomal dominantly inherited cardiac diseases.

2. Are there therapeutic consequences? Is treatment available and what is its effectiveness? The value of identification of a LQTS gene mutation carriers is generally not disputed, because the disorder can have severe consequences (sudden cardiac death) and effective therapy is available (depending on the type of LQTS), like beta blockade, avoiding certain types of medication, life style advises, implantation of an ICD or pacemaker. In other disorders there is more debate on the effectiveness of therapy like e.g. DCM.

Social, psychological and ethical issues

In addition to the elements mentioned above, other issues play an important role in deciding whether or not to perform genetic testing. Because a person is symptomless, the identification of a mutation may lead to a reduced well being, increased anxiety, diminished self-esteem and self worth, which may even lead to declining prophylactic medication. Also social effects like problems obtaining life or health insurance may play a role in someone's decision to undergo predictive screening. Effects on the relationships with other family members can be anticipated: some family members don't want to participate in the testing, while others do not understand their motives to refrain from testing. Another example is the situation in which an individual refuses a genetic test, while that person's adult child chooses the undergo testing. This might influence the relationship in different ways: the child might reproach the parent who declines the test, and if the child turns out to be mutation carrier, this automatically means that that parent is a mutation carrier as well. This parent gets information that he did not want to have.

Family dynamics also have to be kept in mind when someone turns out to be a non-carrier of the disease. The feelings of relief, one would expect, are sometimes not present (survivor's guilt) and the affected family members may treat the non-carrier different.

Privacy

Information on results of genetic tests should only be accessible to the person tested and the physician or counsellor discussing the test results. Disclosure of genetic test results to employers, insurance companies or other people can lead to discrimination, restrictions in insurance and is in conflict with the physicians' duty to confidentiality.

Predictive testing in children

A special category is parents who want predictive genetic testing for their minor

children. One has to keep in mind that genetic testing in minors could theoretically be performed for disorders occurring later in life or for disorders which first manifestations can occur at a young age like e.g. long QT syndrome. Predictive or presymptomatic testing in children is only acceptable if onset can occur in childhood or if interventions (medication, diet) can be offered. It is generally accepted that one refrains from testing for adult-onset disorders in children, unless direct medical benefit will accrue to the child and waiting until the child has reached adulthood would lose this benefit.
Psychological investigations revealed that a high percentage of parents who have their minors tested for heritable cardiac arrhythmia syndromes have high levels of depression and anxiety and coping problems [7]. Special care has to be provided for this category of patients. After the diagnosis is made, overprotectiveness can occur, leading to behavioural problems or a lower self-esteem. Special attention has to be made to this point by the physician who takes care of the patient or family. Identifying a genetic disorder in a child can lead to feelings of failure or guilt in the transmitting parent or negative feelings for the affected child (or transmitting parent).

Informed consent

Because the cardiovascular genetic disorders have great impact on someone's physical and psychological well-being and because important (irreversible) decisions have to be made on e.g. genetic testing with consequences in all kinds of fields described before, clinical geneticists provide written information on all elements of the genetic counselling process . This written information enables the counselee/patient to make proper decisions. It is important that counselees do not feel any obligation to participate in genetic testing. Informed consent is gathered before the actual testing takes place.

Non-directiveness

In reproductive genetic counselling and in presymptomatic genetic counselling for non-treatable late onset disorders in clinical genetics, non-directiveness is always a paradigm. Non-directiveness in genetic counselling for treatable heritable cardiac disorders like LQTS is less defendable. Nevertheless families and counselees should never be obliged to participate in genetic testing.

Cardiovascular medicine is weathering multiple challenges on multiple fronts. Clinical genetics is one of them. This requires from the cardiologist to take on new responsibilities. One of them is to discuss different genetic tests with patients, to explain the possible advantages and limitations, to interpret results in lay terms and to assist patients in understanding the implications of the results for the patients and his families. This is a huge undertaking and a challenge for physicians who are not always familiar with the elements discussed in this chapter.

References

1. Giardello FM. Genetic testing in hereditary colorectal cancer JAMA 1997; 278:1278-81.
2. Harper PS, Clarke AJ Genetics, Society and Clinical Practice. Bios, Oxford 1997.
3. Pronk JC (red) Leerboek medische genetica, Elsevier/Bunge, Maarssen 1998.
4. Baker DL Schuette JL., Uhlmann WR., A Guide to Genetic Counseling. Wiley-Liss, New York 1998.
5. Genetic Counseling Am J Hum Gen 1975; 27:240-1.
6. Lashley FR Genetic Testing, Screening, and Counseling Issues in Cardiovascular Disease J Cardiovasc Nurs 1999; 13:110-26.
7. Hendriks KSWH, Grosveld FJM, van Tintelen JP, van Langen IM, Wilde AAM, ten Kroode HFJ Psychological distress in persons undergoing predictive DNA-diagnostics for an autosomal dominant inherited cardiac arrhythmia syndrome Eur J Human Genet 2000; 8 suppl p.175.

3. GENETICS OF CONGENITAL HEART DISEASE

P. Grossfeld

Introduction

Congenital heart disease is the most common birth defect, affecting 0.7% of liveborn infants [1]. There is overwhelming evidence supporting a genetic etiology for most congenital heart defects in humans [2]. This includes familial occurrences and a high recurrence rate, an association with specific chromosomal disorders, and the high occurrence rate of congenital defects in dysmorphic syndromes. To date, there is a limited number of genes that has been demonstrated to cause congenital heart defects in humans. That number is bound to increase rapidly with the completion of the human genome sequencing project. In this review, congenital heart defects are defined as those defects that are present and can be diagnosed at birth. Other structural heart defects in which specific genes have been identified, including cardiomyopathies, long QT syndrome and Marfan syndrome, are discussed in separate chapters.

Approach to identification of genes causing congenital heart disease

Depending on the criteria, a large number of genes have been identified as "candidates" for causing specific heart defects, but much fewer have been proven to cause congenital heart defects. For diseases with high penetrance in large kindreds, linkage analysis has been used to associate specific chromosomal loci with a congenital heart defect [3,4]. Identification of known genes and/or expressed sequence tags at the associated locus helps to identify possible candidate genes. Alternatively, a balanced translocation in a patient with a congenital heart defect whose breakpoint disrupts a gene can also be used to identify a candidate gene [5].

Once a candidate gene is identified, there remains the formidable task of proving it causes a specific heart defect. Two complementary approaches can be employed. First, mutation screening in isolated human patients with a congenital heart defect can be performed. For non-familial cases, identification of mutations in the patient population not found in controls is usually considered to support causality. In large kindreds with high penetrance, this entails demonstrating cosegregation of the mutant allele with the

PA Doevendans and AA Wilde (eds.), Cardiovascular genetics, 29-34.

disease. DNA sequence analysis can be performed by analyzing PCR products derived from the individual exons, along with the flanking splice site sequences, for a particular gene.

This requires only a small amount of blood from which total genomic DNA is extracted from peripheral blood lymphocytes. Although currently this is only performed in research laboratories, the development of high throughput DNA sequencing techniques makes it likely that mutation screening will become widely available in clinical laboratories for patient diagnosis.

The second approach for proving a gene causes a congenital heart defect involves the use of genetically engineered animal models. For example, gene-specific knockouts can be performed in the mouse in order to attempt to recapitulate the heart defects observed in humans. Gene-specific knockouts can be restricted to specific chambers of the heart at specific developmental times [6]. Generation of a specific cardiac phenotype due to a gene-specific knockout is sufficient proof of causality.

Both human mutation screening and mouse knockouts can have pitfalls. For example, mutation screening will only identify point mutations or tiny deletions/insertions . If the mechanism of mutation is predominantly microdeletions, in which one copy of the gene is completely deleted, this will not be detected by standard DNA sequencing techniques.

In this case, DNA sequencing will only identify the sequence of the retained, normal copy of the gene and, therefore, could not be distinguished from normal, unaffected individuals that have two identical copies of that gene. If polymorphisms exist in the disease-causing gene, then microdeletion may result in the loss of heterozygosity for polymorphic markers in the gene. However, for polygenic disorders, it can be extremely difficult to demonstrate a statistically significant loss of heterozygosity for a specific gene in a group of patients with a specific heart defect. For example, if a particular gene caused a heart defect in a small minority of all patients with that defect, and that gene does not have a high degree of polymorphism, then it would be difficult to demonstrate a statistically significant loss of heterozygosity at that gene locus in the overall population of patients with that heart defect. In that case, the small number of patients that have the disease due to a loss of heterozygosity at the disease-causing gene's locus would be obscured by the high frequency of individuals with the heart defect that are homozygous for that gene.

When performing mouse knockout studies, the generation of a phenotype may be dependent on genetic background. Thus, whether or not the gene-specific knockout produces a phenotype may depend upon which mouse strain is used. The mechanisms underlying strain-dependent phenotypes in the mouse may also provide insight into the basis for incomplete penetrance that can occur in human genetic disorders. Gene knockouts may also cause an early embryonic-lethal phenotype in which the mechanism of lethality can be extremely difficult to prove.

Genes Causing Specific Congenital Heart Defects

To date only a limited number of genes causing congenital heart defects in humans has been identified (table). Many of the heart defects caused by these genes are part of a constellation of problems comprising a dysmorphic syndrome
Understanding the function of these genes has already had an impact on clinical practice.

Holt-Oram syndrome is chararacterized by heart defects, most commonly atrial and ventricular septal defects, in association with limb anomalies. Recently, this syndrome was found to be caused by mutations in the gene TBX-5, a member of the T-box family of transcription factors [7,8]. Studies in large kindreds with atrial septal defects have led to the identification of a second gene, NKX2.5 [9]. This gene also encodes a transcription factor that is involved in cardiac development, and is expressed in the atrial septum as well as the cardiac conduction tissue. It has been shown that patients with atrial septal defects and mutations in the NKX2.5 gene have a lifelong risk for the development of conduction heart block and sudden death. Some patients with Holt-Oram syndrome have also been reported to develop heart block. Thus, ALL patients with atrial septal defects need to be followed serially for the development of arrhythmias. Future studies will be aimed at determining if these factors may interact, and if they share common pathways in cardiac development.

Williams syndrome is a rare dysmorphic syndrome characterized by heart defects, most commonly supravalvar aortic stenosis, peripheral pulmonary stenosis and in 5-10% of cases, life-threatening coronary artery obstructive lesions, in association with elfin facies, mental retardation, neonatal hypercalcemia, and a so-called "cocktail party" personality. This disorder is caused by a microdeletion at 7q11. Studies of patients with isolated supravalvar aortic stenosis and/or pulmonic stenosis have demonstrated that mutations in the gene encoding the structural protein elastin, which is located within the region deleted at 7q11, are responsible for these cardiac defects [5]. Mutations in elastin causing these heart defects are inherited in an autosomal dominant mode. Microdeletions can be detected with FISH using commercially available probes contained within 7q11, although screening for elastin point mutation is only performed in research laboratories.

Alagille syndrome is a rare disorder characterized by heart defects, most commonly peripheral pulmonic stenosis and tetralogy of Fallot, in association with neonatal jaundice caused by a deficiency of intrahepatic bile ducts. Recently, mutations in the Jagged1 gene, which encodes the ligand for the Notch receptor that is involved in signaling pathways in cell fate determination early in development, were found to cause this disorder [10]. Inheritance is autosomal dominant, and to date, mutation screening is only performed in research laboratories.

DiGeorge syndrome is characterized by conotruncal heart defects, including truncus arteriosus, type B interruption of the aortic arch, tetralogy of Fallot with pulmonary atresia, absent pulmonary valve, and right aortic arch, in association with mental retardation, dysmorphic facies, cleft palate, hypoparathyroidism and thymic hypoplasia. This constellation of defects is due to abnormal development of the third and fourth embryonic branchial pouches. The majority of patients with DiGeorge syndrome carry a microdeletion at 22q11, and 18% of all patients with isolated conotruncal defects carry a 22q11 microdeletion. [11]. Identification of the causative gene (s) has been difficult. Most recently, mouse knockouts of at least two genes in the mouse in the region corresponding to 22q11 seem to recapitulate the syndrome: TBX-1, another member of the T-box family of transcription factors which may be essential for cardiac neural crest development [12-14], and CRKL, which is involved in growth factor and focal adhesion signaling [15]. To date, point mutations in either of these genes in patients with conal truncal mutations have not been identified. The 22q11 deletion is transmitted in autosomal dominant mode. Diagnosis is established by Fluorescent In Situ Hybridization with a probe located within the DiGeorge critical region in 22q11.

Char Syndrome is a rare disorder characterized by patent ductus arteriosus and craniofacial abnormalities. Both of these structures are derived from the neural crest. Recently, mutations in the gene TFAP2B, which encodes a transcription factor that is expressed in the neural crest, have been identified [16]. This disorder is inherited as autosomal dominant and to date, mutation screening is only performed in research laboratories.

Summary

There is strong evidence for a genetic etiology underlying most congenital heart defects. To date, only a limited number of genes have been found to cause specific heart defects. The majority of these genes encode transcription factors involved in cardiac development, and most of these genes were detected in association with dysmorphic syndromes characterized by a multitude of other non-cardiac anomalies in addition to heart defects. Currently, mutation screening for most patients with congenital heart defects is not performed routinely and is cost-prohibitive. As more disease-causing genes are identified and high throughput DNA sequencing techniques are incorporated into clinical genetic laboratories, mutation screening for patients with congenital heart disease should become available. This will allow for improvement in predicting recurrences of congenital heart disease in families in which there is an affected child. In addition, as more children with congenital heart disease live to reproductive age, identification of disease-causing mutations will be necessary for the determination of risk of transmission to their offspring. Finally, earlier detection by prenatal diagnosis in the overall population will be possible. The human genome sequencing project promises to expedite the identification of most if not all of the remaining genes that cause congenital heart defects, ultimately allowing for improved diagnosis, treatment and, hopefully, prevention of this catastrophic group of childhood disorders.

Table

Heart Defect	Associated Syndrome: non-cardiac defects	Gene	Locus	Fam. Occurrence
ASD (A)	Holt-Oram: radial, ulnar defects	TBX-5	12q12	
	-	NKX2-5	5q35	
Pulmonic Stenosis (A) Extremely Rare	Williams: neonatal hypercalcemia, elfin facies, "cocktail party" personality, mental retardation	Elastin	7q11.23	
Pulmonic Stenosis, Tetralogy of fallot (A)	Alagille: Liver dysfunction	Jagged1	20p12	Yes
Patent Duct. Arteriosus B)	Char: craniofacial abnormalities	TFAP2B	6p12	Yes
Truncus Arteriorsus, Type B Interruption of the Aortic Arch, Tetralogy of fallot (A)	DiGeorge: cleft palate, abnormal facies, thymic dysplasia. hypocalcemia	TBX-1, CRKL	22q11	Yes
Heterotaxy	----	Connexin-43	6q22.3	
	----	ZIC3	Xq26.2	

References

1. Ferencz C, Loffredo CA, Correa-Villasenor A, Wilson PD (eds.) Perspectives in pediatric cardiology, Vol. 5, Genetic and environmental risk factors of major cardiovascular malformations.The Baltimore-Washington Infant Study 1981-1989. Futura: Armonk, NY, 1997.
2. Grossfeld, PD; Rothman A, Gruber P; Chien KR. Molecular genetics of congenital heart disease, in "Molecular Basis of Cardiovascular Disease" (Ed. Chien KR) WB Saunders 1999; 135-65.
3. Geisterfer-Lowrance, AA; Kass, S; Tanigawa, G; Vosberg, HP; McKenna, W; Seidman, CE; Seidman, JG. A molecular basis for familial hypertrophic cardiomyopathy: a beta cardiac myosin heavy chain gene missense mutation. Cell, 1990; 62:999-1006.
4. Tsipouras, P; Del Mastro, R; Sarfarazi, M; et al and international Marfan syndrome Collaborative Study: Genetic linkage of the Marfan syndrome, ectopia lentis, and congenital contractural arachnodactyly to the fibrillin genes on chromosomes 15 and 5. N Engl J Med 1992; 326: 905-90.
5. Morris, CA; Loker, J; Ensing, G; Stock, AD. Supravalvular aortic stenosis cosegregates with a familial 6; 7 translocation which disrupts the elastin gene. Am J Med Genet 1993; 4:737-44.
6. Chen, J; Kubalak, SW; Chien, KR. Ventricular muscle-restricted targeting of the RXR alpha gene reveals a non-cell-autonomous requirement in cardiac chamber morphogenesis. Development 1998; 125:1943-49.
7. Li, QY; Newbury-Ecob, RA; Terrett, JA; Wilson, DI; Curtis, AR; Yi, CH; Gebuhr, T; Bullen, PJ; Robson, SC; Strachan, T; Bonnet, D; Lyonnet, S; Young, ID; Raeburn, JA; Buckler, AJ; Law, DJ; Brook, JD. Holt-Oram syndrome is caused by mutations in TBX5, a member of the Brachyury (T) gene family. Nat Genet 1997; 1:21-9.
8. Basson, CT; Bachinsky, DR; Lin, RC; Levi, T; Elkins, JA; Soults, J; Grayzel, D; Kroumpouzou, E; Traill, TA; Leblanc-Straceski, J; Renault, B; Kucherlapati, R; Seidman, JG; Seidman, CE. Mutations in human TBX5 cause limb and cardiac malformation in Holt-Oram syndrome Nature Genetics, 1997; 1:30-5.
9. Schott, JJ; Benson, DW; Basson, CT; Pease, W; Silberbach, GM; Moak, JP; Maron, BJ; Seidman, CE; Seidman, JG. Congenital heart disease caused by mutations in the transcription factor NKX2-5 Science, 1998; 5373:108-11.
10. Oda, T; Elkahloun, AG; Pike, BL; Okajima, K; Krantz, ID; Genin, A; Piccoli, DA; Meltzer, PS; Spinner, NB; Collins, FS; Chandrasekharappa, SC. Mutations in the human Jagged1 gene are responsible for Alagille syndrome. Nat Genet 1997; 3:235-42.
11. Goldmuntz, E; Clark, BJ; Mitchell, LE; Jawad, AF; Cuned, BF; Reed, L; McDonald-McGinn, D; Chien, P; Feuer, J; Zackai, EN; Emanuel, BS; Driscoll, DA. Frequency of 22q11 deletions in patients with conotruncal defects. JACC, 1998; 32:492-8.
12. Jerome, LA; Papaioannou, VE. DiGeorge syndrome phenotype in mice mutant for the T-box gene, Tbx1. Nat Genet 2001; 3: 286-91.
13. Merscher, S; Funke, B; Epstein, JA; Heyer, J; Puech, A; Lu, MM; Xavier, RJ; Demay, MB; Russell, RG; Factor, S; Tokooya, K; Jore, BS; Lopez, M; Pandita, RK; Lia, M; Carrion, D; Xu, H; Schorle, H; Kobler, JB; Scambler, P; Wynshaw-Boris, A; Skoultchi, AI; Morrow, BE; Kucherlapati, R. TBX1 is responsible for cardiovascular defects in velo-cardio-facial/DiGeorge syndrome. Cell 2001; 104:619-29.
14. Lindsay, EA; Vitelli, F; Su, H; Morishima, M; Huynh, T; Pramparo, T; Jurecic, V; Ogunrinu, G; Sutherland, HF; Scambler, PJ; Bradley, A; Baldini, A. Tbx1 haploinsufficieny in the DiGeorge syndrome region causes aortic arch defects in mice. Nature, 2001; 410:97-101.
15. Guris, DL; Fantes, J; Tara, D; Druker, BJ; Imamoto, A. Mice lacking the homologue of the human 22q11.2 gene CRKL phenocopy neurocristopathies of DiGeorge syndrome. Nat Genet 2001; 3: 293-8.
16. Satoda, M; Zhao, F: Diaz, GA; Burn, J; Goodship, J; Davidson, R; Pierpoint, MEM; Gelb, BD; Mutations in TFAP2B cause Char syndrome, a familial form of patent ductus arteriosus. Nat Genet 2000; 25:42-6.

4. GENETICS OF HYPERTENSION

A.A. Kroon, W. Spiering, P.W. de Leeuw

Introduction

High blood pressure is a common and major risk factor for cardiovascular disease. Still, the pathogenesis of essential hypertension remains incompletely understood. It is generally felt that different factors may contribute in an individual patient. Among those that have been intensively studied are salt intake, obesity and insulin resistance, the renin-angiotensin system, and the sympathetic nervous system. In the past few years, research has been increasingly directed towards the genetics of hypertension.

Recent advances in molecular genetics such as the polymerase chain reaction, micro array techniques, and the concerted effort of the Human Genome Mapping Project, enable research into the genetic basis of common diseases to become a tangible prospect (See also chapter 1 and 18). A dense map of genetic markers is being developed, providing one marker for, on average, every 700.000 base pairs. This permits the demonstration of links between regions of the genome and common human disorders [1]. The genetic markers exhibit high interindividual variation or polymorphisms and may be based on single nucleotide variations, simple sequence repeats (microsatellites), or upon repetitive segments of tens or hundreds of bases (minisatellites) [2].

Although various individual genes and genetic factors have been linked to the development of essential hypertension, a combination of multiple genes most likely contributes to the development of the disorder in a particular patient. It is therefore extremely difficult to accurately determine the relative contributions of each of these genes. Moreover, it is now recognised that many common disorders, such as hypertension, arise from complex interactions between genes and environmental factors. The understanding of the molecular basis of hypertension may provide us with new and more specific pharmacological targets and perhaps the ability to individualise antihypertensive treatment and maximise reduction in risk of morbidity and mortality from cardiovascular disease.

Genetic strategies for hypertension

Normal blood pressure is maintained by the physiological interaction of cardiac output and peripheral resistance, and by control of salt and water balance by the kidney.

PA Doevendans and AA Wilde (eds.), Cardiovascular genetics, 35-49.

Despite identification and understanding of the physiological systems involved in the regulation of blood pressure, it remains unclear which systems are causative in essential hypertension. Traditional linkage studies reveal tracking of a genetic variation through a family with the trait of interest [1]. The analyses are based upon logarithmic odds ratios (LOD scores) that express the likelihood of linkage divided by the likelihood of non-linkage. A LOD score of 3 is conventionally accepted as evidence in favour of linkage and means that the odds are 1000 to 1 in favour of linkage rather than non-linkage of the particular genetic marker. Such studies have proven to be successful in rare hypertensive syndromes with a Mendelian mode of inheritance. These hypertensive traits may be identified by a specific response to drugs, e.g. corticosteroids in glucocorticoid-remediable aldosteronism, or an associated biochemical phenotype, e.g. hypokalaemia in Conn's syndrome.

These types of model-specific pedigree analyses are less likely to be successful in the general, complex trait of essential hypertension where Mendelian modes of inheritance cannot be assigned because there may be variable penetrance of susceptibility genes. In addition, age at onset of the trait may be variable, or the presence or absence of environmental stimuli or other genetic interactions may be necessary to disclose the phenotype [1].

Several strategies have been followed to determine the genetic basis of essential hypertension. Among these are (model-free) linkage studies, discordant sibling pair analysis, association studies, and family-based association studies [1]. Other approaches involve the assessment of candidate genes and genome screens. In the former, candidate genes and/or genetic polymorphisms of a specific gene are chosen on the basis of systems which are physiologically involved in blood pressure regulation, e.g. the renin-angiotensin system. Ideally, it may be possible to demonstrate biochemical or functional differences in the gene products which track with blood pressure levels through families, and it may also be possible to identify genetic variations that are associated with the trait. Genome screens utilise a dense map of highly polymorphic markers that are spread evenly throughout the human genome, to test for linkage of chromosomal regions to blood pressure [3]. The advantage of this approach is that it may identify chromosomal regions, which harbour susceptibility genes that are not suspected beforehand to contribute to hypertension [4].

Essential hypertension: a complex trait

Hypertension affects approximately 20% of the adult population in Westernised society, and contributes significantly to morbidity and mortality from cardiovascular disease including stroke, myocardial infarction and end-stage renal disease [5]. Human essential hypertension has a multifactorial origin and is thought to arise from an interaction between susceptibility genes and environmental factors. Twin and family studies suggest that approximately 30% of blood pressure variation arises from genes [6]. Multiple transplantation studies in animals and in humans have shown that the inherited tendency to hypertension primarily resides in the kidney [7,8]. These findings have led to the study of genes that affect renal function, leading to the discovery of prohypertensive single gene mutations in a few, rare forms of hypertension [5].

Since blood pressure adopts a normal distribution in the general population and is defined on the basis of thresholds, there will be several genes involved in the genetic susceptibility to this multifactorial or 'complex trait' [1,5]. It is possible that genetic variation within an individual gene may have only modest effects on blood pressure unless combined with anomalies within other genes or with environmental factors such as high sodium in the diet. These interactions may be additive or synergistical. The inter-relationships may, however, prove difficult to establish for both gene-gene or gene-environment interactions [1].

Hypertension due to single gene abnormalities

Glucocorticoid-remediable aldosteronism (GRA)

This is a rare Mendelian (autosomal dominant) form of hypertension associated with both an excess of cerebral haemorrhage and Celtic ancestry [9]. The hypertension, in these cases with a high penetrance in families and a typical onset before age 21, is caused by excessive secretion of aldosterone, which is regulated by adrenocorticotrophic hormone (ACTH) rather than by angiotensin II [1]. Kindred from GRA demonstrate a novel, chimeric gene on chromosome 8 that represents duplication arising from unequal crossover between the aldosterone synthase and 11β-hydroxylase genes, such that regulatory sequences of 11β-hydroxylase are fused with coding sequences of aldosterone synthase. Aldosterone activity is therefore brought under the control of ACTH. Typically, plasma renin activity and angiotensin II production are decreased, and 18-OH cortisol and aldosterone levels are increased. The plasma potassium concentration is normal in more than one-half of cases of GRA in contrast to the hypokalaemia usually seen in primary hyperaldosteronism due to an adrenal adenoma [11]. The main clinical clues suggesting GRA in the normokalaemic patient are the family history of early hypertension and the frequent development of marked hypokalaemia after the administration of a thiazide diuretic. Hypertension in GRA arises from increased water and salt retention. Blood pressure lowering treatment is performed by administration of physiological doses of glucocorticoids, which suppress ACTH secretion and thereby suppress expression of the mutant gene (Category A) [10]. Affected individuals can now be detected by using a simple genetic test rather than extensive biochemical phenotyping [12].

Syndrome of apparent mineralocorticoid excess (AME)

This is an autosomal recessive disorder that produces moderate-to-severe hypertension of early onset. Characteristically, very low levels of renin and aldosterone are found in combination with hypokalaemic alkalosis [13]. Hypertension is caused by stimulation of the mineralocorticoid receptor in the distal convoluted tubule of the kidney by normal circulating concentrations of cortisol due a mutation in the gene encoding for the enzyme 11β-hydroxysteroid dehydrogenase (11β-HSD) type 2. In normal circumstances cortisol and aldosterone have equal affinity for the mineralocorticoid receptor. To prevent cortisol from acting at the mineralocorticoid receptor 11β-HSD metabolises cortisol to cortisone. The latter is incapable of stimulating the receptor,

resulting in the usual selective effect of aldosterone. The human HSD11B2 gene is localised on chromosome 16q22 and spreads over 5 exons (6 kb). In AME, several mutations have been observed which result in loss of the 11β-HSD enzyme activity [14,15]. There is a rough correlation between the severity of the enzymatic defect induced by these mutations and the clinical findings; however, the small number of patients reported precludes thorough analysis [15]. Insufficient 11β-HSD activity to metabolise cortisol has also been proposed to explain the hypertension seen in Cushing's syndrome.
Therapy most commonly includes spironolactone, potassium supplements, and a low-salt diet. Suppression of ACTH with dexamethasone is theoretically possible since it suppresses endogenous cortisol production. However, clinical observations suggest that dexamethasone only occasionally corrects the hypokalaemia and hypertension [16].

Pseudohypoaldosteronism type I (Liddle's syndrome)

This syndrome is also a rare autosomal dominant trait, which is phenotypically characterised by early onset of hypertension with hypokalaemia, suppressed renin activity and low aldosterone levels, all of which respond to amiloride, an inhibitor of the distal renal epithelial sodium channel [17]. Hypertension is caused by enhanced renal reabsorption of salt and water, due to increased activity of epithelial sodium channels (ENaC) in the distal convoluted tubule of the kidney. Mutations in the genes encoding for the β or γ subunits of the ENaC's have been found, leading to a marked increase in sodium transport and loss of inhibition of channel activity by elevated levels of intracellular sodium [18]. In some cases, the defect prevents downregulation of the sodium channels, leading to an increase in the number or in the openness of these channels. This genetic trait is localised on chromosome 16p. Specific markers are used to test the presence of the syndrome in kindred. Several mutations have been observed which either lead to truncation of the protein due to the presence of stop codons (R564X, F589X) or frame-shifts due to deletion or insertion of nucleotides (delC, insG), or missense mutations caused by aminoacid substitutions (616L and Y618H), all leading to increased activity of the β and/or γ subunits causing increased sodium reabsorption in the distal convoluted tubule [19].

Pseudohypoaldosteronism type II (Gordon's syndrome)

This autosomal dominant form of hypertension and hyperkalaemia, which is very responsive to thiazide diuretics, has recently been mapped to two distinct sites on chromosome 1 and 17 [20,21]. This suggests that there may be more than one cause for this disorder, which includes a renal ion channel abnormality [21]. In this context, it is interesting that rat and human comparative mapping studies have identified a locus on the long arm of chromosome 17 which maps to the same region as one of the loci for Gordon's syndrome [22]. As yet, the precise cause of Gordon's syndrome has not been defined, however (Category E). Identifying the abnormality would be beneficial as a marker of thiazide drug responsiveness.

Hypertension due to interaction of different genetic polymorphisms

Because of the observations with the single gene abnormalities and hypertension, numerous studies have assessed any possible linkage between essential hypertension and other mutations in these same genes. However, conflicting results have been published thus far. In an Australian study among 290 families a significant link has been observed between chromosome 16p12, the location for the β and γ subunits of the epithelial sodium channel, and systolic blood pressure [23]. Ambrosius et al., have shown that ENaC activity is higher in blacks than in whites, and that this activity may contribute to racial differences in sodium retention and the subsequent risk of development of low-renin hypertension [24]. Contradictory, a Swedish study did not find any relation with essential hypertension and mutations in the sodium channel responsible for Liddle's syndrome [25]. As a result, additional studies in larger numbers of patients are required to determine whether mutations in the ENaC genes are associated with essential hypertension [26].

As discussed above, candidate genes can also be selected from systems which are physiologically involved in blood pressure regulation. Among these are genes associated with salt-sensitivity, the sympathetic nervous system, and endothelial function. The latter system is increasingly being recognised as a major player in blood pressure variations. Unfortunately, polymorphisms associated with the activity of endothelial nitric oxide synthase (eNOS) could not be associated with high blood pressure until now [27]. Over and above these, the renin-angiotensin system (RAS) has been indicated as very important since it controls blood pressure and sodium balance, and is a major target for antihypertensive therapy. Several polymorphisms have been identified within genes encoding for the RAS which may contribute to the development and/or maintenance of hypertension, and which may influence therapeutic responses to blood pressure-lowering therapy. Some of these will now be discussed in more detail.

Genetic polymorphisms and the renin-angiotensin system

The angiotensinogen polymorphism:

Angiotensin is formed from a precursor, angiotensinogen (AGT), which is produced by the liver and found in the alpha-globulin fraction of plasma. The lowering of blood pressure is a stimulus to secretion of renin by the kidney into the blood. Renin cleaves from angiotensinogen a terminal decapeptide, angiotensin I. This is further altered by the enzymatic removal of a dipeptide to form angiotensin II (Ang II). Cleavage of AGT by renin is the rate-limiting step in the formation of Ang II. By 3 sets of observations (genetic linkage, allelic associations, and differences in plasma angiotensinogen concentrations among AGT genotypes) in a sample of families from 2 different populations, Salt Lake City and Paris, Jeunemaitre et al. demonstrated involvement of the AGT gene in essential hypertension. Hypertension showed association with 2 distinct amino acid substitutions, Met235Thr and Thr174Met. The 2 variants showed complete linkage disequilibrium; Thr174Met occurred on a subset of the haplotypes carrying the Met235Thr variant, and both haplotypes were observed at higher frequency among hypertensives [31]. The M235T variant may be a marker for blood pressure variation [28], coronary atherosclerosis [29], and preeclampsia [30]. Linkage and association studies have been performed, demonstrating higher blood pressure levels, especially at younger age, and higher AGT concentrations in subjects with one or two T-alleles [31-34]. However, presumably due to the heterogeneity of hypertension these results have not been confirmed in some other studies [35]. Another variant, located just next to the initial transcription site, which changes a guanine to adenine at position –6 (G-6A) also showed a strong association to hypertension [36]. It has been suggested that this variant may be more functional, since it increases the level of AGT by altering the transcription rate within the regulatory region of this gene, and has shown to determine the blood pressure response to sodium reduction [37,38]. However, neither the regulation nor the importance of the expression of this gene in various tissues is fully understood and, moreover, a large European study could not find any support for a role of the AGT gene in essential hypertension [39].

With respect to treatment of hypertension, until now, no association has been shown between the AGT genotype and blood pressure reduction induced by a calcium antagonist or a β-blocker [40]. Data with regard to blood pressure reduction by an ACE-inhibitor are inconclusive, although it has been suggested that the greatest efficacy of ACE-inhibitor treatment was present in subjects with the T235 allele [40,41].

Thus, in general, the AGT polymorphism emphasizes the need to analyse combinations of genetic variants, which may alter blood pressure. So far, the polymorphisms of AGT gene have no implications for treatment and risk counselling in essential hypertension (Category D).

The ACE insertion/deletion polymorphism (ACE I/D)

In intron 16 of chromosome 17 the presence (I) or absence (D) of a 287 base pair Alu repeat DNA fragment has been described [42]. This polymorphism correlates with higher plasma ACE activity in subjects with one or two D-alleles. It has been shown that almost 50% of the interindividual variation in plasma ACE levels is determined by the ACE genotype [43]. Numerous studies investigating the association between this polymorphism and blood pressure variation are conflicting. In meta-analyses, a correlation has been found with macro- and microvascular (renal) atherosclerotic complications but not with hypertension [44,45]. A more recent meta-analysis has confirmed this observation, although, the association between the D-allele and ischaemic heart disease could only be shown in smaller studies, using selected subgroups. Large studies failed to demonstrate this association, indicating the importance of the selection of subjects with the same genetic background [46]. Whether there is a causal relationship between the presence of atherosclerotic disease and higher circulating ACE levels, or even more important, tissue ACE levels, is still a matter of debate.

The prediction of patient responses to antihypertensive drugs using genetic polymorphisms has become an important issue (pharmacogenetics) [40]. Although data with respect to the I/D polymorphism are conflicting again, several studies indicate a greater improvement in left ventricular hypertrophy and diastolic function in patients with the DD genotype [47]. However, in larger studies no association has been found between the ACE genotype and responses to antihypertensive therapy, especially ACE-inhibitors [40,41].

The angiotensin II type 1 receptor polymorphism (AT1R)
This single nucleotide polymorphism where cytosine is substituted for adenine (A1166C) at position 1166 of the AT1 receptor gene has been associated with essential hypertension and aortic stiffness [41,48,49]. Furthermore, the presence of the C-allele coincides with an increased sensitivity to Ang II [50]. AT1 receptor expression was higher in hypertensive patients than in normotensive volunteers, and a positive correlation with plasma renin activity was found [51,52]. Although a significant interaction between ACE en AT1 receptor gene loci has been observed in terms of blood pressure variation, the synergistic relation between the presence of a D-allele of the ACE I/D gene and one or two C-alleles of the AT1R gene with regard to an increased risk for myocardial infarction has recently been disputed [41,46]. Only few studies have addressed the response to antihypertensive drugs: no association was found between the AT1R polymorphism and blood pressure reduction by different classes of drugs, although subjects homozygous for the C1166 variant exhibited a 3-fold greater reduction in pulse wave velocity as a measure for arterial compliance when treated with an ACE-inhibitor [41,53].

The aldosterone synthase gene polymorphism (CYP11B2)
The cytochrome P450, CYP11B1, a steroid 11ß-hydroxylase, catalyses the terminal step of cortisol biosynthesis. The CYP11B2, aldosterone synthase, is a related enzyme which also has 11ß-hydroxylase activity as well as the 18-hydroxylase and 18-oxidase activities required for the terminal steps of aldosterone biosynthesis [54,55]. Expression of this latter enzyme is limited to the adrenal zona glomerulosa, where it is principally regulated by serum levels of potassium and Ang II. The two genes encoding these enzymes are located on chromosome 8q22, approximately 40 kb apart [56,57]. Congenital adrenal hyperplasia, which is caused by 11ß-hydroxylase deficiency and characterised by congenital abnormalities and hyperandrogenism, is only rarely associated with hypertension and in those cases is due to the accumulation of 11-deoxycorticosterone and its metabolites, which have mineralocorticoid activity [58,59]. This occurs mainly in the milder, late-onset variants in young adults. On the other hand, several lines of argument have designated the aldosterone synthase gene (CYP11B2) as a major candidate gene for predisposition to essential hypertension. Recently, Brand et al., have shown that the presence of a T-allele of the C-344T polymorphism of the regulatory part of the CYP11B2 gene was significantly more frequent in hypertensives than in controls, especially when the onset of hypertension occurred before the age of 45 years [54,55]. Whether the C-344T polymorphism represents a functional variant of the CYP11B2 gene, modulating the expression of the gene, is still a matter of debate. Nonetheless, plasma levels of aldosterone are higher in subjects with one or two T-alleles [60]. The C-344T polymorphism may also be directly implicated in transcriptional control, or it could be a marker for an as-yet-unidentified other polymorphism. Moreover, the possibility exists that the blood pressure effect of the CYP11B2 gene is more prominent in subjects with a high-sodium or low-potassium diet.

So, although there is a significant association of the aldosterone synthase gene with hypertension, data do not support a major role for this gene in essential hypertension.

Genetic polymorphisms and salt-sensitivity of hypertension

The renin-angiotensin system polymorphisms

The RAS is also implicated in the blood pressure response to variations in salt intake. Low-renin hypertensives show an increased blood pressure response to NaCl load, and salt-sensitive individuals exhibit a blunted response of the RAS when they switch from low to high salt intake compared with salt-resistant subjects [61,62]. Although data are conflicting, there is reason to believe that there is an association with the presence of one or two I-alleles of the ACE I/D polymorphism and salt-sensitivity, and not with the M235T AGT and the A1166C AT1R polymorphism [63]. The mechanism behind this apparent contradiction with regard to the ACE I/D gene polymorphism is not understood, since the presence of a D-allele has been associated with higher cardiovascular risk. A clue may lie in possible combinations with other variants associated with salt-sensitivity.

The α-adducin polymorphism

A polymorphism (ADDU1) which exchanges tryptophan for glycine at position 460 (Gly460Trp) in the gene encoding for the α-subunit in the actin cytoskeleton is associated with an increased tubular sodium reabsorption via stimulation of the renal Na^+-K^+-ATPase [64,65]. This polymorphism is associated with the blood pressure response to sodium loading and depletion, both in the animal model and in humans [66] . In addition, the Gly460Trp mutation may influence the response to thiazide therapy: patients who were heterozygous for the T-allele exhibited a greater blood pressure response than those who were homozygous for the glycine variant [67]. Although there is remarkable heterogeneity within different ethnic populations with respect to the association of this polymorphism with blood pressure [68,69], recent data from our group suggest that in subjects with familial combined hyperlipidaemia the presence of both a T-allele and insulin-resistance induce favourable circumstances for the development of hypertension [70].

G-protein β3 subunit polymorphism (GNB3)

The C825T polymorphism in the gene encoding for the β3-subunit of the guanine nucleotide binding regulatory protein linked to the Na^+-H^+-exchanger in the proximal tubules of the kidney has been shown to be associated with a substantially enhanced activity of the Na^+-H^+-exchanger [71]. The substitution of cytosine by thymidine at position 825 causes a truncation in the β subunit of the GNB3 protein, which is associated with increased activity. Recently, the complete human GNB3 gene and its promoter region were characterised, which will enable refined epidemiological and biochemical investigations of GNB3 in hypertension [72]. Although data are not uniform, several studies suggest an association between the presence of the 825T-allele and hypertension, left ventricular hypertrophy, and obesity [73-75].

No data are available yet with regard to effectiveness and/or predictability of diuretic-induced responses of blood pressure.

Genetic polymorphisms and the sympathetic nervous system

The sympathetic nervous system is involved in blood pressure regulation through its effect on cardiac output, peripheral vascular tone, renal sodium reabsorption, and renin release. Genetic variants may affect blood pressure by modulation of vascular responsiveness through an increased α-adrenoceptor-mediated vasoconstrictor response, an attenuation of β-adrenoceptor-mediated vasodilatation, or an increased central sympathetic drive. Indeed, it has been shown that polymorphisms of the α_2- and β_2-adrenergic receptor were significantly associated with hypertension in African-Americans and white Americans [76,77].

Several polymorphisms of the β_2-adrenergic receptor (ADRB2) have been observed [78]. Expression of the ADRB2 gene may be in linkage disequilibrium with the so-called Gly 16 pro-downregulatory polymorphism on chromosome 5. This genetic variation encodes glycine (Gly) instead of arginine (Arg) at position 16 within the β_2-adrenoceptor and exhibits exaggerated agonist mediated receptor downregulation, which in itself causes increased peripheral vascular resistance and is associated with increased blood pressure [79]. This observation may also account for the impaired vasodilatation in people of African ancestry as observed in studies that assessed forearm blood flow in response to the β_2-adrenoceptor agonist isoproterenol [80]. However, the association between the Gly 16 β_2-adrenoceptor genotype and hypertension has to be proven in further studies.

Pharmacogenomics

Despite the availability of a variety of effective antihypertensive drugs, inadequate control of blood pressure is common in hypertensive patients, and responsible for a large proportion of the burden of stroke and myocardial infarction in the population [81,82]. Although there are some weak predictors of response to antihypertensive drugs, individualization of treatment is mostly done empirically [83]. This situation may be improved by a better knowledge of the mechanisms underlying individual variation in the effectiveness of drugs. As discussed in the foregoing, the phenotype of hypertension of most of the subjects in the general population is the result of multiple genes interacting with various environmental factors. Whereas the contribution of many of these environmental factors has been identified, the opposite is true for genetic factors. It has been assumed that the genetic contribution to blood pressure is approximately 30%. As was shown above, several candidate genes have been associated with essential hypertension, such as AGT, AT1R, and ADDU1. Although many findings of the genetic aetiology of hypertension are still controversial, the role of genetic variability as a determinant of drug response still remains to be elucidated [5]. However, identification of genes, which modify the response to antihypertensive drugs, provides the opportunity to optimise safety and efficacy of the available antihypertensive drugs [84].

Studies of drug-gene interactions may be conducted from a pharmacokinetic and from a pharmacodynamic perspective [85]. From a pharmacokinetic perspective, the potentially important genes include those related to various transporter systems, such as the multidrug resistance (MDR1) gene, and enzymes involved in drug metabolism such as the cytochrome P-450 (CYP) enzyme system (e.g. CYP2D6, CYP2C9,CYP3A4). However, the clinical relevance of variations in these genes and their association with cardiovascular outcomes of antihypertensive therapy remains to be determined. From a pharmacodynamic perspective, several small studies have evaluated the influence of polymorphisms of the renin-angiotensin system genes, the salt-sensitivity genes, and the sympathetic nervous system genes on the response to antihypertensive drugs, mercly by focusing on surrogate endpoint measures like blood pressure reduction after salt-restriction, left ventricular hypertrophy and arterial stiffness [41,47,53,67,77]. Although some studies suggested the existence of drug-gene interactions, in general results have been inconsistent and evaluation in large population-based studies, in which hard endpoints will be determined, are necessary. The importance of these studies finds its explanation in the suggestion that different antihypertensive drug classes have similar effects on short- and intermediate-term outcomes [86], but may have different effects on cardiovascular disease incidence [87]. Understanding the association between antihypertensive drug-gene interactions and various cardiovascular outcomes may eventually help the physician to tailor antihypertensive drug therapy to the individual patient.

Conclusions

This chapter discussed several possible associations of genetic variants with hypertension. Further research is necessary to determine the role of these polymorphisms in risk stratification and treatment (Table). It is likely that significant progress towards the genetic basis of complex diseases such as hypertension will be made in the next few years. Further research is also necessary to establish interactions between genetic polymorphisms and their impact on the final phenotype. Because of the complex character of hypertension, it is likely that different genetic variants act in concert with environmental factors to produce a continuum in blood pressure levels. The relations between genotypes and drug responses wil have to be explored in more detail. This may not only provide insight into the cause of hypertension in specific subgroups, but may also be a way of defining which antihypertensive agent will be most effective in a particular hypertensive patient.

Summary Table

Disorders	Chromosome	Variant	Category *
Mendelian forms of hypertension			
GRA	8	Chimeric gene	A, B
AME	16	HSD11B2	A, B
Liddle	16	/ EnaC	A, B
Gordon	1,17	---	E
Essential hypertension			
AGT	1	M235T	D
	1	G-6A	D
ACE	17	I/D	D
AT1R	3	A1166C	D
CYP11B2	8	C-344T	D
ADDU1	4	Gly460Trp	D
GNB3	12	C825T	D
ADRB2	5	Arg16Gly	D

*A, molecular diagnostics available and diagnosis is relevant for treatment; B, molecular diagnostics available and relevant for genetic counselling; D, polymorphism with implications for predisposition, but minor phenotypic consequences.

References

1. Lander ES, Schork NJ. Genetic dissection of complex traits . Science 1994; 265:2037-48.
2. Dykes CW. Genes, disease and medicine. Br J Clin Pharmacol 1996; 42:683-95.
3. Reed PW, Davies JL, Copeman JB, et al. Chromosome-specific microsatellite sets for fluorescence-based, semi-automated genome mapping. Nat Genet 1994; 7:390-5.
4. Todd JA. Genetic analysis of type 1 diabetes using whole genome approaches. Proc Nat Acad Sci USA 1995; 92:8560-5.
5. Lifton RP. Molecular genetics of human blood pressure variation . Science 1996; 272:676-80.
6. Kaplan NM. Primary hypertension: pathogenesis. In: Kaplan NM (ed). Clinical Hypertension, 7th ed. Baltimore, Williams & Wilkins, 1998, p. 42.
7. Woolfson RG, de Wardener HE. Primary renal abnormalities inhereditary hypertension. Kidney Int 1996; 50:717-31.
8. Guidi E, Menghetti d, Milani S, et al. Hypertension may be tranplanted with the kidney in humans: A long-term historical perspective follow-up of recipients grafted with kidneys coming from donors with or without hypertension in their families. J Am Soc Nephrol 1996; 7:1131-8.
9. Sutherland DJ, Ruse JL, Laidlaw JC. Hypertension, increased aldosterone secretion and low plasma renin activity relieved by dexamethasone. Can Med Assoc J 1996; 95: 1109-19.
10. Lifton RP, Dluhy RG, Powers M, et al. A chimaeric 11 beta-hydroxylase/aldosterone synthase gene causes glucocorticoid-remediable aldosteronism and human hypertension. Nature 1992; 355:262-5.
11. Litchfield WR, Coolidge C, Silva P, et al. Impaired potassium-stimulated aldosterone production: A possible explanation for normokalemic glucocorticoid-remediable aldosteronism. J Clin Endocrinol Metab 1997; 82:1507-10.
12. Jonsson JR, Klemm SA, Tunny TJ, et al. A new genetic test for familial hyperaldosteronism type I aids in the detection of curable hypertension. Biochem Biophys Res Comm 1995; 207:565-71.
13. White PC. Inherited forms of mineralocorticoid hypertension. Hypertension 1996;28:927-36.
14. Mune T, Rogerson FM, Nikkila H, et al. Human hypertension caused by mutations in the kidney isozyme of 11 beta-hydroxysteroid dehydrogenase. Nat Genet 1995; 10:394-9.
15. Dave-Sharma S, Wilson RC, Harbison MD, et al. Examination of genotype and phenotype relationships in 14 patients with apparent mineralocorticoid excess. J Clin Endocrinol Metab 1998; 83:2244-54.
16. White PC, Mune T, Agrawal AK. 11 -Hydroxysteroiddehydrogenase and the syndrome of apparent mineralocorticoid excess. Endocr Rev 1997; 18:135-56.
17. Liddle GW, Bledsoe T, Coppage WS. A familial renal disorder simulating primary aldosteronism but with negligible aldosterone secretion. Trans Assoc Am Physicians 1963; 76:199-213.
18. Kellenberger S,Gautschi I, Rossier BC, Schild L. Mutations causing Liddle syndrome reduce sodium-dependent downregulation of the epithelial sodium channels in the Xenopus oocyte expression system. J Clin Invest 1998; 101:2741-50.
19. Shimkets R, Warnock DG, Bositis CM, et al. Liddle's syndrome: heritable human hypertension caused by mutations in the beta subunit of the epithelial sodium channel. Cell 1994; 79:407-14.
20. Gordon RD, Geddes RA, Pawsey CG, et al. Hypertension and severe hyperkalaemia associated with supression of renin and aldosterone and completely reversed by dietary sodium restriction. Austral Ann Med 1970; 19:287-94.
21. Mansfield TA, Simon DB, Farfel Z, et al. Multilocus linkage of familial hyperkalaemia and hypertension, pseudohypoaldosteronism type II, to chromosomes 1q31-42 and 17p11-q21. Nat Genet 1997; 16:202-5.
22. Julier C, Delepine M, Keaveney B, et al. Genetic susceptibility for human familial essential hypertension in a region of homology with blood pressure linkage on rat chromosome 10. Hum

Mol Genet 1997; 6:2077-85.
23. Wong Y, Stebbing M, Ellis JA, et al. Genetic linkage of beta and gamma subunits of epithelial sodium channel to systolic blood pressure. Lancet 1999; 353:1222-5.
24. Ambrosius WT, Bloem LJ, Zhou L, et al. Genetic variants in the epithelial sodium channel in relation to aldosterone and potassium excretion and risk for hypertension. Hypertension 1999; 34:631-7.
25. Melander O, Orho M, Fagerudd J, et al. Mutations and variants of the epithelial sodium channel gene in Liddle's syndrome and primary hypertension. Hypertension 1998; 31:1118-24.
26. Warnock DG. Aldosterone-related genetic effects in hypertension. Curr Hypertens Rep 2000; 2:295-301.
27. Bonnardeaux A, Nadaud S, Charru A, et al. Lack of evidence fr linkage of the endothelial nitric oxide synthase gene to essential hypertension. Circulation 1995; 91:96-102.
28. Staessen JA, Kuznetsova T, Wang JG, et al. M235T angiotensinogen gene polymorphism and cardiovascular renal risk. J Hypertens 1999; 17:9-17.
29. Ishigami T, Umemura S, Iwamoto T, et al. Molecular variant of angiotensinogen gene is associated with coronary atherosclerosis. Circulation 1995; 91:951-4.
30. Ward K, Hata A, Jeunemaitre X, et al. A molecular variant of angiotensinogen associated with preeclampsia. Nat Genet 1993; 4:59-61.
31. Jeunemaitre X, Soubrier F, Kotelevtsev YV, et al. Molecular basis of hypertension: role of angiotensinogen. Cell 1992; 71:169-80.
32. Caulfield M, Lavender P, Farrall M, et al. Linkage of the angiotensinogen gene to essential hypertension. N Engl J Med 1994; 330:1629-33.
33. Caulfield M, Lavender P, Newell-Price J, et al. Linkage of the angiotensinogen gene locus to human essential hypertension in African Caribbeans. J Cin Invest 1995; 96:687-92.
34. Schunkert H, Hense H-W, Gimenez-Roqueplo A, et al. The angiotensinogen T235 variant and the use of antihypertensive drugs in a population-based cohort. Hypertension 1997; 29:628-33.
35. Hingorani AD, Sharma P, Jia H, et al. Blood pressure and the M235T polymorphism of the angiotensinogen gene. Hypertension 1996; 28:907-11.
36. Jeunemaitre X, Inoue I, Williams C, et al. Haplotypes of angiotensinogen in essential hypertension. Am J Hum Genet 1997; 60:1448-60.
37. Inoue I, Nakajima T, Williams C, et al. A nucleotide substitution in the promotor of human angiotensinogen is associated with essential hypertension and affects basal transcription in vitro. J Clin Invest 1997; 99:1786-97.
38. Hunt SC, Cook NR, Oberman A, et al. Angiotensinogen genotype, sodium reduction, weight loss, and prevention of hypertension (Trials of Hypertension Prevention, phase II). Hypertension 1998; 32:393-401.
39. Brand E, Chatelain N, Keavney B, et al. Evaluation of the angiotensinogen locus in human essential hypertension: a European study. Hypertension 1998; 31:725-9.
40. Dudley C, Keavney B, Casadei B, et al. Prediction of patient responses to antihypertensive drugs using genetic polymorphisms: investigation of renin-angiotensin system genes. J Hypertens 1996; 14:259-62.
41. Hingorani AD, Jia H, Stevens P, et al. Renin-angiotensin system gene polymorphisms influence blood pressure and the response to angiotensin converting enzyme inhibition. J Hypertens 1995; 13:1602-9.
42. Tiret L, Rigat B, Visvikis S, et al. Evidence, from combined segregation and linkage analysis, that a variant of the angiotensin I-converting enzyme (ACE) gene controls plasma ACE levels. Am J Hum Genet 1992; 51:197-205.
43. Cambien F, Alhenc-Gelas F, Herbeth B, et al. Familial resemblance of plasma angiotensin-converting enzyme levels: the Nancy study. Am J Hum Genet 1988; 43:774-80.
44. Staessen JA, Wang JG, Ginocchio G, et al. The deletion/insertion polymorphism of the angiotensin converting enzyme gene and cardiovascular-renal risk. J Hypertens 1997; 15:1579-92.

45. Agerholm-Larsen B, Nordestgaard BG, Tybjærg-Hansen. ACE gene polymorphism in cardiovascular disease. Meta-analyses of small and large studies in whites. Arterioscler Thromb Vasc Biol 2000; 20:484-92.
46. Keavney B, McKenzie C, Parish S, et al. Large-scale test of hypothesised associations between the angiotensin-converting-enzyme insertion/deletion polymorphism and myocardial infarction in about 5000 cases and 6000 controls. International Studies of Infarct Survival (ISIS) Collaborators. Lancet 2000; 355:434-42.
47. Sasaki M, Takashi O, Luchi A, et al. Relationship between the angiotensin converting enzyme gene polymorphism and the effects of enalapril on left ventricular hypertrophy and impaired diastolic filling in essential hypertension: M-mode and pulsed doppler echocardiographic studies. J Hypertens 1996; 14:1403-8.
48. Bonnardeaux A, Davies E, Jeunemaitre X, et al. Angiotensin II (type I) receptor gene polymorphisms in human essential hypertension. Hypertension 1994; 24:63-9.
49. Benetos A, Topouchian J, Ricard S, et al. Influence of angiotensin II type I receptor polymophism on aortic stiffness in never-treated hypertensive patients. Hypertension 1995; 26:44-7.
50. Spiering W, Kroon AA, Fuss-Lejeune MMJJ, et al. Sensitivity, but not reactivity to angiotensin II is associated with the angiotensin II type 1 receptor A1166C polymorphism. Hypertension 2000; 36:411-16.
51. Diegeuz-Lucena JL, Aranda-Lara P, Ruiz-Galdon M, et al. Angiotensin I-converting enzyme genotypes and angiotensin II receptors – respons to therapy. Hypertension 1996; 28:98-103.
52. Staessen JA, Kuznetsova T, Wang JG, et al. M235T angiotensinogen gene polymorphism and cardiovascular renal risk. J Hypertens 1999; 17:9-17.
53. Benetos A, Cambien F, Gautier S, et al. Influence of angiotensin II type I receptor gene polymorphism on the effects of peridopril and nitrendipine on arterial stiffness in hypertensive individuals. Hypertension 1996; 28:1081-4.
54. Kawamoto T, Mitsuuchi Y, Toda K, et al. Role of steroid 11ß-hydroxylase and steroid 18-hydroxylase in the biosynthesis of glucocorticoids and mineralocorticoids in humans. Proc Natl Acad Sci U S A 1992; 89:1458–62.
55. Curnow KM, Tusie-Luna MT, Pascoe L, et al. The product of the CYP11B2 gene is required for aldosterone biosynthesis in the human adrenal cortex. Mol Endocrinol 1991; 5:1513–22.
56. Chua SC, Szabo P, Vitek A, et al. Cloning of cDNA encoding steroid 11ß-hydroxylase (P450c11). Proc Natl Acad Sci U S A 1987; 84:7193–7.
57. Wagner MJ, Ge Y, Siciliano M, Wells DE. A hybrid cell mapping panel for regional localization of probes to human chromosome 8. Genomics 1991; 10:114–25.
58. White PC, New MI, Dupont B. Congenital adrenal hyperplasia. Part 1. N Engl J Med 1987; 316:1519-24.
59. White PC, New MI, Dupont B. Congenital adrenal hyperplasia. Part 2. N Engl J Med 1987; 316:1580-6.
60. Brand E, Chatelain N, Mulatero P, et al. Structural analysis and evaluation of the aldosterone synthase gene in hypertension. Hypertension 1998; 32:198-204.
61. Weinberger MH, Miller JZ, Luft FC, Grim CE, Fineberg NS. Definitions and characteristics of sodium sensitivity and blood pressure resistance. Hypertension 1986; 8(suppl II):127-34.
62. De la Sierra A, Luch MM, Coca A, et al. Fluid, ionic and hormonal changes induced by high salt intake in salt-sensitives and salt-resistant hypertensive patients. Clin Sci 1996; 91:155-61.
63. Giner V, Poch E, Bragulat E, et al. Renin-angiotensin system genetic polymorphisms and salt-sensitivity in essential hypertension. Hypertension 2000; 35:512-7.
64. Matsuoka Y, Hughes CA, Bennet V. Adducin regulation. Definition of the calmodulin-binding domain and sites of phosphorylation by protein kinases A and C. J Biol Chem 1996; 271:25157-66.
65. Huges CA, Bennett V. Adducin: a physical model with implications for function in assembly of spectrin-actin complexes. J Biol Chem 1995; 270:18990-6.

66. Ferrandi M, Salardi S, Tripodi G, et al. Evidance for an interaction between adducin and Na(+)-K(+)-ATPase : relation to genetic hypertension. Am J Physiol 1999; 277:H1338-49.
67. Cusi D, Barlassina C, Azzani T, et al. Polymorphisms of alpha adducin and salt sensitivity in patients with essential hypertension. Lancet 1997; 349:1353-7.
68. Kamitani A, Wong ZY, Frasser R, et al. Human alpha-adducin gene, blood pressure, and sodium metabolism. Hypertension 1998; 32:138-43.
69. Kato N, Sugiyama T, Nakiba T, et al. Lack of association between the alpha-adducin locus and essential hypertension in the Japanese population. Hypertension 1998; 32:730-3.
70. Beeks E, Janssen RGJH, Kroon AA, et al. Association between the alpha-adducin Gly460Trp polymorphism and blood pressure in familial combined hyperlipidemia. Hypertension 2000; 36:668 (abstract).
71. Siffert W, Rosskopf D, Siffert G, et al. Association of a human G-protein 3 subunit variant with hypertension. Nat Genet 1998; 18:45-8.
72. Rosskopf D, Busch S, Manthey I, Siffert W. G protein beta 3 gene: structure, promoter, and additional polymorphisms. Hypertension. 2000; 36:33-41.
73. Siffert W, Forster P, Jockel KH, et al. Worldwide ethnic distribution of the G protein beta3 subunit 825T allele and its association with obesity in Caucasian, Chinese, and Black African individuals. J Am Soc Nephrol 1999; 10:1921-30.
74. Brand E, Herrmann SM, Nicaud V, et al. The 825C/T polymorphism of the G-protein subunit beta3 is not related to hypertension. Hypertension. 1999; 33:1175-8.
75. Poch E, Gonzalez D, Gomez-Angelats E, et al. G-Protein beta(3) subunit gene variant and left ventricular hypertrophy in essential hypertension. Hypertension. 2000; 35(1Pt2):214-8.
76. Sevetkey LP, Timmons PZ, Emovon O, et al. Association of hypertension with $beta_2$- and $alpha_2$-adrenergic receptor genotype. Hypertension 1996; 27:1210-5.
77. Jia H, Hingorani AD, Sharma P, et al. Association of the G_s gene with essential hypertension and response to -blockade. Hypertension 1999; 34:8-14.
78. Bray MS, Boerwinkle E. The role of $_2$-adrenergic receptor variation in human hypertension. Curr Hypertens Rep 2000; 2:39-43.
79. Kotanko P, Binder A, Tasker J, et al. Essential hypertension in African Caribbeans associates with a variant of the $beta_2$-adrenoceptor. Hypertension 1997; 30:773-6.
80. Lang CC, Stein M, Brown M, et al. Attenuation of isoproterenol-mediated vasodilatation in blacks. N Engl J Med 1995; 333:155-60.
81. Klungel OH, Stricker BHC, Paes AHP, et al. Excess stroke among hypertensive men and women due to undertreatment of hypertension. Stroke 1999; 30:1312-8.
82. Kaplan RC, Psaty BM, Heckbert SR, et al. Blood pressure level and incidence of myocardial infarction among patients treated for hypertension. Am J Public Health 1999; 89:1414-7.
83. Weder AB. Selecting the right drug for initial antihypertensive therapy. Curr Hypertens Rep 2000; 2:13-5.
84. Drews J. Drug discovery: a historical perspective. Science 2000; 287:1960-4.
85. Evans WE, Relling MV. Pharmacogenomics: translating functional genomics into rational therapeutics. Science 1999; 286:487-91.
86. Neaton JD, Grimm RH Jr., Prineas RJ, et al. Treatment of Mild Hypertension Study. Final results Treatment of Mild Hypertension Study Group. JAMA 1993; 270:713-24.
87. Blood Pressure Lowering Treatment Trialists' Collaboration. Effects of ACE inhibitors, calcium antagonists, and other blood-pressure-lowering drugs: results of prospectively designed overviews of randomised trials. Lancet 2000; 355:1955-64.

5. LIPOPROTEINS AND ATHEROSCLEROSIS

J. C. Defesche, J. J.P. Kastelein

Introduction

New developments in molecular biology have directed research of human disease etiology towards its genetic basis. The understanding of the genetic basis, or the molecular origin, of a disorder and the insight into the way genetic information is expressed or modulated by the environment, will have a major impact on treatment and prevention of disease. This approach, complete elucidation of the molecular basis, unequivocal diagnosis, optimized treatment and prevention of the disorder, is referred to as disease management. Cardiovascular disease, as a result of the atherosclerotic process, can serve as a model for disease management. It is estimated that more than 400 genes are involved in the regulation of processes such as endothelial function, lipoprotein metabolism, coagulation, inflammation and carbohydrate and amino acid metabolism [1]. Of these, lipoprotein metabolism is probably best understood. Many genes involved in lipoprotein metabolism have been identified, some of which are strongly related to atherosclerosis or cardiovascular disease. Nonetheless, atherosclerosis is a multifactorial disease with clear environmental determinants, but also with a strong and unavoidable genetic basis. In many cases the outcome of the atherosclerotic process is the result of the interaction between the environment and the genetic make-up of each individual. Therefore, intervention should be directed towards both environmental and genetic risk factors. Whereas the role of environmental risk factors for atherosclerosis such as smoking, diet, obesity or lack of exercise is recognized, only a limited number of genetic risk factors have been elucidated. The major genes, leading to atherosclerosis by themselves, and minor genes, causing disease only in interaction with other genes or environmental factors, are reviewed in this chapter.

The LDL-receptor gene

The gene coding for the low-density lipoprotein (LDL) receptor has been extensively characterized. Mutations in this gene cause an inherited disorder called Familial Hypercholesterolemia (FH). FH is a very common disease. With an incidence of one in 500 persons in Western societies, FH is one of the most frequent autosomal dominant

PA Doevendans and AA Wilde (eds.), Cardiovascular genetics, 51-58.

inherited disorders. Because of a diminished number of active LDL-receptors on the liver cell surface, in case of the heterozygous form, or a complete absence of LDL-receptors in the homozygous form, the LDL fraction in plasma is severely elevated from birth onwards. The markedly increased cholesterol levels in the LDL fraction in plasma, predispose for premature atherosclerosis [2]. Diagnosis of FH can be confirmed by demonstration of a mutation in the LDL-receptor gene. Today, more than 600 different mutations, all leading to FH, have been identified [3].

FH is sometimes difficult to differentiate from hypercholesterolemias of other origin, such as familial combined hyperlipidemia or polygenic hypercholesterolemia. The clinical characteristics, such as the elevated LDL-cholesterol levels and the typical tendon xanthomas, may facilitate the diagnosis. However, in many cases the diagnosis can not be made unequivocal. In young FH patients not necessarily all clinical signs may have developed and cholesterol levels in the lower range for FH patients may coincide with the higher cholesterol levels observed within the general population. Moreover, another inherited disorder, familial defective apolipoprotein B (Familial Defective apolipoprotein B, FDB), produces a clinical picture similar to FH [4].
A highly accurate diagnosis of FH can be established by molecular diagnosis: characterization of the molecular defect in the LDL-receptor gene which causes the disorder. Since clinical expression of FH and the cardiovascular risk is in part related to the nature of the mutation in the LDL-receptor gene, medical management can be optimized.
Once a LDL-receptor gene mutation in a patient with FH has been detected, the diagnostic tools are available to examine all family members of the (index) patient, for the presence of the same mutation. Due to the autosomal dominant mode of inheritance of FH, all first degree relatives of an index case run a chance of 50% of having the same mutation and are therefore at high risk of developing cardiovascular disease at young age. Good treatment modalities, in the form of inhibitors of cholesterol synthesis (Hydroxymethylglutaryl-CoA reductase inhibitors, statins), are available and have been shown to reduce cardiovascular morbidity and mortality by reduction of cholesterol levels [5,6]. In this view, active case finding by means of family investigation and DNA-analysis becomes of great importance for the prevention and early treatment of cardiovascular disease in FH (category B).

Other genes causing inherited hypercholesterolemia

A second gene leading to a phenotype resembling FH, is the gene coding for apolipoprotein B (apoB), the structural protein moiety of the LDL-particle. Structural alterations in part of this protein, which interacts with the LDL-receptor, lead to hypercholesterolemia, because of decreased uptake of the defective LDL-particles. This disorder is referred to as FDB [4].
So far 4 mutations have been characterized in the apoB gene, of which the amino acid change of glutamine for arginine at position 3500 (R3500Q- variant) is the most frequent. In a given cohort of clinically diagnosed FH patients 2 to 4% can be attributed to FDB. In many cases no detectable mutations can be found after complete analysis of

the LDL-receptor gene (FH1) and the apoB gene (FH2). This indicates that other genes must be involved in inherited hypercholesterolemia. Recent evidence supports the existence of a third gene, located on the short arm of chromosome 1 that produces a somewhat milder but definite FH-like phenotype [7,8]. Although this gene has not been fully characterized, the existence of this so-called FH3 gene further enlarges the genetic heterogeneity of FH. The distribution of FH-causing genes may vary between populations of different origin, i.e. mostly LDL-receptor mutations in Iceland [9], mostly apoB mutations in the Swiss [10] and mostly FH3 mutations in Southeast Asian patients [11].
Recently, an autosomal recessive form of familial hypercholesterolemia (ARFH) has been described. In such cases, the patient has inherited two, hitherto unknown, mutations from the unaffected and asymptomatic parents, which lead to severe hypercholesterolemia and xanthomatosis and consequently to cardiovascular disease at a very young age [12].

The Lipoprotein Lipase gene

Lipoprotein lipase (LPL) is a key lipolytic enzyme in the turnover of triglyceride-rich lipoproteins, such as chylomicrons and very-low-density lipoproteins (VLDL) in plasma. Reduced activity of LPL results in elevated levels of triglycerides and reduced levels of HDL-cholesterol, both risk factors for cardiovascular disease. Subtle combined hyperlipidemia can be caused by mutations in the LPL gene, such as N291S or D9N. Mutations in the LPL gene confer an elevated risk for cardiovascular disease. The frequency of certain mutations in this gene was higher in patients with cardiovascular disease than in healthy controls [13]. Frequencies of LPL-mutations can be up to two-fold higher in patients with Familial Hypercholesterolemia, Familial Combined Hyperlipidemia or Dysbetalipoproteinemia, that have manifest cardiovascular disease [14,15]. In these patients, the already increased risk is further elevated by raised levels of triglycerides and decreased levels of HDL-cholesterol, conferred by mutations in the LPL-gene [16,17]. These variants provide an example of how genetic variation can contribute to the disease. However, not every individual with an unfavorable LPL gene develops atherosclerosis, indicating the modest role of mutations in this gene, and their interaction with environment. Some mutations in the LPL gene have been shown to decrease the risk of myocardial infarction, for instance a mutation at the 3'-end of the gene. This mutation involving amino acid 447 results in a stop-codon instead of serine (S447X), and hence in a truncated protein, missing the last few amino acids at the carboxy-terminal end [18]. This mutation appears to be protective, mediated by less postprandial increases in triglyceride levels.

Apolipoprotein E-gene

Apolipoprotein E (apoE) is the ligand protein via which triglyceride-rich lipoproteins such as chylomicron-remnants, VLDL and VLDL-remnants are cleared by a B,E-receptor on the liver cell, which is in fact the LDL-receptor. Natural variants of the gene coding for apoE give rise to the occurrence of three isoforms of apoE: E2, E3 and E4. As every individual inherits 2 alleles of every gene, six combinations are possible. The affinity of these E-isoforms for the B,E-receptor differs: E2 has the lowest affinity and E4 the highest. Consequently, cholesterol levels are (to a minor extent) determined by the apoE-genotype. However, homozygosity for E_2 can lead to a serious dyslipidemic condition. Binding capacity of lipoproteins with the E_2/E_2 phenotype is reduced to 1% of that of E3/E3. Only a small part (1-4%) of E_2-homozygous individuals ultimately develops a disorder known as Familial Dysbetalipoproteinemia, characterized by dramatically elevated cholesterol and triglyceride levels in the VLDL-fraction. When untreated, the rate of the atherosclerotic process is enhanced significantly, resulting in premature cardiovascular disease. The clinical expression of the E2-type is strongly dependent on aggravating environmental factors such as obesity, diabetes, diet rich in fat and alcohol abuse [19]. Apparently, these factors interfere with alternative pathways for clearance of apoE-containing lipoproteins. Elimination of these aggravating factors leads to normalization of lipid levels, even without drug therapy.

Lipoprotein(a)

Plasma levels of lipoprotein(a) [Lp(a)] are genetically determined. The gene that codes for apolipoprotein(a), the main protein constituent of this particle, is highly polymorphic. The gene contains a varying number of specific protein domains the so-called Kringle IV repeats [20]. The number of Kringle IV repeats (12 to over 50) in each gene is inherited in a Mendelian mode, and the number of repeats directly determines the levels of Lp(a), in an inverse fashion: the more Kringle IV repeats, the lower the plasma level of Lp(a). Over a level of approximately 300 mg/L, Lp(a) is an independent risk factor for cardiovascular disease [20,21]. Lp(a) concentrations in the general population can vary from below 1 mg/L to over 1000 mg/L. Although Lp(a) levels remain constant during life, some conditions are known to influence plasma levels: pregnancy and renal disease increase Lp(a) and liver disease, alcohol abuse and steroid hormones decrease Lp(a) levels. Therefore, also the proatherogenic effects of Lp(a) depend on environmental influences. Thus far the cholesterol-lowering drugs have not been shown to be effective in reducing Lp(a) levels [22]. DNA-analysis can be used to determine the number of Kringle IV repeats in order to confirm the cause of an elevated Lp(a) level. But since this has no therapeutic consequences, such an analysis is not performed in clinical practice.

HDL-cholesterol

Where elevated LDL-cholesterol levels, acquired or genetically determined, constitute a major risk factor for atherosclerosis, a decreased level of high density lipoprotein (HDL)-cholesterol, also acquired or genetically determined, is a risk factor of at least similar importance. Smoking and lack of exercise are environmental factors known to reduce HDL-cholesterol. Genetic conditions leading to reduced or deficient HDL-cholesterol levels are not well known. Disorders such as hypo-alphalipoproteinemia, Tangier disease, Fish-Eye disease and deficiency of lecithin-cholesterol-acyl transferase (LCAT) are very rare genetic traits associated with HDL deficiency [23].

For both Fish-Eye disease and Tangier disease, and recently for hypo-alphalipoproteinemia the molecular genetic basis has been identified [24-27].

Gene based response to treatment

As discussed above unfavorable mutations in the LPL gene can predispose for premature atherosclerosis. The deleterious effects of these specific mutations in the LPL gene could be totally reversed by statin therapy [15]. This is a good example of the importance of knowledge on the genetic make-up to predict the outcome of pharmacological treatment.
Recently, a significant relation was described between a polymorphism in the gene locus of cholesterylester transfer protein (CETP) and the progression of CAD. CETP is involved in reversed cholesterol transport, reducing HDL-cholesterol levels and thus may be involved in the atherosclerotic process. This common CETP-gene variant (Taq1b) appeared to predict, independent of plasma cholesterol, whether men with CAD would benefit from lipid lowering treatment to delay the progression of coronary atherosclerosis [34]. Patients at high risk of progression (b1/b1 genotype) largely benefited from pravastatin therapy. Patients at intermediate risk of progression (b1/b2 genotype) had intermediate benefit, whereas patients at low risk of progression (b2/b2 genotype), which represented 16% of the cases, had no apparent benefit from pravastatin with regard to disease progression, suggesting that this latter group might be better off with a different or even no medical intervention (see also chapter 8). Although these results are very intriguing the relevance with respect to clinical outcome remains to be established. The importance of the CETP polymorphism is currently being analyzed in larger patient cohorts.

Atherosclerosis: genes and environment

It is well known that a family history of CAD is associated with increased risk for development of CAD and its clinical sequelae. Studies in twins have revealed a greater genetic risk in monozygotic than dizygotic twins, and adoption studies have shown that most of the excess risk is genetic rather than environmental. However, the mechanism through which a family history of CAD increases risk is still largely unknown. Atherosclerosis is a multifactorial disease with clear environmental factors, but also with a strong and unavoidable genetic basis. In many cases the outcome of the atherosclerotic process is the result of the interaction between the environment and the genetic make-up of each individual. Therefore, intervention should be directed towards both environmental and genetic risk factors. Where the role of environmental risk factors for atherosclerosis such as smoking, diet, obesity or lack of exercise is recognized, only a limited number of genetic risk factors have been elucidated. With regard to atherosclerosis and cardiovascular disease, regulation of blood pressure, lipoprotein and homocysteine metabolism, coagulation, fibrinolysis and endothelial function, are known to play a pivotal role.

Patient selection for DNA analysis in clinical practice

DNA-analysis is still a specialized laboratory procedure that is not available in every hospital or clinical chemistry laboratory. Informativity of DNA-analysis is in first instance dependent on the quality of the clinical diagnosis. For instance, when the clinical diagnosis of Familial Hypercholesterolemia is uncertain, and DNA-analysis is requested to confirm the diagnosis, the probability that DNA-analysis will reveal a LDL-receptor gene mutation is very low. If no mutations are encountered the diagnosis FH can not be excluded. With regard to lipoproteins and cardiovascular disease a limited number of DNA-analyses is available. Correct phenotyping is essential to direct genotyping. To select patients eligible for DNA-analysis, careful assessment of the lipid profile is required, and subsequently DNA-analysis of the gene or genes directly related to specific lipoprotein disorders can be indicated (Table 1).

Table 1: criteria for the selection of patients with lipoprotein disorders, eligible for DNA-doagnosis

	Disorder/trait	lipoproteins affected	gene	variants	classification
•	Familiar Hypercholesterolemia	LDL↑↑	LDL-receptor	>700 mutations	B [3]
•	Familiar Defective apolipoprotein B	LDL↑↑	apolipoprotein B	R3500Q frequent, 3 rare variants	B [4]
•	Familiar combined Hyperlipidemia	LDL↑, TG↑	not known	not known	F [8]
•	Familiar Dysbetalipoproteinemia	VLDL↑↑	apolipoprotein E	E2, E3, E4, rare variants	B [19]
•	Hypo-alphalipoproteinemia and	HDL↓	ABC1-transporter	C1417R, Q537R, delCTT2017	B, C [27]
	Tangier disease	HDL↓↓		delG1764, ins110bp ex.12	
•	LCAT deficiency and	HDL↓	LCAT	>25 mutations	B, C [25]
	Fish Eye disease	HDL↓↓			
•	Elevated triglycerides, low HDL	TG↑, HDL↓	LPL	D9N, N291S, rare variants	D [15]
•	Elevated lipoprotein(a)	Lp(a)↑	apo(a)	number of Kringle IV repeats	C [21]
•	Response to statins and	HDL↓	CETP	Taq1B polymorphism	D [34]
	progression of athersclerosis				
•	Autosomal recessive hypercholesterolemia	LDL↑↑	not known	not known	E [12]
•	Non-LDL receptor, non-apo B linked	LDL↑↑	FH3	not known	F [7]
	hypercholesterolemia				
•	Hyperhomocysteinemia	homocysteine	MTHFR	C677T	D [31]

References

1. Funke H, Assmann G. Strategies for the assessment of genetic coronary artery disease risk. Curr Opin Lipidol. 1999; 10:285-91.
2. Goldstein JL, Brown MS. The LDL receptor locus and the genetics of familial hypercholesterolemia. Ann Rev Genet. 1979; 13:259-89.
3. Day INM. LDL receptor mutation catalogue. http://www.ucl.ac.uk/fh/
4. Defesche JC, Pricker KL, Hayden MR, Van den Ende AE, Kastelein JJP. Familial Defective Apolipoprotein B_{100} is clinically indistinguishable from Familial Hypercholesterolemia. Arch Int Med 1993; 153:2349-56.
5. Randomised trial of cholesterol lowering in 4444 patients with coronary heart disease: the Scandinavian Simvastatin Survival Study (4S). Lancet 1994; 344:1383-89.
6. Pedersen TR, Olsson AG, Faergeman O et al. Lipoprotein changes and reduction in the incidence of major coronary heart disease events in the Scandinavian Simvastatin Survival Study (4S). Circulation 1998; 97:1453-60.
7. Varret M, Rabes JP, Saint-Jore B. A third locus for autosomal dominant hypercholesterolemia maps to 1p3.1-p32. Am J Hum Genet 1999; 64:1378-87.
8. Hunt SC, Hopkins PN, Bulka K. Genetic localisation to chromosome 1p32 of the third locus for familial hypercholesterolemia in a Utah kindred. Arterioscler Thromb Vasc Biol 2000; 20: 1089-93.
9. Gudnason V, Sigurdsson G, Nissen H, Humphries SE : Common founder mutation in the LDL receptor gene causing familial hypercholesterolemia in the Icelandic population. Hum Mutat 1997; 10:36-44.
10. Miserez AR, Laager R, Chiodetti N, Keller U: High prevalence of familial defective apolipoprotein B-100 in Switzerland. J Lipid Res 1994; 35:574-83.
11. Khoo KL, Van Acker P, Defesche JC, Tan H, Van de Kerkhof L, Heijnen-Van Eijk SJ, Kastelein JJP, Deslypere JP: Low-density lipoprotein receptor gene mutations in a Southeast Asian population with familial hypercholesterolemia. Clin Genet 2000; 58:98-105.
12. Ciccarese M, Pacifico A, Tonolo G. A new locus for autosomal recessive hypercholesterolemia maps to human chromosome 15q25-26. Am J Hum Genet 2000; 66:453-60.
13. Mailly F, Tugrul Y, Reymer PW et al. A common variant in the gene for lipoprotein lipase (Asp9-->Asn). Functional implications and prevalence in normal and hyperlipidemic subjects. Arterioscler Thromb Vasc Biol. 1995; 15:468-78.
14. Pimstone SN, Gagne SE, Gagne C et al. Mutations in the gene for lipoprotein lipase. A cause for low HDL cholesterol levels in individuals heterozygous for familial hypercholesterolemia. Arterioscler Thromb Vasc Biol. 1995; 15:1704-12.
15. Jukema JW, van Boven AJ, Groenemeijer B et al. The Asp9 Asn mutation in the lipoprotein lipase gene is associated with increased progression of coronary atherosclerosis. REGRESS Study Group, Interuniversity Cardiology Institute, Utrecht, The Netherlands. Regression Growth Evaluation Statin Study. Circulation 1996; 94:1913-8.
16. Wittekoek ME, Pimstone SN, Reymer PWA. Circulation 1998; 97:729-35. A common mutation in the lipoprotein lipase gene (Asn^{291} Ser) alters the lipoprotein phenotype and risk for coronary artery disease in patients with Familial Hypercholesterolemia. Wittekoek ME, Pimstone SN, Reymer PWA. Circulation 1998; 97:729-35.
17. Wittekoek ME, Moll E, Pimstone SN. Arterioscl Thromb Vasc Biol 1999; 19:2708-13. A frequent mutation in the lipoprotein lipase gene (D9N) deteriorates the biochemical and clinical phenotype of familial hypercholesterolemia.
18. Hokanson JE. Lipoprotein lipase gene variants and risk of coronary disease: a quantitative analysis of population-based studies. Int.J.Clin.Lab Res. 1997; 27:24-34.
19. Mahley RW, Rall SC. Type III hyperlipidemia (dysbetalipoproteinemia): the role of apolipoprtein E in normal and abnormal lipoprotein metabolism. The metabolic basis of

inherited disease. Scriver CR, Beaudet AL, Sly WS, eds. New York NY, McGraw-Hill, 1989: 1195-213.

20. Van den Ende A, van der Hoek YY, Kastelein JJ, Koschinsky ML, Labeur C, Rosseneu M. Lipoprotein [a]. Adv.Clin.Chem. 1996; 32:73-134.
21. Matsumoto Y, Daida H, Watanabe Y et al. High level of lipoprotein(a) is a strong predictor for progression of coronary artery disease. J Atheroscler Thromb. 1998; 5:47-53.
22. Kronenberg F, Kronenberg MF, Kiechl S et al. Role of lipoprotein(a) and apolipoprotein(a) phenotype in atherogenesis: prospective results from the Bruneck study. Circulation 1999; 100: 1154-60.
23. Kuivenhoven JA, Weibusch H, Pritchard PH et al. An intronic mutation in a lariat branchpoint sequence is a direct cause of an inherited human disorder (fish-eye disease). J Clin Invest. 1996; 98:358-64.
24. Marcil M, Brooks-Wilson A, Clee SM et al. Mutations in the ABC1 gene in familial HDL deficiency with defective cholesterol efflux. Lancet 1999; 354:1341-6.
25. Kuivenhoven JA, van Voorst tot Voorst EJ, Wiebusch H et al. A unique genetic and biochemical presentation of fish-eye disease. J Clin Invest. 1995; 96:2783-91.
26. Kuivenhoven JA, Stalenhoef AF, Hill JS et al. Two novel molecular defects in the LCAT gene are associated with fish eye disease. Arterioscler Thromb Vasc Biol. 1996; 16:294-303.
27. Brooks-Wilson A, Marcil M, Clee SM et al. Mutations in ABC1 in Tangier disease and familial high-density lipoprotein deficiency. Nat Genet. 1999; 22:336-45.
28. Folsom AR, Nieto FJ, McGovern PG et al. Prospective study of coronary heart disease incidence in relation to fasting total homocysteine, related genetic polymorphisms, and B vitamins: the Atherosclerosis Risk in Communities (ARIC) study. Circulation 1998; 98:204-10.
29. Malinow MR, Duell PB, Hess DL et al. Reduction of plasma homocyst(e)ine levels by breakfast cereal fortified with folic acid in patients with coronary heart disease. N Engl J Med. 1998; 338:1009-15.
30. Rimm EB, Willett WC, Hu FB et al. Folate and vitamin B6 from diet and supplements in relation to risk of coronary heart disease among women. JAMA 1998; 279:359-64.
31. Frosst P, Blom HJ, Milos R et al. A candidate genetic risk factor for vascular disease: a common mutation in methylenetetrahydrofolate reductase. Nat Genet. 1995; 10:111-3.
32. Kluijtmans LA, Kastelein JJ, Lindemans J et al. Thermolabile methylenetetrahydrofolate reductase in coronary artery disease. Circulation 1997; 96:2573-7.
33. Folsom AR, Rosamond WD, Shahar E et al. Prospective study of markers of hemostatic function with risk of ischemic stroke. The Atherosclerosis Risk in Communities (ARIC) Study Investigators. Circulation 1999; 100:736-42.
34. Kuivenhoven JA, Jukema JW, Zwinderman AH et al. The role of a common variant of the cholesteryl ester transfer protein gene in the progression of coronary atherosclerosis. The Regression Growth Evaluation Statin Study Group. N Engl J Med 1998; 338:86-93.

6. HOMOCYSTEINE, GENETIC DETERMINANTS AND CARDIOVASCULAR RISK

F.F. Willems , G.H.J. Boers, H.J. Blom

Introduction

Vascular events due to atherosclerotic disease are the leading cause of death in Western society. Established risk factors as hypercholesterolaemia, hypertension, diabetes mellitus and smoking cannot fully explain the great number of patients with cardiovascular disease. Classic homocystinuria due to a deficiency in cystathionine -synthase (CBS) is a rare inborn error of metabolism resulting in very high blood levels of homocysteine. Such patients suffer from serious vascular disease [1]. Also, a blockade of homocysteine remethylation due to defects of methylenetetrahydrofolate reductase (MTHFR) or methionine synthase (MS) activities can cause very high levels of plasma homocysteine with a high risk of arterial and venous vascular disease [2]. This observation has brought up the hypothesis that homocysteine is toxic to the vascular wall. Next it was postulated that mild hyperhomocysteinemia is a possible risk factor for arterial occlusive disease [3]. Most retrospective and prospective studies have demonstrated an association between mild hyperhomocysteinemia and arterial vascular disease [4]. Until now however it remains unclear whether mildly elevated homocysteine levels itself are causally related to the increased cardiovascular risk [5].

Homocysteine metabolism

Homocysteine is a sulphydryl-containing amino acid derived from the metabolic demethylation of methionine, an essential amino acid which is present in mammalian diets. Two pathways, the transsulphuration pathway and the remethylation pathway are involved in the regulation of homocysteine homeostasis (figure 1). Homocysteine can be irreversibly degraded to cystathionine by CBS which requires pyridoxal-5-phospahate, the active form of vitamin B6 for adequate function [6]. Cystathionine is further converted to cysteine by -cystathionase. Thetranssulphuration pathway has a limited distribution and is found primarily in organs like kidney and liver. Homocysteine can also be metabolised via two methionine conserving remethylation pathways. A substantial portion of homocysteine is remethylated in the liver or kidney using betaine-homocysteine methyltransferase (BHMT) with betaine as methyl donor. The second remethylation pathway uses MS in the conversion of homocysteine to

PA Doevendans and AA Wilde (eds.), Cardiovascular genetics, 59-69.

methylenentetrahydrofolate by MTHFR, serves as methyl donor, cobalamin is required for methyl transport and S-adenosylmethionine activates the enzyme [7]. The MTHFR dependant MS remethylation pathway is located in almost all tissues.

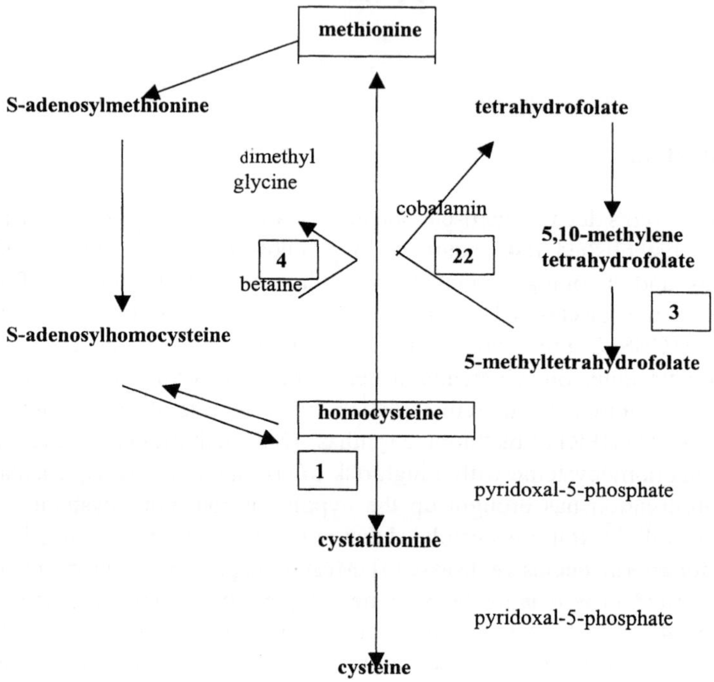

Figure 1. *Homocysteine metabolism*

1) cystathionine -synthase (CBS)
2) methionine synthase (MS)
3) methylenetetrahydrofolate reductase (MTHFR)
4) betaine-homocysteine methyltransferase (BHMT)

Determination of homocysteine levels

Homocysteine levels are determined through analyses of blood plasma. Based on the results of the European COMAC study we consider fasting homocysteine levels of 15 mol/l or more as elevated [8]. In the COMAC study, 14% of the patients with premature vascular disease had normal fasting homocysteine levels while loading with L-methionine, 100 mg/kg revealed a mildly elevated post methionine loading level. However, the relevance of post-load hyperhomocysteinemia as risk factor in premature vascular disease is uncertain.

Table 1

Category A: Moderate and severe hyperhomocysteinemia, fasting homocysteine level > 40 μmol/l

Category C: mild hyperhomocysteinemia, homocysteine levels < 15-40 mol/l

Homocysteine and arterial vascular disease

Until now more than 80 cross-sectional, case-control and prospective cohort studies have been published upon the relationship between homocysteine and arterial vascular disease [4]. In 1976 Wilcken et al. reported for the first time on 25 patients with coronary artery disease in whom 7 patients had homocysteine levels in the range of obligate heterozygotes of cystathionine- -synthase after loading withmethionine [3]. In 1983 and 1985 Boers reported that patients with premature peripheral vascular disease and cerebrovascular arterial occlusive disease had mild post load hyperhomocysteinemia in 28% of the cases [9,10]. These findings were confirmed by Clarke et. al. in 1991 who showed that post-load hyperhomocysteinemia is associated with premature coronary artery disease, cerebrovascular disease and peripheral arterial disease [11]. A meta analysis of 27 reports from 1988 until 1994 on 2500 patients with coronary artery disease, 900 with cerebrovascular disease and 700 with peripheral disease together with several thousands of control subjects showed a calculated summary odds ratio as an estimation of the relative risk in persons with elevated homocysteine levels of 1.7 (95% CI 1.5-1.9) for coronary artery disease, 2.5 (95% CI 2.0-3.0) for cerebrovascular disease and 6.8 (95% CI 2.9-15.8) for peripheral arterial disease [12]. These odds ratio's were calculated from all included homocysteine levels, mainly fasting levels but also post methionine loading levels. The odds ratio's for fasting homocysteine levels were comparable with odds ratio's calculated from post-loading homocysteine levels. Since meta analyses of pooled data have important limitations because of variations in study design, number and definition of patients and controls, differences concerning the measurement of plasma homocysteine levels and the definition of vascular events a systematic review of the data is complicated.

The European Concerted Action Project on hyperhomocysteinemia and vascular disease was initiated in 19 centres in Europe. This multi-centre case control study with a sufficient number of patients and controls was started to provide robust confirmation of mild hyperhomocysteinemia being associated with arterial occlusive disease and to determine possible interactions with the established risk factors [8]. Fasting and post-load homocysteine levels in the upper quintile of the distribution of levels were considered hyperhomocysteinemic. These low cut-off points, 12 mol in the fasting state and 38 mol/l after methionine loading, defined mild hyperhomocysteinemia as a common factor in the general population. In this population with relative low cut-off points the odds ratio for arterial occlusive disease was 2.2 (95% CI 1.7-2.7) of fasting plasma homocysteine levels and 2.1 (95% CI 1.7-2.7) of post load hyperhomocysteinemia. These odds ratio's did not change after adjustment for other risk factors suggesting that mild hyperhomocysteinemia is an independent risk factor for arterial vascular disease. In contrast to earlier meta analyses the odds ratio's for coronary artery disease, cerebrovascular disease and peripheral disease were not different. Furthermore this project showed that mild hyperhomocysteinemia as a risk factor has equal potentials as hypercholesterolaemia and smoking. In this study hypertension carried a greater risk for vascular disease. Importantly, there was a synergistic interaction between hyperhomocysteinemia and hypertension and smoking which indicates a potentiating effect of these factors if concomitantly present in a patient.

With regard to the consistency of the findings of a positive association between mild hyperhomocysteinemia and premature vascular disease it is important to note that in 3 out of 18 prospective studies reported until now, no association could be established, whereas in 16 there was such association, albeit not statistically significant in 4 [13].

Genetic determinants of hyperhomocysteinemia and cardiovascular risk

Association between CBS deficiency and cardiovascular risk

One of the main regulating enzymes in homocysteine metabolism is CBS. Mutant CBS enzyme is an important determinant of hyperhomocysteinemia and is in homozygous form biochemically characterized by very high levels of plasma homocysteine, homocystinuria, hypermethionemia and hypocysteinemia. This inborn error of metabolism is the most common cause of homocystinuria with a worldwide incidence of 1:344.000 living births with the highest incidence in Ireland at 1:65.000 and is inherited as an autosomal recessive trait [14]. The reported world wide incidence has been based on newborn screening and may be an underestimation of the true incidence. A recent study showed that the incidence of mutated CBS gene in homozygous form may be as high as 1:20.500 in a Danish population [15]. Until now 92 different mutations have been described in the CBS gene [16] which is located on chromosome 21q22.3 [17,18]. Relatively common mutations in homozygous form responsible for the classical homocystinuric phenotype are 833T C (I278T), amino acid substitution isoleucine to threonine, which confers vitamin B6 responsiveness(category A) and 919G A (G307S), amino acid change glycine to serine, which represents severe pyridoxine non-responsiveness (category A) both together present in almost 75% of the homocystinuric alleles analysed [16]. Approximately 50% of the patients who are CBS deficient respond to pyridoxine, and this responsiveness is constant within sibships [1]. Patients who are homozygous for CBS deficiency have a very high risk for arterial and venous vascular disease. Pooled data on homozygous CBS deficient patients showed that before the age of 30 years more than half of the patients has had a severe vascular event [1]. Recent studies revealed that homocysteine lowering therapy in these patients reduces the risk on a major vascular event with 90 % [19].

In two early studies, CBS activity was studied in cultured fibroblasts of mild hyperhomocysteinemic patients with vascular disease [9,10]. In these patients a reduced activity in CBS activity was found resembling heterozygosity for classical homocystinuria and it was proposed that such carriership was the cause of mild hyperhomocysteinemia. In later studies the association between reduced activity of CBS and vascular patients with mild hyperhomocysteinemia could not be reproduced [20-22]. Also, molecular genetic studies demonstrated that heterozygosity for mutant CBS is at the most a very minor cause for mild hyperhomocysteinemia in vascular patients [22-25]. Furthermore, the calculated number of individuals heterozygote for CBS deficiency is shown to be too low to account for the high incidence of hyperhomocysteinemia in patients with premature vascular disease [26].

Association between MTHFR deficiency and cardiovascular risk

Patients with severe deficiencies of MTHFR display a wide range of clinical features such as neurological abnormalities, mental retardation and premature vascular disease [2]. Severe MTHFR deficiency is the most common inborn error in folate metabolism, still very rare with an estimated world wide incidence of 1:3.000.000 living births [2]. This inborn error of folate metabolism is inherited as an autosomal recessive trait (Category A). Severe MTHFR deficiency is biochemically characterized by hyperhomocysteinemia and homocystinuria in the presence of hypomethionemia. The MTHFR gene has been mapped to 1p36.3 and in homocystinuric patients until now 24 mutations of MTHFR have been identified [27-29].

In 1988 Kang demonstrated a new MTHFR variant that is very sensitive to heating at 46 C [30]. In 1995 Frosst et al. identified a very common thermolabile mutation in the MTHFR gene, 677 C T converting analanine to a valine codon [31]. Subjects who are homozygous for this mutation have residual activities after heating that are approximately 30% of those for controls. It is important to note that this mutation also decreases specific activity of MTHFR at normal body temperature. Prevalence of this polymorphism in homozygous form is between 10 to 25% depending upon the population in which prevalence was determined [32]. Kluijtmans demonstrated that thermolabile MTHFR was associated with elevated fasting homocysteine levels [22,33]. Kang et.al were the first who demonstrated that thermolabile MTHFR enzyme was more common among patients with coronary artery disease compared to controls [34]. If elevated homocysteine levels are responsible for the increased risk for vascular disease than the thermolabile MTHFR genotype, accompanied by higher homocysteine levels, should lead to an increased risk for vascular disease. In one of the largest case-control studies on 735 patients with coronary artery disease and 1250 controls the calculated odd's ratio was 1.21 (95% CI: 0.87-1.68) suggesting that the risk for premature vascular disease is not associated with the MTHFR TT genotype [33]. A

recent meta analysis of 23 studies indeed revealed no significant increased risk of vascular disease among subjects with the TT genotype compared to subjects with the CC genotype (Category D) [35]. The calculated odd's ratio was 1.12 (95% CI 0.92-1.37). Nevertheless, patients with TT genotype had a plasma homocysteine concentration of 2.6 μmol/l higher than patients with CC genotype. The expected odds ratio for vascular disease of patients with TT genotype compared to CC genotype based on their homocysteine levels therefore, should be about 1.26. This is well within the confidence interval of the calculated odds ratio in the above mentioned meta-analysis. It is remarkable that the association of this mutation with an increased risk of vascular disease differs between continents. Among the European studies, 6 out of 11 report an odds ratio more than 1 compared to only 2 out of 8 studies in the United States and Canada. A possible explanation can be that it is much more common to fortify grain products and to take multivitamin supplements in the United States and Canada [36]. As shown by several studies, the mutation is associated with moderate hyperhomocysteinemia mainly in subjects with low-normal folate status which makes it likely that the TT genotype emerges as a risk factor for vascular disease mainly in populations with a low-normal folate intake.
Homozygosity for another MTHFR 1298A C mutation, converting glutamate toalanine, in the population is also very common with a prevalence of 10%, however an association between hyperhomocysteinemia and this mutation was not found [37,38].

Association between other enzymes involved in homocysteine metabolism and cardiovascular risk

Until now seven mutations of MS have been described [39-41]. There is however little evidence that MS polymorphisms play an important role in hyperhomocysteinemia. Methionine synthase reductase (MTR), a recently identified enzyme, is involved in homocysteine metabolism by reductive activation of MS [42]. Recently a very common missense mutation has been identified in the MTR gene. Homozygosity for this mutation, MTR 66 A G, amino acid substitutionisoleucine to methionine, is prevalent in 25-30 % and is associated with an increased risk for spina bifida. An association with hyperhomocysteinemia or vascular disease has not been observed [43]. Until now 13 mutations of MTR are identified [42,44].
So far, 3 mutations have been described in the betaine homocysteine methyltransferase (BHMT) gene [45] but mutant BHMT which remethylation reaction is limited to liver and kidney seems not associated with hyperhomocysteinemia (Category D) [45].

Table 2

Gene	locus	mutation	category ref.
CBS	21q22.3 919 G A	A	[16]
CBS	21q22.3 833 T C	A	[16]
MTHFR 1p36.3	several mutations	A	[27-29]
MTHFR 1p36.3	677 C T	C	[31]

Treatment of inborn errors of metabolism leading to severe and moderate hyperhomocysteinemia

Severe hyperhomocysteinemia

Homozygous CBS deficiency and homozygosity for severe MTHFR mutations will lead to severe hyperhomocysteinemia, with fasting homocysteine levels above 50 μmol/l in children and 100 μmol/l in adults and cause, irrespectively of the underlying enzymatic defect, a very high risk on premature arteriosclerotic and thrombotic events. Clinical treatment of patients, homozygous for CBS deficiency, should aim on reduction of the major biochemical abnormalities in these patients. For the 50% of the patients that are vitamin B6 responsive, vitamin B6 in pharmacological doses in combination with folic acid or vitamin B12 or both is the treatment of choice. Patients who are non-pyridoxine responsive are advised to use a methionine restricted, cysteine supplemented diet mostly in combination with some pyridoxine, folic acid and vitamin B12 supplementation. In the treatment of the latter patients, also the use of betaine is an option, especially when maintaining a dietary restriction is not achievable [46].

Patients with severe MTHFR deficiency are treated with the high doses of folate and riboflavin, a co-factor in MTHFR activity [47] and patients with folate non-responsiveness MTHFR deficiency with large doses betaine [48].

It is therefore obvious that for patients with severe hyperhomocysteinemia genetic diagnosis in addition to assessment of enzymatic activity is imperative for adequate tailoring of treatment and for genetic counselling.

Moderate hyperhomocysteinemia

Moderate hyperhomocysteinemia can be the result of mutated genotypes which cause a less severe enzyme deficiency with homocysteine levels between 40 μmol/l and 100 μmol/l in adults often combined with a reduced folate status [49]. Also combinations of heterozygosity for mutant CBS and mutant MTHFR can cause moderate elevated homocysteine levels with a high risk on premature vascular disease. In patients with moderate hyperhomocysteinemia, it is therefore advisable to perform genetic diagnosis and assess enzymatic activity for optimal treatment and for genetic counselling.

Mild hyperhomocysteinemia

There is convincing evidence that mild hyperhomocysteinemia with fasting homocysteine levels of 15 mol/l or more is a risk factor for premature vascular disease. It is important to note that mildly elevated homocysteine levels can be caused by genetic as well as environmental factors. Several lifestyle determinants like folate intake, smoking and coffee intake can modulate homocysteine levels causing mildly elevated plasma homocysteine levels. It is therefore inaccurate to assume that the increased risk for premature vascular disease associated with mild hyperhomocysteinemia can always be attributed to a single genetic mutation. A meta-analysis of 12 studies revealed that folic acid lowered total plasma homocysteine levels by 25% [50]. Addition of vitamin B12 led to a further reduction of 7%. Vitamin B6 did not lower fasting homocysteine levels but uncontrolled studies showed that post-load homocysteine levels were reduced 21% to 42 % [51,52]. It might therefore be useful to add vitamin B6 in case of elevated post-load homocysteine levels. Since the treatment of mildly elevated homocysteine levels does not depend on a possible underlying genetic defect, genetic diagnosis is not indicated. Ongoing trials still have to prove a clinically beneficial effect of homocysteine-lowering intervention in vascular patients. Since the effect of homocysteine-lowering treatment in healthy family members of mildly hyperhomocysteinemic patients is unclear, until results of primary prevention trials are published in the future, it does not seem indicated for the moment to screen for genetic defects in patients with mild hyperhomocysteinemia for genetic counselling reasons.

Summary

We suggest that genetic investigation in patients with premature vascular disease should depend on the patient's homocysteine level. Only in the case of fasting homocysteine levels higher than 40µmol/l, molecular genetic and enzymatic diagnosis is relevant both for the selection of the most appropriate treatment for these patients and for genetic counselling.

References

1. Mudd SH, Skovby F, Levy HL, et al. The natural history of homocystinuria due to cystathionine -synthase deficiency. Am J Hum Genet 1985; 37:1-31.
2. Rosenblatt DS. Inherited disorders of folate transport and metabolism. In the metabolic and molecular basis of inherited disease. CR Scriver, AL Beaudet, WS Sly, and D Valle. Mc Graw-Hill, New York 1995; 3111-28.
3. Wilcken DEL, Wilcken B. The pathogenesis of coronary artery disease. A possible role for methionine metabolism. J Clin Invest 1976; 57:1079-82.
4. Refsum H, Ueland PM, Nygård O, et al. Homocysteine and cardiovascular disease. Annu Rev Med. 1998; 49:31-62.
5. Welch GN, Loscalzo J. Homocysteine and atherothrombosis. N Engl J Med. 1998; 338:1042-50.
6. Finkelstein JD. The metabolism of homocysteine: pathways and regulation. Eur J Pediatrics 1998; 157 : S40-4.
7. BanerjeeRV, Matthews RG. Cobalamin dependant methionine synthase . FASEB J 1990; 1450-9.
8. Graham, Daly LE, Refsum HE, et al. Plasma homocysteine as a risk factor for vascular disease. The European Concerted Action Project. JAMA 1997; 277:1775-81.
9. Boers GHJ, Schoonderwaldt HC, Schulte BPM, et al. Heterozygosity for homocysteinuria, a risk factor for occlusive cerebrovascular disease. Clin Genet 1983; 24:300-1.
10. Boers GHJ, Smals AGH, Trijbels JMF, et al. Heterozygosity for homocysteinuria in premature peripheral and cerebral occlusive arterial disease. N Engl J Med 1985; 313: 709-15.
11. Clarke R, Daly L, Robinson K, et al. Hyperhomocysteinemia, an independent risk factor for vascular disease. N Engl J Med 1991; 324: 1149-55.
12. Boushey CJ, Beresford SAA, Omenn GS, et al. A quantitative assessment of plasma homocysteine as a risk factor for vascular disease. JAMA 1995; 274:1049-57.
13. Boers GH. Mild hyperhomocysteinemia is an independent risk factor for arterial vascular disease. Sem Thromb Heamost. 2000; 26:291-5.
14. Mudd SH, Levy HL, Skovby F, Disorders of transsulphuration. In The metabolic and molecular basis of inherited disease. CR Scriver, AL Beaudet WS Sly and D. Vall, editors, McGraw-Hill Inc. New York. 1995; 1279-327.
15. Gaustadnes M, Rudiger N, Rasmussen K, et al. Familial thrombophilia associated with Homozygosity for cystathionine synthase 833T T mutation.Arterioscler Thromb Vasc Biol 2000; 20:1392-5.
16. Kraus JP, Miroslav J, Viktot K, et al. cystathionine-b-synthase mutations in homocysteinuria. Hum Mutat 1999; 13: 362-75.
17. Skovby F, Krassikoff N, Francke U. Assignment of the gene for cystathionine-b-synthase to human chromosome 21 in somatic cell hybrids. Hum Genet 1984; 65:291-4.
18. Muncke M, Kraus JP, Ohura T, et al. The gene for cystathionine-b-synthase maps to the subtelomeric region on human chromosome 21q and the proximal mouse chromosome 17. Am J Hum Genet 1988; 42:550-9.
19. Yap S, Naughten ER, wilcken B, et al. Vascular complications of severe hyperhomocysteinemia in patients with homocysteinuria due to cystathionine-b-synthase deficiency: effects of homocysteine lowering therapy. Thromb Haemost 2000; 26:335-40.
20. Engbersen AM, Franken DG, Boers GHJ, et al Thermolabile 5,10 methylenentetrahydrofolate reductase as a cause of mild hyperhomocysteinemia. Am J Hum Genet 1995; 56:142-50.
21. Dudman NP, Wilcken DE, Wang J, et.al. Disordered methionine/homocysteine metabolism in premature vascular disease. Arterioscler Thromb 1993; 13:1253-60.
22. Kluijtmans LA, Van Den Heuvel LP, Boers GHJ, et al. Molecular genetic analysis in mild hyperhomocysteinemia: a common mutation in the methylenetetrahydrofolate reductase gene is a genetic risk factor for cardiovascular disease. Am J Hum Genet 1996; 58:35-41.

23. Folsom AR, Nieto FJ, McGovern, et al. Prospective study of coronary heart disease incidence in relation to fasting total homocysteine, related genetic polymorphism and B-vitamins. The atherosclerotic Risk in Communities study. Circulation 1998; 98:204-10.
24. Whitehead AS, Ward P, Tan S, et al. The molecular genetics of homocistinuria, hyperhomocysteinemia, and premature vascular disease in Ireland: 1994; 81-3.
25. Kozich V, Kraus E, de Franchis R, et al. Hyperhomocysteinemia in premature arterial disease: examination of cystathionine synthase alleles at the molecular level. Hum Mol Genet 1995; 4:623-9.
26. Daly R, Robinson K, Tan KS, et al. Hyperhomocysteinemia: a metabolic risk factor for coronary heart disease determined by both genetic and environmental influences? QJ Med 1993; 86:685-9.
27. Sibani S, Christensen B, O'Ferrell, et al. Characterization of six novel mutations in the methylenetetrahydrofolate reductase gene in patients with Homocystinuria. Human mutation 2000; 15:280-7.
28. Goyette P, Frosst P, Rosenblatt DS, et al. Seven novel mutations in the methylenentetrahydrofolate reductase gene and genotype/fenotype correlatios in severe MTHFR deficiency. Am J Hum Genet 1995; 56:1052-9.
29. Kluijtmans LA, den Heijer J, Reitsma PH, et al. Thermolabile methylenetetrahydrofolate reductase and factor V Leiden in the risk of deep vein thrombosis. Thromb Haemost 1998; 79:254-8.
30. Kang S, Zhou PWK, Wong J, et al. Intermediate homocysteinemia: a thermolabile variant of methylenentetrahydrofolate reductase. Am J Hum Genet 1988; 43: 414-21.
31. Frosst P, Blom HJ, Milos R, et al. A candidate genetic risk factor for vascular disease: a common mutation in methylenentetrahydrofolate reductase. Nat Genet 1995; 10:111-3.
32. Rozen R. Genetic modulation of homocysteinemia. Sem Throm Hemos 2000;26:255-61.
33. Kluijtmans LAJ, Kastelein JJP, Lindemans J, et al. Thermolabile methylenetetra-hydrofolate reductase in coronary artery disease. Circulation 1997; 96:2573-7.
34. Kang SS, Wong PW, Susmano A, et al. Thermolabile defect of methylenetetra-hydrofolate reductase: an inherited risk factor for coronary artery disease. Am J Hum Genet 1991; 48:536-45.
35. Brattstrom L, Wilcken DE, Ohrvik J, et al. Common methylenetetrahydrofolate reductase gene mutation leads to hyperhomocysteinemia but not to vascular disease: the result of a meta-analysis. Circulation 1998; 98:2520-6.
36. De Bree A, van Dusseldorp M, Brouwer IA, et al. Folate intake in Europe: recommended, actual, and desired intake. Eur J Clin Nutr 1997; 51: 643-60.
37. Weisberg I, Tran P, Christensen B, et.al. A second genetic polymorphism in methylenetetrahydrofolate reductase associated with decreased enzyme activity. Mol Genet Metab 1998; 64:169-72.
38. Van der Put NMY, Gabreels F, Stevens EMB, et.al. A second common mutation in the methylenetetrahydrofolate reductase gene. An additional risk factor for neural tube defects. Am J Hum Genet 1998; 62:1044-51.
39. Leclerc D,Campeau E, Goyette P, et al. Human methionine synthase:cDNA cloning, chromosomal localisation and identification of mutations in patients of the cb/G complementation group of folate/cobalamin disorders. Hum Mol Genet 1996; 5:1867-74.
40. Gulati S, Baker P, Yunan LN, et al. Defects in human methionine synthase in cb1G patients. Hum Mol Genet 1996; 5:1859-65.
41. Wilson A, Leclerc D, Saberi F, et al. Functionally null mutations in patients with the cb1G variant from methionine synthase Am J Hum Genet 1998; 63:409-14.
42. Leclerc D, Wilson A, Dumas R, et.al. Cloning and mapping of a cDNA for methionine synthase reductase, a flavaprotein defective in patients with homocysteinuria. Proc Natl Acad Sci USA 1998; 95:3059-64.

43. Wilson A, Platt R, Wu Q, et al. A common variant in methionine synthase reductase combined with low cobalamin increases risk for spina bifida. Mol Genet Metab 1999; 67:317-23.
44. Wilson A, Leclerc D, Rosenblatt DS, et al. Molecular basis for methionine synthase reductase deficiency in patients belonging to thecblE complementation group of disorders in folate/cobalamin metabolism. Hum Mol Genet 1999; 8:2009-16.
45. Heil SG, Lievers KJA, Boers GH, et al. Betaine homocysteine methyltransferase: genomic sequencing and relevance to hyperhomocysteinemia and vascular disease in humans. Mol Genet Metab 2000; 71:511-9.
46. Boers GHJ, Yap S, Naughten E, et al. The treatment of high homocysteine concentration in homocysteinuria. Biochemical control in patients and their vascular outcome. In: Robinson K ed. Homocysteine and vascular disease. Dordrecht, The Netherlands: Kluwer Academic Publishers, 2000; 387-409.
47. Freeman JN, Finkelstein JD, Mudd SH. Folate responsive homocystinuria and "schizophrenia". A defect in methylation due to deficient 5,10-methylenetetra-hydrofolatereductase activity. N Engl J Med 1975; 292:491-6.
48. Wendel U, Bremer HJ. Betaine in the treatment of homocysteinuria due to 5,10-methylenetetrahydrofolate reductase deficiency. Eur J Pediatrics 1984;142 :147-50.
49. Guttormsen AB, Ueland PM, Nesthus I, et al. Determinants and vitamin responsivness of intermediate hyperhomocysteinemia (> 40 mol/l) The HordalandHomocysteine Study. J Clin Invest 1996; 98:2174-83.
50. Homocysteine Lowering Trialist Collaboration. Lowering blood homocysteine with folic acid based supplements. BMJ;1998; 316:894-8.
51. Franken DG, Boers GHJ, Blom HJ, et al. Effects of various regimens of vitamin B6 and folic acid on mild hyperhomocysteinemia in vascular patients. J Inherit Metab Dis 1994; 17:159-62.
52. Berg van den, Franken DG, Boers GH, et al. Combined vitamin B6 and folic acid therapy in young patients with arteriosclerosis and hyperhomocysteinemia. J Vasc Surg 1994; 20:933-40.

7. GENETIC MARKERS OF HEMOSTATIC FACTORS

D. Girelli, O. Olivieri, R. Corrocher

Introduction

Thrombosis underlies most acute manifestations of coronary atherosclerotic disease, including myocardial infarction (MI) [1]. In this setting, the rupture of an atherosclerotic plaque, endothelial cell damage, or both, are the key events that trigger the thrombotic process. Plaque disruption is followed by the exposure of blood flow to tissue factor (TF), a glycoprotein elaborated by several cells infiltrating the plaque, which is accumulated especially in the lipid-rich core [2]. TF forms a high-affinity complex with coagulation factor VII [3], which initiates a cascade of enzymatic reactions resulting in the local generation of thrombin and deposition of fibrin. The evolution to occlusive thrombus or resolving lesion is depending on a delicate equilibrium between thrombosis and endogenous thrombolysis. As part of the response to any type of endothelial wall disruption, platelet adhesion occurs through the binding of the glycoprotein (Gp) Ib/IX/V platelet receptor to von Willebrand Factor (vWF) and/or direct binding of platelets by means of their collagen receptor (Gp Ia/IIa complex). These reactions determine a conformational change in the platelet Gp IIb/IIIa integrin, from a ligand-unreceptive state to a ligand-receptive state. Ligand-receptive Gp IIb/IIIa receptors bind fibrinogen molecules, which form bridges between adjacent platelets, facilitating platelet aggregation and propagation of thrombus [4,5].

Thus, thrombosis is a complex, multifactorial, condition involving several interrelated systems such as the coagulation and the fibrinolytic pathways, and the platelet integrins. Perturbation of each of these systems may be genetically determined, and, when this is the case, its influence is potentially profound because of its life-long presence. On the other hand, it is well-known that the hemostatic balance is strongly influenced by a number of life-style and environmental factors, and this points to the importance of gene-environment interactions in modulating the thrombotic risk.

This review will focus on common variations in the genes for blood coagulation factors, fibrinolytic factors and platelet-membrane receptors, which may influence the hemostatic balance (table 1). In spite of a rapidly growing literature in this field, our understanding is only primitive and mainly based on the results of association studies.

PA Doevendans and AA Wilde (eds.), Cardiovascular genetics, 71-87.

Table 1. Common variations in genes for hemostatic factors

GENE	***LOCUS***	**POLYMORPHISM**	**FUNCTION**	***CATEGO.***
Fibrinogen	4q28	455 G/A	high fibrinogen levels in carriers, especially in smokers and males	D
Factor VII	13q34	Arg353Gln	low factor VII levels in carriers of Gln allele	D
		A1/A2	low factor VII levels in carriers of A2 allele	D
		H5/H6/H7/H8	low factor VII levels in carriers of H7 allele	D
Prothrombin	11p11-q12	20210 G/A	high prothrombin levels in carriers of A allele	D
Factor V	1q23	Arg506Gln (Leiden mutation)	APC-resistance	D
		His1299Arg (R2 polymorphism)	Carriers have low factor V levels and an imbalance between the two different FV isoforms normally present in plasma, with a relative increase of the more thrombogenic FV_1 isoforms	D
Factor XIII	Subunit A: 6p25-p24	Val34Leu	Unclear	D
Plasminogen activator inhibitor-1 (PAI-1)	7q21.3-q22	4G/5G	Subjects with 4G/4G genotype have plasma PAI-1 concentration approximately 25% higher than subjects with 5G/5G genotype	D
Gp IIb/IIIa	17q21.32	Leu33Pro (in Gp IIIa)	Pro33 allele is associated to an increased binding of fibrinogen to platelets and increased epinephrine-induced aggregation	D
Gp Ib-IX-V complex	Ib: 22q11.2	A/B/C/D	Unclear	D
		Thr145Met	Unclear	D
Gp Ia/IIa complex	IIa: 5q23-q31	807 C/T	T allele is associated with a high-receptor density	D

Coagulation factors

Fibrinogen

Fibrinogen has been indicated as an independent predictor for MI and stroke in several prospective studies [6-8], with an effect size similar to cholesterol [9]. The causal relationship has been questioned since fibrinogen is an acute-phase marker which may merely reflect the inflammatory nature of the atherosclerotic process. Also, increased fibrinogen is associated with other cardiovascular risk factors [10], especially with smoking [11]. On the other hand, the presence of fibrinogen in the atherosclerotic plaques in proportion to circulating levels [12,13], and its influence on platelet aggregation and plasma viscosity, are biologically plausible factors supporting a direct role for fibrinogen in atherosclerosis.

Fibrinogen is a 340-kd glycoprotein consisting of 3 non-identical chains (Aα, Bβ and γ) linked by disulfide bonds. The 3 polypeptides are encoded by 3 genes in close proximity on the long arm of chromosome 4 [14]. All of them contain several sequence elements that are known to regulate gene expression. Particularly important are considered the interleukin-6 (IL-6)-responsive elements located in the 5' region of all genes, which are thought to mediate the behaviour of fibrinogen as an acute-phase reactant. This interaction explains the elevated levels of fibrinogen found in response to environmental risk factors such as smoking or infections.

Multiple polymorphisms have been described in the 3 fibrinogen genes. Most studies have focused on two polymorphism of the Bβ-chain gene, the *Bcl*I polymorphism located in the 3' region, and the -455 G/A polymorphism located in the 5' promoter region. The two polymorphisms are in strong linkage disequilibrium, so that the analysis are frequently restricted to the -455 G/A transition, supposed to be functional because of its proximity to the IL-6-responsive element. Several large studies have confirmed a consistent association between the -455 G/A transition and its intermediate phenotype, with elevated plasma fibrinogen levels in mutation carriers [15-19]. This association was generally more evident in smokers and/or males [15,16]. Notwithstanding this evidence, the relationship between fibrinogen polymorphisms and coronary disease is not clear. Some studies suggested an association, especially with the severity of coronary atherosclerosis [15,19,20]. An unambiguous association with MI was found only in a highly selected population of Italian patients with "familial" cardiovascular disease (i.e. having at least one first-degree relative who had MI or stroke before 65 years of age), in which the *Bcl*I polymorphism was investigated [21]. By contrast, other studies failed to show any association between fibrinogen genotypes and either coronary artery disease or MI [17,18].

Another polymorphism of potential interest is the amino acid Thr312Ala mutation in the coding region of the α-chain [22]. It is located within the region close to the factor XIII cross-linking site at position 328 [23,24]. These findings have suggested a role of the Ala312 allele in influencing clot stability. However, in a recent case-control study no difference was found in the frequency of the genotypes between MI survivors and controls [25].

It should be stressed that family studies designed to assess heritability of fibrinogen have estimated a contribution of genetic factors to the variability of circulating levels near to 50% [26-28]. The above mentioned polymorphisms in the Bβ chain have been shown to account for minor contributions (about 5%) to variations in concentrations, suggesting that there is still a substantial genetic effect on fibrinogen concentrations which is yet to be identified.

Factor VII

Coagulation factor VII (FVII) is a vitamin K-dependent protease secreted by the liver as a single-chain inactive zymogen of 48 kD. FVII is the first protease to be activated in the extrinsic pathway of blood coagulation. As mentioned above, the disruption of an atherosclerotic plaque is followed by the formation of the TF/FVII complex, with subsequent activation of factor X and IX, ultimately leading to thrombin generation. During the past two decades, there has been substantial interest in investigating the role of FVII levels in coronary disease. The Northwick Park Heart Study investigators reported that a high plasma level of FVII was a predictor of death due to coronary disease [6]. The trend was similar in some other studies [8, 29], but not all [30, 31]. Control of plasma levels of FVII is multifactorial, with both genetic and environmental influences [32]. Non-genetic factors known to be important are diet, hyperlipidemia, diabetes, and inflammation. The human FVII gene spans 13 kB on chromosome 13. At least three common polymorphisms have been identified on this gene [33,34]: 1) a 10-bp insertion in the promoter region (5'F7), where allele A1 corresponds to the absence of the decamer (10 bp) and allele A2 to its insertion; 2) the substitution of adenine for guanine in the codon for residue 353 in the catalytic domain of exon 8, which results in the substitution of glutamine (Q) for arginine (R), i.e. the Arg353Gln or R353Q polymorphism; 3) a variable number (five to eight) of 37-bp tandem repeats in intron 7, where allele "a" (also called H7) corresponds to the presence of seven monomers, "b" (H6) the presence of six monomers, "c" (H5) the presence of five monomers, and "d" (H8) the presence of eight monomers. The first two polymorphisms are in strong linkage disequilibrium [35], with a degree of allelic association of more than 80 percent. Many studies in different populations have confirmed that these polymorphisms account for a substantial part of the variance in the circulating levels of FVII, estimated to be near 30% [36]. Interestingly, the rare alleles of each polymorphism, i.e. the A2, Q, and H7 alleles, are associated with decreased levels of FVII, indicating possible *protective* variants. Up to now, this issue remains controversial. A first Italian study of 165 subjects with familial MI and 225 controls found that homozygosity for the Q allele was associated to a strong and significant protection against MI (OR = 0.08; 95% CI, 0.01 to 0.9) [37]. Other studies in patients from Northern Europe, failed to detect an influence of the R353Q polymorphism on the risk of MI [38, 39]. Also, Wang et al. [20] found no association between the R353Q polymorphism and the angiographically documented severity of coronary atherosclerosis. On the other hand, it is biologically plausible that FVII does not influence the development of coronary atherosclerosis, but only its thrombotic complications, i.e.MI. A more recent study [40] investigated all the three FVII gene polymorphisms mentioned above in 444 Italian subjects with coronary angiography documentation. Each of the polymorphisms significantly influenced FVII levels. Patients with the A2A2 and QQ genotypes had the lowest levels of activated FVII (66 percent and 72 percent lower, respectively, than the levels in patients with the A1A1 or RR genotypes). When a comparison was made between patients with or without coronary disease (CAD vs CAD-free), none of the polymorphisms was associated to the atherosclerotic phenotype. On the other hand, in the CAD group with severe, multi-vessel CAD, there were significantly more heterozygotes and homozygotes for the A2 and Q alleles among those who had not suffered a MI than among those who had an infarction. The adjusted odds ratio (OR) for MI among the patients with the A1A2 or RQ genotype was 0.47 (95 percent confidence interval, 0.27 to 0.81). Another recent study found a reduced procedural risk for coronary catheter intervention in carriers of the Q allele from a population of 666 patients with angiographically documented CAD [41]. Taken together, the data available so far suggest that in certain well-characterized subgroups of CAD patients, i.e. with angiographically documented multi-vessel disease and/or homogeneous ethnic background, FVII gene markers may help to predict the risk of thrombotic complications. It has been recently suggested that low-dose regimens of oral anticoagulants independently reduce the rate of death due to coronary heart disease in subjects at high risk for cardiovascular events [42]. Remarkably, the low-normal FVII levels resulting from low-dose warfarin treatment substantially overlap those associated with the *protective* FVII genotypes [43]. Thus, in the future, such a pharmacologic approach could be effectively restricted to persons with "unfavorable" genotypes; those with the protective genotypes could be excluded because of the low probability of benefit and increased risk of bleeding.

Prothrombin

Prothrombin is the 72-kD zymogen precursor of the serine protease thrombin, a key enzyme acting both as procoagulant through platelet activation and the generation of fibrin, factor Va, VIIIa and XIIIa, and subsequently as anticoagulant, by activating circulating protein C [44]. Regulation of thrombin activity is therefore crucial to maintain hemostatic balance.

Prothrombin, is synthesized in the liver from a 2-kB mRNA, which in turn is generated from a genomic locus of 20 kB on chromosome 11. In 1996, Poort et al. described a variant in the 3'-untranslated region of the prothrombin gene, i.e. a guanine to adenine substitution at position 20210, that was associated with an increased risk of venous thrombosis [45]. Several other studies have been reported afterwards that confirm the role of the G20210A mutation as a risk factor for thrombosis in the venous system [46-49]. The 20210 A allele has a peculiar geographic distribution, being more common in southern than in northern Europe (incidence approximate 3% and 1.7%, respectively), and quite rare among individuals of Asian and African descent [50]. Importantly, this polymorphism, outside of the coding region, does not affect thrombin structure or function. On the other hand, the heterozygosity for the 20210A allele is associated to plasma prothrombin levels about 20% higher than those found in subjects with the GG genotype. As the mutation is located at or near the cleavage and polyadenylation site, it has been postulated that it may induce a higher translation efficiency or higher stability of the messenger RNA. Indeed, a very recent report strongly supports the view that G20210A represents a functional polymorphism [51]. An excessive thrombin generation has been described in individuals at high risk of fatal CAD [52]. It seems biologically plausible that the higher prothrombin levels related to the 20210A variant may also confer an increased risk of arterial vascular disease. To date, however, studies on the role of this mutation in CAD have given conflicting results. In some reports, carriership of the mutation was associated to an increased risk of MI [53, 54], especially when other major risk factors are also present [55-57]. Notably, the US Physicians Health Study, the only prospective study published thus far, did not identify an association of the 20210A allele with either MI or stroke [58], whereas several ethnic, demographic and methodological differences may account for the null findings in this highly selected population [59]. Recently, a case-control study performed on 436 patients with angiographically documented severe CAD, and 224 controls with normal coronary angiography, suggested that elevated prothrombin levels may be associated *per se* with CAD. Subjects with prothrombin activity in the upper tertile, compared with the lower tertile, had an OR for coronary atherosclerosis of 1.86 (95% CI, 1.01 to 3.40) [60]. Heterozygosity for the 20210 A allele was higher in patients than in controls (5.3% vs 3.1%, respectively), but the difference did not reach statistical significance. On the other hand, it contributed significantly to high prothrombin levels, with an increased number of carriers in the group with prothrombin activity in the upper tertile. This suggests that the 20210A allele may be only one of the factors (genetic or environmental) which contribute to the risk of CAD by means of increased prothrombin levels. The genetic heritability of plasma prothrombin levels has been demonstrated to be high (greater than 50%), also independently of the effect of the 20210A allele [51]. This indicates that a substantial portion of the phenotypic variation in plasma prothrombin levels is due to the additive effects of yet unknown genetic factors.

Factor V

Coagulation factor V (FV), a large (330-kD) and asymmetric glycoprotein mainly synthesized by the liver and megakaryocytes, circulates in plasma and is partially stored in platelets. The protein has a multi-domain structure which shares several homologies with factor VIII. When activated by limited proteolysis (release of the B-domain→ FVa) it participates as an essential co-factor in the activation of prothrombin by activated factor X. On the other hand, FVa is inactivated by activated protein C (APC), an anticoagulant proteinase also able to inactivate factor VIIIa [61].

Human FV is encoded by a gene localized on chromosome 1q21-25, spanning more than 80 kb, and comprising 25 exons and 24 introns [62]. An exon 10 mutation (G1691A) gives rise to a FV molecule not properly inactivated by APC [63,64], which causes the so-called APC-resistance. In fact, the mutation results in the substitution of an arginine with a glutamine at position 506 (Arg506Gln), which is one of the two primary cleavage inactivation sites by APC (the other is Arg 306). As a consequence, the APC-induced cleavage is delayed [65,66]. This polymorphism, also known as factor V Leiden (FVL), is an established risk factor for venous thrombosis. FVL arose from a common source 20,000 to 30,000 years ago (founder effect) [67].

The potential role of this mutation in arterial thrombosis and disease has been evaluated in several large studies. The majority of them gave negative results [68-74].

Interestingly, whereas most cases of APC-resistance in subjects with thrombophilia are explained by the FVL mutation, it is well-known that there are subjects with the APC-resistance phenotype but who do not carry the FVL mutation [75]. Several acquired conditions, i.e. pregnancy [76], oral contraceptive use [77], the presence of lupus anticoagulant [78] or high FVIII levels [79,80] are associated with a reduced sensitivity to APC. APC-resistance could also theoretically result from a variety of other mutations on critical sites in FV or FVIII, yet unknown. A recent large population study on 826 subjects who underwent ultrasound imaging of femoral and carotid arteries, demonstrated an independent and gradual association between low sensitivity to APC and advanced atherosclerosis [81]. In this sample form the general population, fewer than 50% of APC-resistant subjects actually had the FVL mutation. This study emphasizes the need to characterize further genetic determinants of APC. A recently described polymorphism in the FV gene is being studied. In 1996, Lunghi et al. [82] first described the A4070G mutation in the large exon 13 (2.8 kb), which replaces His by Arg at position 1299 of the B domain. Because of the susceptibility to the RsaI restriction enzyme, this polymorphism is generally designed as "R2". Actually, the R2 polymorphism is linked to many other mutations, mostly in exon 13, so that it is more correct to speak of the R2 haplotype, a very ancient gene dating back to a time antecedent the migration of man out of Africa [83], especially common in southern Europe (approximately 12% are carriers). The R2 haplotype has been shown to influence plasma FV levels and contribute to the APC-resistance phenotype [84]. Biochemical studies have shown that the R2 haplotype is associated to an imbalance between the two different FV isoforms normally present in plasma, which differ in the degree of glycosylation and affinity for phosphatidylserine-containing membranes [85]. Indeed, carriership of the R2 haplotype is associated with a relative increase of the more glycosylated and more thrombogenic FV_1 isoform [86,87]. Because of these functional implications, studies are in progress to evaluate the role of this haplotype as a possible risk factor for arterial disease.

Fibrinolysis

The formation of stable, fibrinolysis-resistant, cross-linked fibrin is the ultimate step in coagulation and occurs as a result of thrombin-induced cleavage of fibrinogen, with concurrent activation of coagulation factor XIII and the generation of cross-linked fibrin polymers. There are several inhibitors of fibrinolysis in the circulation. Among the most important is the Plasminogen Activator Inhibitor-1 (PAI-1), a fast-acting inhibitor of tissue plasminogen activator (t-PA) [88]. At least theoretically, a decrease in fibrinolysis due to high plasma PAI-1 concentrations might be expected to result in an increase in the deposition of fibrin and subsequent formation of a thrombus.

Plasminogen Activator Inhibitor-1 (PAI-1)

PAI-1 is a 50-kd linear glycoprotein that is composed of 379 amino acids [89]. High concentrations of PAI-1 occur in the atheromatous plaque [90,91], and elevated circulating concentrations of PAI-1 have been associated to the risk of arterial disease in a number of studies [92,-95]. On the other hand, it is well-known that PAI-1 is an acute phase reactant and that high PAI-1 levels are strongly related to the metabolic features of the insulin resistance syndrome [96,97]. Thus, it remains to be determined whether the association of PAI-1 levels with vascular risk is causal or not.

Though the insulin resistant state has been estimated to account for about 49% of PAI-1 levels [98], genetic influences are also known to be important in determining PAI-1 variance. The human PAI-1 gene is located on chromosome 7 and contains nine exons [99]. Several polymorphic loci have been described within the gene, including a common single-base-pair polymorphism (four or five guanine bases) in the promoter region of the gene, 675 bp upstream of the transcriptional start site (4G/5G) [100]. Increased gene transcription has been associated to the 4G allele, since it only binds a transcriptional activator, whereas the 5G allele binds also a repressor protein that decreases the binding of the activator [100]. Indeed, subjects who are homozygous for the 4G allele (4G/4G genotype) have plasma PAI-1 concentrations that are approximately 25 percent higher than those of subjects who are homozygous for the 5G allele (5G/5G genotype) [101]. Because of these functional implications, the identification of the 4G/5G polymorphism was followed by intensive clinical investigations with a mixture of results. Some studies reported a positive association with MI [101-103] or CAD [104], whereas others did not [105-107]. A meta-analysis suggested a weak, but significant effect of PAI-1 genotype on MI [108]. Interestingly, some in vitro studies led support to the hypothesis of a triglyceride/genotype specific interaction. A very-low-density lipoprotein triglyceride-sensitive site has been identified in the promoter region adjacent to the 4G/5G site [109]. Furthermore, triglycerides increase the production of PAI-1 by hepatocytes in vitro, an effect that is mediated by the low-density lipoprotein receptor and increased in the presence of insulin [110]. Thus it is tempting to speculate that the interaction between the 4G allele and other genetic and/or environmental determinants of the insulin resistance syndrome is required for the full expression of a phenotype at vascular risk.

Moreover, a gene-gene interaction between the PAI-1 4G/5G and a polymorphism in the FXIII gene has been described. **Coagulation factor XIII** is a 320 kd, tetrameric (2 "A" subunits plus 2 "B" subunits) protransglutaminase that has a crucial role in clot stabilisation [111]. When activated by thrombin (at position Arg37-Gly38 in the A subunit), it facilitates the cross-linking of fibrin chains, leading to resistance of the clot to fibrinolysis. Several mutations in the FXIII gene have been related to FXIII deficiency, a severe bleeding disorder.

A common G-to-T point mutation in codon 34, exon 2, of the FXIII A-subunit gene that codes for a valine-to-leucine change (FXIII Val34Leu) close to the site of thrombin activation has been recently found to be protective against MI [112,113], though the mechanism is unclear. However, the protective effect of FXIII Val34Leu was lost in subjects with high plasma PAI-1 concentrations, in whom the prevalence of the 4G/4G genotype was increased [114]. These findings suggest that FXIII Val34Leu interferes beneficially in some way with the formation of fibrin, an effect that is canceled out in the presence of increased PAI-1 concentrations associated with 4G/4G genotype and/or the insulin resistance. Future studies to clarify the role of the 4G/4G genotype in modulating the risk of arterial disease should take into account these gene-gene and gene-environmental interactions.

Platelet-membrane glycoproteins

Several platelet-membrane glycoproteins play a crucial role in platelet adhesion and aggregation [115,116]. Inherited polymorphisms within their genes have attracted considerable interest because of their profound impact on the antigenic makeup of platelets, their involvement in platelet disorders with bleeding tendency, and, more recently, for their possible role in regulating the risk of arterial thrombosis.

Gp IIb/IIIa

Gp IIb is a disulfide-linked protein of 150-kd that associates with the 90-kd polypeptide Gp IIIa. Many coding polymorphisms in Gp IIb/IIIa have been identified in normal populations and approximately 18 mutations are involved in the pathogenesis of Glanzmann thrombasthenia, a bleeding disorder. A common point mutation in Gp IIIa results in the substitution of proline for leucine at codon 33. The pro33 allele, also known as PLA2, is found in approximately 15% of the white population [117]. It has been associated to an increased binding of fibrinogen to platelets [118], and increased epinephrine-induced aggregation [119].

In 1996, a small study on 71 patients with acute coronary syndrome first reported an association between the PLA2 allele and risk for MI [120]. The risk was high especially in a subgroup of subjects younger than 60, in whom an OR of 6.2 was reported. Some studies that concentrated on young survivors of MI confirmed an increased risk in carriers of the PLA2 allele [121,122]. Also, a positive interaction with smoking was described [122]. However, several large studies yielded negative reports [123, 124]. Similarly, conflicting results have been reported on the association between the PLA2 allele and either the extent of coronary atherosclerosis estimated by coronary angiography [121,125,126] or the outcome of patients undergoing coronary artery procedures [127, 128].

Gp Ib-IX-V complex

The Gp Ib-IX-V complex mediates the initial and transient tethering of platelets to the extracellular matrix under a wide range of flow conditions via the binding of vWF to the amino-terminal domain of glycoprotein Ibα. The deficiency of the Gp Ib-IX-V complex is associated to the Bernard Soulier syndrome. This receptor is composed of four proteins that are the products of distinct genes: Gp Ibα, approximately 140-kd, Gp Ibβ, approximately 25-kd, Gp IX, approximately 22-kd and Gp V, approximately 82-kd [129]. The complex is an heptamer in which one molecule of Gp V is noncovalently associated with two molecules each of GpIb and Gp IX. Two polymorphisms have attracted interest for their potential role as thrombotic risk factors. A length polymorphism in Gp Ib results from a variable number of tandem repeats of 39-bp coding for 13 amino acids in the glycosylated region (macroglycopeptide). Four polymorphic alleles (1, 2, 3, or 4 repeats; designated D, C, B, A, respectively) have been described. The C/B genotype has been associated to arterial disease (coronary and cerebrovascular), with an OR of 2.8 [130]. The second polymorphism, C to T at position 3550, results in a Thr145Met substitution and is linked to the HPA-2 alloantigen system. It is located close to the vWF and the high-affinity thrombin binding sites. The Met145 variant was also associated with CAD in one study [130] but not in a case-control study of 200 young MI survivors [122].

Gp Ia/IIa complex

This complex, also known as integrin α2/β1, consists of an approximately 167-kd (α2) and an approximately 130-kd (β1) polypeptide. It is a collagen receptor which plays a fundamental role in adhesion of platelets to both fibrillar and nonfibrillar collagen. It is deficient in patients with mild bleeding disorders characterized by an impaired response to collagen [131,132]. Noteworthy, the expression of this receptor on platelet surface varies markedly (by approximately a 10-fold order of magnitude) among normal persons, resulting in different in vitro response to collagen [133]. This density variation is associated with a silent exonic dimorphism at position 807, C/T. A large study (n = 2237) of male patients undergoing coronary angiography found an association between the T allele (predicting high-receptor density) and MI in patients younger than 62 years [134]. Conversely, a case-control study was unable to establish an association between the T allele and MI, even for homozygous carriers [135].

Perspectives

At present, the role of the above-mentioned genetic markers of hemostatic factors as potential contributors to the risk of arterial disease is matter of discussion. This is not surprising, since atherosclerosis is a complex disease in which a myriad of genetic and environmental factors are involved, so that it is highly unlikely that single genetic polymorphisms will be the sole determinants of disease. In many occasions, initial studies yielded promising results which were not subsequently confirmed. Several factors may account for these discrepancies. The clinical endpoints are highly heterogenous (i.e.: MI, unstable angina, CAD, progression of arterial disease), so that a comparison among different investigations lacking a common definition of the clinical phenotype is often not feasible. Also, insufficient attention to minimize bias in the selection of controls is a common problem, especially if coronary atherosclerosis is the phenotype of interest. Subjects from the general population are often used as controls, without objective information about their coronary arteries. By this approach, one is never sure about the extent of the coronary narrowing, since those controls might have substantial, though not yet clinically manifest, coronary atherosclerosis. This in turn contributes to attenuate the association between the polymorphism(s) under investigation and CAD. Substantial variations of the frequencies of certain polymorphisms among different ethnic groups is another possible explanation. It should be stressed that the effect on the intermediate phenotype (i.e. the concentrations of certain coagulation factors) of the currently known polymorphisms is often mild and mediated by the interaction with environmental factors. Future studies should be specifically addressed to investigate these interactions, as well as to the identification of the yet unknown major genetic determinants of coagulation factors concentrations. Since our understanding in this field has to be considered only primitive, at present there is no specific advice for patients with arterial thrombosis and MI.

References

1. Fuster V, Badimon L, Badimon J and Chesebro JH. The pathogenesis of coronary artery disease and the acute coronary syndromes. N Engl J Med 1992; 326:242-50.
2. Wilcox JN, Smith KM, Schwartz SM, Gordon D. Localization of tissue factor in the normal vessel wall and in the atherosclerotic plaque. Proc Natl Acad Sci USA 1989; 86:2839-43.
3. Rao LV, Rapaport SI. Activation of factor VII bound to tissue factor: a key early step in the tissue factor pathway of blood coagulation. Proc Natl Acad Sci USA 1988; 85:6687–91.
4. Madan M, Berkowitz SD, Tcheng JE. Glycoprotein IIb/IIIa integrin blockade. Circulation 1998; 98:2629-35.
5. Lefkovits J, Plow EF, Topol EJ. Platelet glycoprotein IIb/IIIa receptors in cardiovascular medicine. N Engl J Med 1995; 332:1553-9.
6. Meade TW, Mellows S, Brozovic M, et al. Haemostatic function and ischaemic heart disease: prinicipal results of the Northwick Park Heart Study. Lancet. 1986; 2:533-7
7. Wilhelmsen L, Svardsudd K, Korsan-Bengtsen K, Larsson B, Welin L, Tibblin G. Fibrinogen as a risk factor for stroke and myocardial infarction. N Engl J Med. 1984; 311:501-505.
8. Heinrich J, Balleisen L, Schulte H, Assmann G, van de Loo J. Fibrinogen and factor VII in the prediction of coronary risk: results from the PROCAM study in healthy men. Arterioscler Thromb 1994; 14:54-9.
9. Maresca G, Di Blasio A, Marchioli R, Di Minno G. Measuring plasma fibrinogen to predict stroke and myocardial infarction: an update. Arterioscler Thromb Vasc Biol 1999; 19: 1368-77.
10. Lee AJ, Lowe GDO, Woodward M, Tunstall Pedoe H. Fibrinogen in relation to a personal history of prevalent hypertension, diabetes, stroke, intermittent claudication, coronary heart disease and family history: the Scottish Heart Health Study. Br Heart J. 1993; 69:338-42.
11. Meade TW, Imeson J, Stirling Y. Effects of changes in smoking and other characteristics on clotting factors and the risk of ischaemic heart disease. Lancet. 1987; 986-8.
12. Bini A, Kudryk B. Fibrinogen in human athrosclerosis. Ann N Y Acad Sci 1995; 748:461-71.
13. Smith E, Keen G, Grant A. Fate of fibrinogen in human arterial intimae. Arteriosclerosis 1990; 6:263-75.
14. Kant JA, Furnace AJ, Saxe D, Simon MI, McBride OW, Crabtree GR. Evolution and organization of the fibrinogen locus on chromosome 4: gene duplication accompanied by transcription and inversion. Proc Natl Acad Sci U S A. 1985; 82:2344-8.
15. Behague I, Poirier O, Nicaud V, et al. fibrinogengene polymorphisms are associated with plasma fibrinogen and coronary artery disease in patients with myocardial infarction. Circulation. 1996; 93:440-9.
16. Humphries SE, Ye S, Talmud P, Bara L, Wilhelmsen L, Tiret L. European Athersclerosis Research Study: genotype at the fibrinogen locus (G_{-455}-A gene) is associated with differences in plasma fibrinogen levels in young men and women from different regions in Europe: evidence for gender-genotype-environment interaction. Arterioscler Thromb Vasc Biol. 1995; 15:96-104.
17. Tybjaerg-Hansen A, Agerholm-Larsen B, Humphries SE, Abildgaard S, Schnohr P, Nordestgaard BG. A common mutation (G_{-455}-A) in the -fibrinogen promoter is an independent predictor of plasma fibrinogen, but not of ischemic heart disease: a study of 9,127 individuals based on the Copenhagen City Heart Study. J Clin Invest. 1997; 99:3034-9.
18. Gardemann A, Schwartz O, Haberbosch W, et al. Positive association of the fibrinogen H1/H2 gene variation to basal fibrinogen levels and to increase in fibrinogen concentration during acute phase reaction but not to coronary artery disease and myocardial infarction. Thromb Haemost. 1997; 77:1120-6.
19. de Maat MPM, Kastelein JJP, Jukema JW, et al. -455G/A polymorphism of the -fibrinogen gene is associated with the progression of coronary atherosclerosis in symptomatic men: proposed role for an acute phase reaction pattern of fibrinogen. Arterioscler Thromb Vasc Biol.

1998; 18:265-71.

20. Wang XL, Wang J, McCredie RM, Wilcken DEL. Polymorphisms of factor V, factor VII, and fibrinogen genes: relevance to severity of coronary artery disease. Arterioscler Thromb Vasc Biol 1997; 17:246-51.
21. Zito F, Di Castelnuovo A, Amore C, D'Orazio A, Donati MB, Iacoviello L. Bcl I polymorphism in the fibrinogen -chaingene is associated with the risk of familial myocardial infarction by increasing plasma fibrinogen levels: a case-control study in a sample of GISSI-2 patients. Arterioscler Thromb Vasc Biol. 1997; 17:3489.
22. Baumann RE, Henschen AH. Human fibrinogen polymorphic site analysis by restriction endonuclease digestion and allele-specific polymerase chain reaction amplification: identification of polymorphisms at position A 312 and B 448. Blood. 1996; 82:2117-24.
23. Muszbek L, Adany R, Mikkola H. Novel aspects of blood coagulation factor XIII, I: structure, distribution, activation and function. Crit Rev Clin Lab Sci. 1996; 33:357-421.
24. Credo RB, Curtis CG, Lorand L. -chain domain of fibrinogen controls generation of fibrinoligase (factor XIIIa): calcium ion regulatory aspects. Biochemistry. 1981; 20:3770-8.
25. Curran JM, Evans A, Arveiler D, et al. The -fibrinogen T/A 312 polymorphism in the ECTIM study. Thromb Haemost. 1998; 79:1057-8.
26. Hamsten A, Iselius L, De Faire U, Blomback M. Genetic and cultural inheritance of plasma fibrinogen concentrations. Lancet. 1987; 2:988-91.
27. Friedlander Y, Elkana Y, Sinnreich R, Kark JD. Genetic and environmental sources of fibrinogen variability in Israeli families: The Kibbutzim Study. Am J Hum Genet. 1995; 56:1194.
28. de Lange M, Snieder H, Arlens RAS, Spector TD, Grant PJ. The genetics of haemostasis: a twin study. Lancet 2001; 357:101-5.
29. Redondo M, Watzke HH, Stucki B, et al. Coagulation factors II, V, VII, and X, prothrombin gene 20210G-to-A transition, and factor V Leiden in coronary artery disease: high factor V clotting activity is an independent risk factor for myocardial infarction. Arterioscler Thromb Vasc Biol 1999; 19:1020-5.
30. Folsom AR, Wu KK, Rosamond WD, Sharrett AR, Chambless LE. Prospective study of hemostatic factors and incidence of coronary heart disease: the Atherosclerosis Risk in Communities (ARIC) Study. Circulation 1997; 96:1102-8.
31. Smith FB, Lee AJ, Fowkes FGR, Price JF, Rumley A, Lowe GDO. Hemostatic factors as predictors of ischemic heart disease and stroke in the Edinburgh Artery Study. Arterioscler Thromb Vasc Biol 1997; 17:3321-5.
32. Green FG, Humphries S. Genetic determinants of arterial thrombosis. Baillieres Clin Haematol 1994; 7:675-92.
33. Green F, Kelleher C, Wilkes H, Temple A, Meade T, Humphries S. A common genetic polymorphism associated with lower coagulation factor VII levels in healthy individuals. Arteroscler Thromb. 1991; 11:540.
34. Marchetti G, Patracchini P, Papaschini M, Ferrati M, Bernardi F. A polymorphism in the 5' region of coagulation factor VII gene (F7) caused by an inserted decanucleotide. Hum Genet. 1993; 90:575.
35. Bernardi F, Arcieri P, Bertina RM, et al. Contribution of factor VII genotype to activated FVII levels: differences in genotype frequencies between northern and southern European populations. Arterioscler Thromb Vasc Biol 1997; 17:2548-53.
36. Bernardi F, Marchetti G, Pinotti M, et al. Factor VII gene polymorphisms contribute about one third of the factor VII level variation in plasma. Arterioscler Thromb Vasc Biol 1996; 16:72-6.
37. Iacoviello L, Di Castelnuovo A, de Knijff P, et al. Polymorphisms in the coagulation factor VII gene and the risk of myocardial infarction. N Engl J Med 1998; 338:79-85.
38. Lane A, Green F, Scarabin PY, et al. Factor VII Arg/Gln353 polymorphism determines factor VII coagulant activity in patients with myocardial infarction (MI) and control subjects in Belfast and in France but is not a strong indicator of MI risk in the ECTIM study. Atherosclerosis 1996; 119:119-27.

39. Doggen CJM, Manger Cats V, Bertina RM, Reitsma PH, Vandenbroucke JP, Rosendaal FR. A genetic propensity to high factor VII is not associated with the risk of myocardial infarction in men. Thromb Haemost 1998; 80:281-5.
40. Girelli D, Russo C, Ferraresi P, Olivieri O, Pinotti M, Friso S, Manzato F, Mazzucco A, Bernardi F, Corrocher R. Polymorphisms in the Factor VII gene and the risk of myocardial infarction in patients with coronary artery disease. New Engl J Med 2000; 343:774-80.
41. Mrozikiewicz PM, Cascorbi I, Ziemer S, Laule M, Meisel C, Stangl V, Rutsch W, Wernecke K, Baumann G, Roots I, Stangl K. Reduced procedural risk for coronary catheter interventions in carriers of the coagulation factor VII-Gln353 gene. J Am Coll Cardiol 2000; 36:1520-5.
42. The Medical Research Council's General Practice Research Framework. Thrombosis Prevention Trial: randomised trial of low-intensity oral anticoagulation with warfarin and low-dose aspirin in the primary prevention of ischaemic heart disease in men at increased risk. Lancet 1998; 351:233-41.
43. Iacoviello L, Donati MB. Interpretation of Thrombosis Prevention Trial. Lancet 1998; 351:1205.
44. Jackson CM. Physiology and biochemistry of prothrombin. In Haemostasis and Thrombosis. Bloom A, Forbes CD, Thomas DP, Tuddenham EGD eds. Edinburgh, UK Churchill Livingstone 1994; 397-438.
45. Poort SR, Rosendaal FR, Reitsma PH, et al. A common genetic variation in the 3'-untranslated region of the prothrombin gene is associated with elevated plasma prothrombin levels and an increase in venous thrombosis. Blood 1996; 88: 3698-703.
46. Hillarp A, Zöller B, Svensson PJ, et al. The 20210 A allele of the prothrombin gene is a common risk factor among swedish outpatients with deep verified venous thrombosis. Thromb Haemost 1997; 78: 990-2.
47. Arruda VD, Bizzacchi JM, Goncalves MS, et al. Prevalence of the prothrombin gene variant (nt 20210A) in venous thrombosis and arterial disease. Thromb Haemost 1997; 78:1430-3.
48. Vicente V, Gonzalez-Conejero R, Rivera J, et al. The prothrombin gene variant 20210A in venous and arterial thromboembolism. Haematologica 1999; 84:356-62.
49. Martinelli I, Sacchi E, Landi G, et al. High risk of cerebral-vein thrombosis in carriers of a prothrombin-gene mutation and in users of oral contraceptives. N Engl J Med. 1998; 338: 3562-5.
50. Rosendaal FR, Doggen CJ, Zivelin A, et al: Geographic distribution of the 20210 G to A prothrombin variant. Thromb Haemost 1998; 79:706-8.
51. Soria HM, Almasy L, Souto JC, et al. Linkage analysis demonstrates that the prothrombin G20210A mutation jointly influences plasma prothrombin levels and the risk of thrombosis. Blood 2000; 95: 2780-5.
52. Miller GJ, Bauer KA, Barzegar S, et al. Increased activation of the hemostatic system in men at high risk of fatal coronary heart disease. Thromb Haemost 1996; 75: 767-71.
53. Franco RF, Trip MD, ten Cate H, et al. The 20210 G→A mutation in the 3'untranslated region of the prothrombin gene and the risk for arterial thrombotic disease. Br J Haematol 1999; 104: 50-4.
54. Watzke HH, Schüttrumpf J, Graf S, et al. Increased prevalence of a polymorphism in the gene coding for human prothrombin in patients with coronary heart disease. Thromb Res 1997; 87: 521-6.
55. Doggen CJM, Cats VM, Bertina RM, et al. Interaction of coagulation defects and cardiovascular risk factors. Circulation 1998; 97: 1037-41.
56. Rosendaal FR, Siscovick DS, Schwartz SM, et al. A common prothrombin variant (20210 G to A) increases the risk of myocardial infarction in young women. Blood 1997; 90:1747-50.
57. Gardemann A, Arsic T, Katz N, et al. The factor II G20210A and factor V G1691A gene transitions and coronary heart disease. Thromb Haemost 1999; 81: 208-13.
58. Ridker PM, Hennekens CH, Miletich JP. G20210A mutation in prothrombin gene and risk of myocardial infarction, stroke , and venous thrombosis in a large cohort of US men. Circulation 1999; 99: 999-1004.

59. Andreotti F, Burzotta F, De Stefano V, et al. The G20210A prothrombin mutation and the Physician's Health Study. Ciculation 2000; 101: 207-8.
60. Russo C, Girelli D, Olivieri O, et al. The G20210A prothrombin gene polymorphism and prothrombin activity in subjects with or without angiographically documented coronary artery disease. Circulation 2001, in press.
61. Esmon CT. Protein C: biochemistry, physyology, and clinical implications. Blood 1983; 62:1155-8.
62. Cripe LD, Moore KD, Kane WH. Structure of the gene for human coagulation factor V. Biochemistry 1992; 31:3777-85.
63. Bertina RM, Koeleman BPC, Koster T, Rosendaal FR, Dirven RJ, de Ronde H, van der Velden PA, Reitsma PH: Mutation in blood coagulation factor V associated with resistance to activated protein C. Nature 1994; 369:64.
64. Svensson PJ, Dahlbäck B: Resistance to activated protein C as a basis for vcnous thrombosis. N Engl J Med 1994; 330:517.
65. Nicolaes GAF, Tans G, Thomassen MCLGD, et al. Peptide bond cleavages and loss of functional activity during inactivation of factor Va and factor Va R506Q by activated protein C. J Biol Chem. 1995; 270:158.
66. Rosing J, Hoekema L, Nicolaes GAF, et al. Effects of protein S and factor Xa on peptide bond cleavages during inactivation of factor Va and factor Va R506Q by activated protein C. J Biol Chem. 1995; 270:852.
67. Zivelin A, Griffin JH, Xu X, et al. A single genetic origin for a common Caucasian risk factor for venous thrombosis. Blood. 1997; 89:397.
68. Ridker PM, Hennekens CH, Lindpaintner K, Stampfer MJ, Eisenberg PR, Miletich JP. Mutation in the gene coding for coagulation factor V and the risk of myocardial infarction. N Engl J Med. 1995; 332:912.
69. Ferraresi P, Marchetti G, Legnani C, et al. The heterozygous 20210 G/A prothrombin genotype is associated with early venous thrombophilias and is not increased in frequency in arterial disease. Arterioscler Thromb Vasc Biol. 1997; 17:2418.
70. Emmerich J, Poirier O, Evans A, et al. Myocardial infarction, Arg 506 to Gln factor V mutation, and activated protein C resistance. Lancet. 1995; 345:321.
71. Ardissino D, Peyvandi F, Merlini PA, Colombi E, Mannucci PM. Factor V (Arg506 to Gln) mutation in young survivors of myocardial infarction. Thromb Haemost. 1996; 75:701.
72. Cushman M, Rosendaal FR, Psaty BM, et al. Factor V Leiden is not a risk factor for arterial vascular disease in the elderly: results from the Cardiovascular Health Study. Thromb Haemost. 1998; 79:912.
73. Catto A, Carter A, Ireland H, et al. Factor V Leiden gene mutation and thrombin generation in relation to acute stroke. Arterioscler Thromb Vasc Biol. 1995; 15:783.
74. Longstreth WT, Rosendaal FR, Siscovick DS, et al. Risk of stroke in young women and two prothrombotic mutations: factor V Leiden and prothrombin gene variant (G20210A). Stroke. 1998; 29:577.
75. de Visser MCH, Rosendaal FR, Bertina RM. A reduced sensitivity for activated protein C in the absence of factor V Leiden increases the risk of venous thrombosis. Blood 1999;93:1271-6.
76. Cumming AM, Tait RC, Fildes S, Yoong A, Keeney S, Hay CRM: Development of resistance to activated protein C during pregnancy. Br J Haematol 1995; 90:725.
77. Olivieri O, Friso S, Manzato F, Guella A, Bernardi F, Lunghi B, Girelli D, Azzini M, Brocco G, Russo C, Corrocher R: Resistance to activated protein C in healthy women taking oral contraceptives. Br J Haematol 1995; 91:465.
78. Ehrenforth S, Radtke KP, Scharrer I: Acquired activated protein C-resistance in patients with lupus anticoagulants. Thromb Haemost 1995; 74:797.
79. Henkens CMA, Bom VJJ, van der Meer J: Lowered APC-sensitivity ratio related to increased factor VIII-clotting activity. Thromb Haemost 1995; 74:1198.
80. Laffan MA, Manning R: The influence of factor VIII on measurement of activated protein C resistance. Blood Coagul Fibrinolysis 1996; 7:761.

81. Kiechl S, Muigg A, Santer P, et al. Poor response to activated protein C as a prominent risk predictor of advanced arterial disease. Circulation. 1999; 99:614.
82. Lunghi B, Iacoviello L, Gemmati D, Dilasio MG, Castoldi E, Pinotti M, Castaman G, Redaelli R, Mariani G, Marchetti G, Bernardi F. Detection of new polymorphic markers in the factor V gene: association with factor V levels in plasma. Thromb Haemost 1996; 75:45-48.
83. Faioni EM. Factor V HR2: an ancient haplotype out of Africa. Reasons for being interested. Thromb Haemost 2000; 83: 358-359.
84. Bernardi F, Faioni E, Castoldi E, Lunghi B, Castaman G, Sacchi E, Mannucci PM. A factor V genetic component differing from factor V R506Q contributes to the activated protein C resistance phenotype. Blood 1997; 90: 1552-7.
85. Rosing J, Bakker HM, Thomassen M, Hemker HC, Tans G. Characterization of two forms of human factor Va with different cofactor activities. J Biol Chem 1993; 268:21130-6.
86. Castoldi E, Rosing J, Girelli D, Hoekema L, Lunghi B, Mingozzi F, Ferraresi P, Friso S, Corrocher R, Tans G, Bernardi F. Mutations in the R2 FV gene affect the ratio between the two FV isoforms in plasma. Thrombosis and Haemostasis 2000; 83:362-5.
87. Hoekema L, Castoldi E, Tans G, Girelli D, Gemmati D, Bernardi F, Rosing J. Functional properties of factor V and factor Va encoded by the R2-gene. Thrombosis and Haemostasis 2001; 85:75-81.
88. Sprengers ED, Kluft C. Plasminogen activator inhibitors. Blood 1987; 69:381-7.
89. Kruithof EKO. Plasminogen activator inhibitors. A review. Enzyme 1988; 40:113-21.
90. Lupu F, Bergonzelli GE, Heim DA, et al. Localization and production of plasminogen activator inhibitor-1 in human healthy and atherosclerotic arteries. Arterioscler Thromb. 1993; 13:1090-100.
91. Sobel BE, Woodcock-Mitchell J, Schneider DJ, Holt RE, Marutsuka K, Gold H. Increased plasminogen activator inhibitor type 1 in coronary artery atherectomy specimens from type 2 diabetic compared with non-diabetic patients: a potential factor predisposing to thrombosis and its persistence. Circulation. 1998; 97:2213-21.
92. Hamsten A, de Faire U, Walldius G, et al. Plasminogen activator inhibitor in plasma: risk factor for recurrent myocardial infarction. Lancet 1987; 2:3-9.
93. Juhan-Vague I, Pyke SDM, Alessi MC, Jespersen J, Haverkate F, Thompson SG. Fibrinolytic factors and the risk of myocardial infarction or sudden death in patients with angina pectoris. Circulation 1996; 94:2057-63.
94. Margaglione M, Di Minno G, Grandone E, et al. Abnormally high circulation levels of tissue plasminogen activator and plasminogen activator inhibitor-1 in patients with a history of ischemic stroke. Arterioscler Thromb. 1994; 14:1741-5.
95. Thogersen AM, Jansson JH, Boman K, et al. High plasminogen activator inhibitor and tissue plasminogen activator levels in plasma precede a first acute myocardial infarction in both men and women: evidence for the fibrinolytic system as an independent primary risk factor. Circulation. 1998; 98:2241-7.
96. Juhan-Vague I, Alessi MC, Vague P. Increased plasma plasminogen activator inhibitor 1 levels: a possible link between insulin resistance and atherothrombosis. Diabetologia. 1991; 34:457-62.
97. Juhan-Vague I, Thompson SG, Jespersen J, on behalf of the ECAT Angina Pectoris Study Group I. Involvement of the hemostatic system in the insulin resistance syndrome: a study of 1,500 patients with angina pectoris. Arterioscler Thromb. 1993; 13:1865-73.
98. Henry M, Tregouet DA, Alessi MC, et al. Metabolic determinants are much more important than genetic polymorphisms in determining the PAI-1 activity and antigen plasma concentrations: a family study with part of the Stanislas Cohort. Arterioscler Thromb Vasc Biol. 1998; 18:84-91.
99. Strandberg L, Lawrence D, Ny T. The organization of the human-plasminogen-activator-inhibitor-1 gene: implications on the evolution of the serine-protease inhibitor family. Eur J Biochem 1988; 176:609-16.

100. Dawson SJ, Wiman B, Hamsten A, Green F, Humphries S, Henney AM. The two allele sequences of a common polymorphism in the promoter of the plasminogen activator inhibitor-1 (PAI-1) gene respond differently to interleukin-1 in HepG2 cells. J Biol Chem. 1993; 268:739-45.
101. Eriksson P, Kallin B, van 't Hooft FM, Bavenholm P, Hamsten A. Allele-specific increase in basal transcription of the plasminogen-activator inhibitor 1 gene is associated with myocardial infarction. Proc Natl Acad Sci U S A 1995; 92:1851-5.
102. Ossei-Gerning N, Mansfield MW, Stickland MH, Wilson IJ, Grant PJ. Plasminogen activator inhibitor-1 (PAI-1) promoter 4G/5G genotype and levels in relation to a history myocardial infarction in patients characterised by coronary angiography. Arterioscler Thromb Vasc Biol. 1997; 17:33-7.
103. Margaglione M, Cappucci G, Colaizzo D, et al. The PAI-1 gene locus 4G/5G polymorphism is associated with a family history of coronary artery disease. Arterioscler Thromb Vasc Biol 1998; 18:152-6.
104. Gardemann A, Lohre J, Katz N, Tillmanns H, Hehrlein FW, Haberbosch W. The 4G4G genotype of the plasminogen activator inhibitor 4G/5G gene polymorphism is associated with coronary atherosclerosis in patients at high risk for this disease. Thromb Haemost 1999; 82:1121-6.
105. Ye S, Green FR, Scarabin PY, et al. The 4G/5G genetic polymorphism in the promoter of the plasminogen activator inhibitor-1 (PAI-1) gene is associated with differences in plasma PAI-1 activity but not with risk of myocardial infarction in the ECTIM study. Thromb Haemost. 1995; 74:837-41.
106. Ridker PM, Hennekens CH, Lindpaintner K, Stampfer MJ, Miletich JP. Arterial and venous thrombosis is not associated with the 4G/5G polymorphism in the promoter of the plasminogen activator inhibitor gene in a large cohort of US men. Circulation. 1997; 95:59-62.
107. Doggen CJM, Bertina RM, Manger Cats V, Reitsma PH, Rosendaal FR. The 4G/5G polymorphism in the plasminogen activator inhibitor-1 gene is not associated with myocardial infarction. Thromb Haemost. 1999; 82:115-20.
108. Iacoviello L, Burzotta F, Di Castelnuovo A, Zito F, Marchioli R, Donati MB. The 4G/5G polymorphism of PAI-1 promoter gene and the risk of myocardial infarction: a meta-analysis. Thromb Haemost. 1998; 80:1029-30.
109. Eriksson P, Nilsson L, Karpe F, Hamsten A. Very-low-density lipoprotein response element in the promoter region of the human plasminogen activator inhibitor-1 gene implicated in the impaired fibrinolysis of hypertriglyceridemia. Arterioscler Thromb Vasc Biol 1998;18:20-6.
110. Sironi L, Mussoni L, Prati L, et al. Plasminogen activator inhibitor type-1 synthesis and mRNA expression in HepG2 cells are regulated by VLDL. Arterioscler Thromb Vasc Biol 1996; 16:89-96.
111. Ichinose A. The physiology and biochemistry of factor XIII. In: Bloom AL,Forbes CD,Thomas DP,Tuddenham EGD, eds. Haemostasis and Thrombosis. 3rd ed. Edinburgh: Churchill Livingstone; 1994:53.
112. Kohler HP, Stickland MH, Ossei-Gerning N, Carter A, Mikkola H, Grant PJ. Association of a common polymorphism in the factor XIII gene with myocardial infarction. Thromb Haemost 1998; 79:8-13.
113. Wartiovaara U, Perola M, Mikkola H, et al. Association of FXIII Val34Leu with decreased risk of myocardial infarction in Finnish males. Atherosclerosis 1999; 142:295-300.
114. Kohler HP, Mansfield MW, Clark PS, Grant PJ. Interaction between insulin resistance and factor XIIII Val34Leu in patients with coronary heart disease. Thromb Haemost.1999; 82:1202-3.
115. Peerschke EIB, Lopez JA. Platelet membranes and receptors. In: Loscalzo J,Schafer AI, eds. Thrombosis and Hemorrhage. 2nd ed. Baltimore: Williams & Wilkins; 1998:229.
116. Ruggeri ZM. New insights into the mechanisms of platelet adhesion and aggregation. Semin Hematol. 1994; 31:229-39.

117. Newman PJ. Platelet alloantigens: cardiovascular as well as immunological risk factors. Lancet. 1997; 349:370-1.
118. Goodall AH, Curzen N, Panesar M, et al. Increased binding of fibrinogen to glycoprotein IIIa-proline33 (HPA-1b, Pla2, Zwb) positive platelets in patients with cardiovascular disease. Eur Heart J 1999; 20:742-7.
119. Feng DL, Lindpaintner K, Larson MG, et al. Increased platelet aggregability associated with platelet GPIIIa Pla2 polymorphism. The Framingham Offspring study. Arterioscler Thromb Vasc Biol 1999; 19:1142-7.
120. Weiss EJ, Bray PF, Tayback M, et al. A polymorphism of a platelet glycoprotein receptor as an inherited risk factor for coronary thrombosis. N Engl J Med. 1996; 334:1090-4.
121. Zotz RB, Winkelmann BR, Nauck M, et al. Polymorphism of platelet membrane glycoprotein IIIa: human platelet antigen Ib (HPA-Ib/PlA2) is an inherited risk factor for premature myocardial infarction in coronary artery disease. Thromb Haemost. 1998; 79:731-5.
122. Ardissino D, Mannucci PM, Merlini PA, et al. Prothrombotic genetic risk factors in young survivors of myocardial infarction. Blood. 1999; 94:46-51.
123. Ridker PM, Hennekens CH, Schmitz C, Stampfer MJ, Lindpaintner K. PlA1/A2 polymorphism of platelet glycoprotein IIIa and risks of myocardial infarction, stroke and venous thrombosis. Lancet. 1997; 349:385-8.
124. Herrmann SM, Poirier O, Marques-Vidal P, et al. The Leu 33/Pro polymorphism (PlA1/PlA2) of the glycoprotein IIIa (GPIIIa) receptor is not related to myocardial infarction in the ECTIM Study. Thomb Haemost. 1997; 77:1179-81.
125. Carter AM, Ossei-Gerning N, Wilson IJ, Grant PJ. Association of the platelet Pl(A) polymorphism of glycoprotein IIb/IIIa and the fibrinogen Bb448 polymorphism with myocardial infarction and extent of coronary artery disease. Circulation. 1997; 96:1424-31.
126. Durante-Mangoni E, Davies GJ, Ahmed N, Ruggiero G, Tuddenham EG. Coronary thrombosis and the platelet glycoprotein IIIA gene PlA2 polymorphism. Thromb Haemost. 1998; 80:218-9.
127. Walter DH, Schachinger V, Elsner M, Dimmeler S, Zeiher AM. Platelet glycoprotein IIIa polymorphisms and risk of coronary stent thrombosis. Lancet. 1997; 350:1217-9.
128. Mamotte CD, van Bockxmeer FM, Taylor RR. PlA1/A2 polymorphism of glycoprotein IIIa and risk of coronary artery disease and restenosis following coronary angioplasty. Am J Cardiol. 1998; 82:13-6.
129. Andrews RK, Shen Y, Gardiner EE, Dong JF, Lopez JA, Berndt MC. The glycoprotein Ib-IX-V complex in platelet adhesion and signaling. Thromb Haemost. 1999; 82:357-64.
130. Gonzalez-Conejero R, Lozano ML, Rivera J, et al. Polymorphisms of platelet membrane glycoprotein Iba associated with arterial thrombotic disease. Blood. 1998; 92:2771-6.
131. Moroi M, Jung SM, Okuma M, Shinmyozu K. A patient with platelets deficient in glycoprotein VI that lack both collagen-induced aggregation and adhesion. J Clin Invest. 1989; 84:1440-5.
132. Nieuwenhuis HK, Akkerman JWN, Houdijk WPM, Sixma JJ. Human blood platelets showing no response to collagen fail to express surface glycoprotein Ia. Nature. 1985; 318:470-2.
133. Kunicki TJ, Orchekowski R, Annis D, Honda Y. Variability of integrin a2 b1 activity on human platelets. Blood. 1993; 82:2693-703.
134. Santoso S, Kunicki TJ, Kroll H, Haberbosch W, Gardemann A. Association of the platelet glycoprotein Ia C807T gene polymorphism with nonfatal myocardial infarction in younger patients. Blood. 1999; 93:2449.
135. Croft SA, Hampton KK, Sorrell JA, et al. The GpIa C807T dimorphism associated with platelet collagen receptor density is not a risk factor for myocardial infarction. Br J Haematol. 1999; 106:771.

8. THE PHARMACOGENETICS OF ATHEROSCLEROSIS

J.W. Jukema, W.R.P. Agema

Introduction

Atherosclerosis is the pathophysiological basis of the majority of morbidity and mortality in Western societies. In recent years progression has been made in unraveling the basis of atherosclerosis. Presently, atherosclerosis is considered to have a complex pathophysiology.in which inflammation is most important [1]. Advances also have been made in both primary and secondary prevention of complications of atherosclerosis like myocardial infarction and ischemic cerebrovascular disease. New treatment strategies, incorporating cholesterol lowering therapy, improve survival with increasing financial costs.

Treatment of individuals with cholesterol lowering therapy like 3-hydroxy-3-methyl-glutaryl coenzyme A reductase inhibitors has been shown to effectively reduce coronary events and even reduce the progression of atherosclerosis [2]. However, it remains questionable if all individuals have the same benefit of this medication. Actually, it is very likely that considerable differences between individuals exist in both the effectiveness and the tolerance of chemical interventions.

The contribution of genetic factors to coronary artery disease (CAD) is well illustrated by twin studies. In a study of monogenetic and dizygotic twins, death from CAD at an early age of one twin was a strong predictor of the risk in the other twin. The fact that this risk was greatest in monozygotic compared to dizygotic twins indicates a strong contribution of genes to CAD [3]. The genes that contribute to this common disease are without doubt many and they code for proteins involved in multiple metabolic pathways. Such genes include those controlling lipoprotein metabolism, vascular tone and reactivity, macrophage structure and function, and haemostatic as well as fibrinolytic pathways. The clinical impact of gene polymorphisms in the development of atherosclerosis has been discussed in chapters 4, 5 and 6. It is now clear that much individuality in drug response is also inherited: this genetically determined variance in drug response defines the research area known as pharmacogenetics. In this chapter further clarification of the field of pharmacogenetics focused on atherosclerosis is provided. Furthermore, genetic markers and their relevance to clinical practice are discussed.

PA Doevendans and AA Wilde (eds.), Cardiovascular genetics, 89-100.

Pharmacogenetics: tailored therapy to fit individual profiles

With the Human Genome Project nearing completion genetic association studies are stimulated enormously. The purpose of genetic association studies is to investigate the relation of genetic variations or polymorphisms with disease or environment. Ecogenetics embodies the study of gene-environment interactions in the broadest sense. These environmental factors include amongst others food, chemicals, radiation, smoking and drugs. For example, studies in humans demonstrate dietary hypo- and hyperresponders [4] and the presence of individuals at increased risk of CAD from tobacco smoke due to underlying mutations in the nitric oxide synthase gene [5]. More specific, the study of inheritable responses to pharmaceutical agents is known as pharmacogenetics [6]. The position of pharmacogenetics in the field of genetic testing in general is illustrated in figure 1.

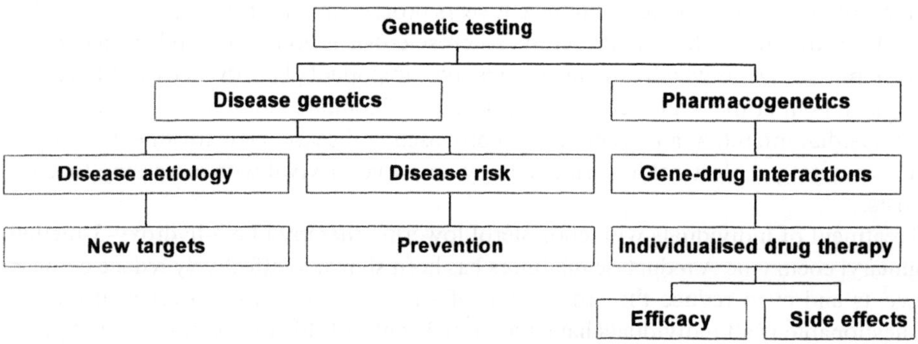

***Figure 1**. The position of pharmacogenetics in the field of genetic testing*

Pharmaceutical treatment in the individual might be either beneficial, have no effect at all or result in toxicity or adverse drug reactions. The first would be the desired effect. Identification of individuals in the second group, the non-responders, would facilitate both a reduction of the costs and of the number of individuals at risk of toxicity. Furthermore, identification of persons at increased risk of adverse reactions to a specific drug or treatment would enable the physician to reduce costs, morbidity and perhaps even mortality due to toxicity. Patterns of genetic markers or polymorphisms are highly individual and thus provide the theoretical possibility to make this distinction.

Genetic markers used in practice most often are single nucleotide polymorphisms (SNPs), variants of a single nucleotide in DNA. SNPs are frequent throughout the genome. It is estimated that there is about one SNP in every 1000 base pairs. These SNPs occur in the coding region (coding region SNP or cSNP), in noncoding regions in or in the immediate vicinity of the gene (perigenic SNP or pSNP) and between the genes (intergenic SNP or iSNP) [6]. Individuals that carry a particular allele of a gene are likely to carry specific variants of several SNP markers, which are not necessarily located in the coding region of the gene. Actually, these SNP markers are close to that allele because of linkage desequilibrium. Linkage desequilibrium is present if certain polymorphisms occur together more frequently than might be expected by chance alone. This suggests that the combination of these polymorphisms is inherited together. Therefore, the association of a certain SNP with disease does not necessarily implicate an association with its mechanism [7]. On the other hand, a marker for disease might still be useful and further study of linked alleles might indicate the key functional mutation.

Although insight in disease mechanisms requires the detection of the actual mutation responsible for the difference in protein levels, this might not be necessary in pharmacogenetics. As long as it is possible to identify individuals with a specific, positive or negative, response to medication the goal of pharmacogenetics can be achieved. On the other hand, a theoretical pathophysiologic link would provide the explanation for gene-environment interactions. In other words, to predict the response of an individual to medication the pattern of SNP markers might suffice [7;8].

Prediction of tolerance by gene polymorphisms

Identifying genetic variants associated with adverse drug reactions is potentially useful. Polymorphisms of genes encoding drug receptors, drug transporters and signaling pathways can determine the clinical response to specific drugs. For example, certain polymorphisms involved in drug metabolizing enzymes (DME) determine the half-life of a number of known drug substrates (see table 1). It is notable that the effects of these polymorphisms are under substantial ethnic influence.

Thiopurine methyltransferase

The enzyme thiopurine methyltransferase (TPMT) is involved in the breakdown of certain antitumor agents used in childhood leukemia. An inherited deficiency of this enzyme results in higher serum levels of the chemotherapeutic agent 6-mercaptopurine and thus increases toxicity, especially on the haematopoeietic system [9-12]. In other individuals, a certain polymorphism at this gene locus is associated with difficulty in achieving an effective dose of these drugs. Although the TPMT polymorphism is exceedingly rare (1% of the white population is homozygous carrier) the importance of the phenotype of TPMT deficiency has persuaded some centers to provide diagnostic services.

The cytochrome P450

An example, which is important for cardiovascular medicine, are mutations encoding the gene for cytochrome P450. The cytochrome P450 system includes a number of enzymes involved in the metabolic elimination of drugs used in medicine today, such those used for treating psychiatric, neurological and cardiovascular diseases. Amiodarone, propafenone, flecainide, propanolol, timolol and mexiletine are examples of drugs used in cardiovascular medicine that are substrates of the cytochrome P450 CYP2D6 system [13;14]. CYP2D6 is highly polymorphic and is inactive in about 6% of white people. Furthermore, some individuals inherit up to 13 copies of the gene. Affected people have

Table1

Table 1

Common pharmacogenetics in human drug metabolizing enzymes

Gene	Phenotype	Frequency in different ethnic groups	Known drug substrates: Total No of drugs	Known drug substrates: Examples
Thiopurine Methyltransferase (S-methylation)	Poor metaboliser	Low in all populations	<10	6-Mercaptopurine, 6-thioguanine, azathioprine
Cytochrome P450 (drug oxidation):				
CYP2D6	Poor metaboliser	White 6%, African American 2%, Oriental 1%	>100	Codeine, nortryptiline, dextromethorphan
	Ultra-rapid metaboliser	Ethiopian 20%, Spanish 7%, Scandinavian 1.5%		
CYP2C9	Reduced activity		>60	Tolbutamide, diazepam, ibuprofen, warfarin
CYP2C19	Poor metaboliser	Oriental 23%, white 4%	>50	Mephenytoin, omeprazole, proguanil, citalopram
N-Acetyl Transferase	Poor metaboliser	White 60%, African American 60%, oriental 20%, Inuit 5%	>15	Isoniazid, procainamide, sulphonamides, hydralazines

(Adapted from Weber, W.W. Pharmacogenetics. Oxford: Oxford University Press, 1997)

a more active drug metabolism so that therapeutic effects cannot be obtained with conventional doses of the prescribed drugs. On the other hand, simultaneously administered drugs inhibiting or competing at the CYP2D6 may render the metabolism non-active. These individuals would turn out to be poor metabolisers and thus are at an increased risk for drug toxicity.

Prediction of efficacy in the treatment of atherosclerosis

Identifying genetic variants associated with drug efficacy can provide simple improvements in patient care. Polymorphisms of genes encoding enzymes involved in the metabolism of lipids can influence the clinical response to cholesterol lowering therapy. For example, certain polymorphisms in the lipoprotein lipase (LPL) gene and the cholesterylesther transfer protein (CETP) gene have been implicated to effect efficacy of statin therapy, as clarified below. However, another example, that of the angiotensin converting enzyme (ACE) insertion/deletion polymorphism, demonstrates the potential fallacy of methodological shortcomings.

Lipoprotein lipase

In most people, plasma triglycerides are in dynamic equilibrium, mediated by a balance between very low-density lipoprotein and chylomicron synthesis, lipolysis of triglyceride (TG)-rich lipoproteins, and by uptake of remnant particles through appropriate receptors. However, with abnormalities involving synthesis, lipolysis, or remnant uptake, hypertriglyceridemia may ensue. LPL is a multifunctional protein. After synthesis in parenchymal cells, primarily in adipose tissue and skeletal muscle, LPL is transported to the intimal surface of the vascular endothelium where it is anchored by the heparin sulfate side chains of membrane proteoglycans. LPL plays a pivotal role in the hydrolysis of lipoprotein triacylglycerols to monoacylglycerols and fatty acids. The enzyme has also been shown to have other important functions where it acts as a ligand for the LDL receptor related protein and influences the secretion and uptake of LDL-cholesterol.

It is possible that mutations of the gene encoding LPL might underlie mild-to-moderate hypertriglyceridemia, but that their phenotype will not be recognized until other environmental or genetic factors are present. We have shown that a mutation in the human LPL gene, Asn291Ser, which results in a partial deficiency of lipolytic activity, is present with increased frequency in patients with angiographically proven premature CAD where it is associated with significantly decreased HDL cholesterol and increased TG levels [15]. An other common mutation in the LPL gene, a C-to-G substitution, results in a truncation of the C-terminal and of the LPL protein by two amino acids (Ser447stop). The presence of the Ser447stop mutation was significantly increased in those in the highest quartile of HDL cholesterol in REGRESS, pointing towards a positive association of this premature stop codon with elevated levels of HDL cholesterol and thus subsequently with protection against the development of CAD [16]. A recent meta-analysis of Wittrup and colleagues of the impact of lipoprotein lipase mutations on risk of CAD underscores the above-described observations [17].

In individuals with combined hyperlipidemia and CAD, another mutation, i.e. an aspartic acid to an asparagine residue at position 9 (Asp9Asn) in the mature LPL protein was also identified. This mutation, too, was accompanied by high-TG/low-HDL cholesterol phenotype [18]. In addition, we investigated whether the presence of this Asp9Asn mutation could confer increased susceptibility to atherosclerosis and therefore be associated with more progression of CAD. The mutation was identified in 4,8% of the patients who participated in the lipid-lowering angiographic clinical study REGRESS [2;19]. Carriers of this Asp9Asn mutation more frequently had a positive family history of CAD and exhibited lower HDL cholesterol levels than non-carriers. Indeed, it could be shown that these patients - with only subtle disturbances of lipoprotein metabolism due to the presence of this mutation - exhibited accelerated progression of coronary atherosclerosis and a diminished clinical event-free survival [19]. Also of specific interest was the observation that the carriers of this mutation seemed particularly sensitive to pravastatin therapy, in that on average progression was abolished in this group.

Cholesterylesther transfer protein

In another exemplary study from the REGRESS trial, we could demonstrate that variation in the CETP gene is associated with changes in CETP activity and changes in lipid and lipoprotein activity [20]. In the placebo arm of this lipid-lowering regression trial it became obvious that homozygosity for a certain genotype (B1,B1) was associated with the highest CETP protein mass and activity and consequently with the lowest HDL cholesterol. In addition, this high activity CETP genotype led to a faster rate of progression of CAD in this particular patient group. The notion that high CETP activity, particularly when genetically determined, confers a high risk for the development of atherosclerosis was recently confirmed by the Framingham Offspring Study (FOS) research group [21]. In the FOS cohort, an affluent Caucasian population, B1,B1 CETP genotype was again associated with low HDL cholesterol and a higher incidence of CAD. The associations, both in CAD and in the general population, suggest that variation at the CETP gene influences the risk for premature CAD, at least in Caucasians living in a affluent society.

Far more important, in the pravastatin arm of the REGRESS trial a different picture emerged. Patients carrying the B1,B1 genotype reacted most favorably to statin therapy when compared to their counterparts with the B2,B2 genotype. This pharmacogenomic observation led to the concept that lowering CETP activity that is already low, i.e. in the case of a B2,B2 genotype, is possibly undesirable and does not lead to regression of coronary atherosclerosis. This notion was strengthened by the observation that pravastatin influenced lipids and lipoproteins to a similar extent in all CETP genotypes and decreased CETP mass activity by approximately 20% in all REGRESS patients [20]. If these data were confirmed in trials with clinical endpoints, CETP genotyping could become an important decision point in the prescription of statins. Variations in genes encoding microsomal triglyceride transfer protein , lecithin:cholesterol acyltransferase , hepatic lipase , and LPL are currently studied to enable extension of these pharmacogenomic observations in those patients eligible for statin therapy.

Angiotensin Converting Enzyme insertion/deletion polymorphism
ACE is the regulating enzyme in the formation of angiotensin II. This protein has numerous effects in vivo. Inhibitors of ACE have been shown to effectively lower blood pressure and improve prognosis in heart failure patients. Furthermore, certain ACE inhibitors seem to have an anti-atherosclerotic effect.

It is not surprising that a polymorphism of the gene encoding ACE has been implicated to affect a number of different phenotypes, which in clinical practice are being treated with ACE inhibitors. In 1992 Cambien et al. reported on an AluI insertion/deletion in intron 16 of the DCP1 or ACE gene [22]. In this polymorphism a fragment of 287 base pair is either present or absent. The DD genotype emerged as a potent risk factor for myocardial infarction. Since than the DD genotype has been implicated as a risk factor for hypertension, ischemic cerebrovascular disease, multivessel coronary artery disease, left ventricular hypertrophy, elite athletic performance, response to physical training and restenosis after percutaneous coronary interventions, particularly after coronary stenting.

Recently, a meta-analysis of the ACE gene polymorphism in cardiovascular disease did not show any association of the DD genotype with myocardial infarction, ischemic heart disease or ischemic cerebrovascular disease [23]. However, the ACE gene did affect plasma ACE activity. Although it seems likely that an effect would be more evident in highly selected subgroups (e.g. young people) much doubt has been generated whether or not this polymorphism is the actual mutation or just a mere genetic marker in linkage desequilibrium with another mutation. In fact, recently Rieder et al. sequenced 24kb of the DCP1 gene in 11 individuals, identifying 78 varying sites in 22 chromosomes. It became evident that 17 variant sites were in absolute linkage desequilibrium with the AluI insertion/deletion polymorphism, implicating that each of these sites might be the actual pathophysiologically important mutation [24]. Thus, cautious interpretation of a phenotypic association with a single SNP is warranted.

Despite the wobbly theoretical basis pharmacogenetic studies have been undertaken to evaluate the efficacy of ACE inhibitors in prevention of in-stent restenosis after percutaneous coronary interventions. A Japanese, a Danish and an Italian study have been presented, in which there was diversity of the genotype exhibiting the highest risk of in-stent restenosis (II genotypes bearing the highest risk in Japanese, DD genotypes in Caucasians) and the efficacy of ACE inhibitors (not effective in Danish, effective in Italians) [25].

It is evident that the insertion/deletion polymorphism of the ACE gene at present is insufficiently well investigated to be used in clinical practice. However, since it has been the subject of such a vast amount of research important lessons can be deducted from its results. These lessons result in the guidelines provided below.

Future expectations

The above mentioned examples are only a few in the rapidly increasing number of candidate genes. Genes involved in different processes like vascular wall homeostasis, inflammation, haemostasis, smooth muscle cell proliferation, extracellular matrix homeostasis and many others will be evaluated in the future. Other interesting aspects of the lipid metabolism like paraoxonase polymorphisms will be part of future pharmacogenetic investigations.

Pharmacogenetics and current practice
What is the current position of pharmacogenetics in clinical practice? This question can be addressed from different viewpoints. Pharmacogenetics set up a blending of medicine and genetics with a twist of ethics and industrial interest. The way to handle current knowledge therefore depends on one's position.

The pharmaceutical industry's view
The current knowledge can be used to make clinical trials more effective. Knowledge of responders would make trials more effective thus increasing cost effectiveness. Identification of drug-sensitive genotypes in phase II studies would enable the design of a phase III study with responders only, thus allowing smaller trials and preventing non-responders to be exposed unnecessary to a risk of adverse drug reactions.
One step further, considering that rare adverse drug reactions frequently emerge after introduction of the medicine to the market, enhanced surveillance systems after market introduction might incorporate DNA storage of all individuals, who receive prescriptions of this newly introduced drug. This would quickly and reliably enable the identification of SNP marker profiles once a rare adverse drug reaction has been encountered [7;8;26].
At present, these stimulating ideas are only theory. Industry, regulatory authorities, and governments should explore the details. As long as the fear for genetic research in medical ethic committees and amongst politicians prevails above the insight that this approach both enhances safety and cost effectiveness, and thus the cost of healthcare, pharmacogenomic clinical trials are elusive.

The geneticist's view
Polymorphisms are frequent throughout the genome and occur in both coding and regulatory segments of a gene as in noncoding areas of which the significance is unknown (junk-DNA) [6]. Multiple single gene disorders have been identified in which a certain nucleotide variance is associated with a change in transcription of RNA, either quantitatively or qualitatively. This results in alternations in protein levels or structure leading to the disorder. In multifactorial or multigenetic disorders like atherosclerosis the impact of a single polymorphism might be small. However, the same rules of genetics should apply as outlined below. In some genetic association studies confusing results have been found, not in concurrence with accepted genetic theories. To overcome these drawbacks in genetic epidemiological research criteria have been suggested to be met in establishing useful links between genetic variations and diseases [27;28]. First, the change in the gene must cause a relevant alteration in the function or level of a gene product (which is always a protein). However, it is not always possible to measure protein levels, since some relevant proteins are only present in tissue and not in serum. Furthermore, effects of genetic variance in inhibitors of certain proteins are not necessarily reflected by serum protein levels. Second, the beneficial and harmful

phenotypes must have apparent clinical differences. Third, the hypothesis linking the genotype to disease must be physiological plausible. Fourth, the number of cases investigated in an individual study linking a genotype to disease must be sufficient to detect even small relative risks. These small differences may still be important since this is the case over a lifetime.
In practice it is not always possible to follow these guidelines. For example, following these criteria the study of the impact of the nitric oxide synthase gene in the development of atherosclerosis requires the measurement of nitric oxide (NO).[29] NO is immediately degraded and can not be measured. However, associations of a single polymorphism with a phenotype should always evoke caution, since linkage desequilibrium with other alleles might obfuscate the actual mechanism. In the near future haplotype analysis and SNP marker patterns in concert with the above mentioned guidelines will without doubt enable useful pharmacogenetic associations in clinical practice.

The clinician's view

Until now pharmacogenetics is merely a fascinating field of research. The examples presented above are exemplary studies, which need to be extended into clinical trials and to clear phenotypic endpoints like death, myocardial infarction or need for revascularisation [30]. A summary of the practical status of these gene polymorphisms is provided in table 2.
The clinician should be aware of the promises and above all the drawbacks of pharmacogenetic and genetic association studies in general. Regretfully, numerous reports of interesting observations evoke enthusiasm among physicians and their patients and relatives. At present, technology does not provide the capacity or the cost effectiveness to test complete patient populations. However, technological advances like high-throughput sequencing studies and the development of DNA-microarray analysis with computerized detection methods will soon facilitate the implementation of genome-wide SNP marker screening in clinical trials [31].
Furthermore, development of bioinformatics programs will allow combined marker analysis in patients who differ in their response to therapy, both in a positive and negative way.

The power of genetic techniques, enabling cloning of mammals, and possible implications in assurances demand strict guidelines for the use of genetic specimen and profound ethical consideration. Coding of databases and other safety features to warrant privacy to the individual are of paramount importance. Therefore, genetic studies are frequently hampered by difficult negotiations with ethical committees. The lack of an effective treatment is a frequent argument for limiting diagnostic and prognostic tests. However, disease susceptibility gene polymorphisms are much less discussed and certainly do not have the same impact. Moreover, restrictive regulations for genetic studies might inadvertently impede our ability to prescribe safe and effective medication. Therefore, clinicians should understand the importance to stress the necessity of pharmacogenetic research and use their influence in making laymen like politicians and perhaps ethic committees aware of its enormous potential.

Table 2

Practical use of pharmacogenetics and atherosclerosis treatment.

Enzyme	Polymorphism	Allele Frequency in Healthy Caucasians	Classification*	
			Atherosclerosis	Other diseases
Thiopurine Methyltransferase	TPMT-Low	<1%	D	A†
Cytochrome P450	CYP2D6	6%	D	A‡
	CYP2C9	6%	D	
	CYP2C19	4%	D	
N-Acetyl Transferase		60%	D	
Lipoprotein Lipase	Asn291Ser	1-7%	D	
	Asp9Asn	2-4%	D	
	Ser447stop	17-22%	D	
Cholesterylesther Transfer Protein	TaqIB (B1 allele)	59.4%	D	
Angiotensin Converting Enzyme	Deletion allele	52-61%	D	D

* See introduction for clarification. "A" denotes molecular diagnostics available and diagnosis relevant for treatment. "D" denotes polymorphism with implications for predisposition, but minor phenotypic consequences.
†To indentify children at increased risk of toxic responses to chemotherapeutics for childhood leukemia.
‡ To aid individual dose selection for drugs used to treat psychiatric illnesses.

References

1. Ross R. Atherosclerosis--an inflammatory disease. N.Engl.J.Med. 1999; 340:115-26.
2. Jukema JW, Bruschke AV, van Boven AJ et al. Effects of lipid lowering by pravastatin on progression and regression of coronary artery disease in symptomatic men with normal to moderately elevated serum cholesterol levels. The Regression Growth Evaluation Statin Study (REGRESS). Circulation 1995; 91:2528-40.
3. Marenberg ME, Risch N, Berkman LF, Floderus B, de Faire U. Genetic susceptibility to death from coronary heart disease in a study of twins. N.Engl.J.Med. 1994; 330:1041-6.
4. Katan MB, Beynen AC, de Vries JH, Nobels A. Existence of hypo- and hyperresponders to dietary cholesterol in man. Am.J.Epidemiol. 1986; 123:221-34.
5. Wang XL, Sim AS, Badenhop RF, McCredie RM, Wilcken DE. A smoking-dependent risk of coronary artery disease associated with a polymorphism of the endothelial nitric oxide synthase gene. Nat.Med. 1996; 2:41-5.
6. Nebert DW. Suggestions for the nomenclature of human alleles: relevance to ecogenetics, pharmacogenetics and molecular epidemiology. Pharmacogenetics 2000; 10:279-90.
7. Roses AD. Pharmacogenetics and future drug development and delivery. Lancet 2000; 355:1358-61.
8. Wilkins MR, Roses AD, Clifford CP. Pharmacogenetics and the treatment of cardiovascular disease. Heart 2000; 84:353-4.
9. McBride KL, Gilchrist GS, Smithson WA, Weinshilboum RM, Szumlanski CL. Severe 6-thioguanine-induced marrow aplasia in a child with acute lymphoblastic leukemia and inhibited thiopurine methyltransferase deficiency. J.Pediatr.Hematol.Oncol. 2000; 22:441-5.
10. McLeod HL, Pritchard SC, Githang'a J et al. Ethnic differences in thiopurine methyltransferase pharmacogenetics: evidence for allele specificity in Caucasian and Kenyan individuals. Pharmacogenetics 1999; 9:773-6.
11. McLeod HL, Coulthard S, Thomas AE et al. Analysis of thiopurine methyltransferase variant alleles in childhood acute lymphoblastic leukaemia. Br.J.Haematol. 1999; 105:696-700.
12. McLeod HL, Krynetski EY, Relling MV, Evans WE. Genetic polymorphism of thiopurine methyltransferase and its clinical relevance for childhood acute lymphoblastic leukemia. Leukemia 2000; 14:567-72.
13. Mikus G, Gross AS, Beckmann J, Hertrampf R, Gundert-Remy U, Eichelbaum M. The influence of the sparteine/debrisoquin phenotype on the disposition of flecainide. Clin.Pharmacol.Ther. 1989; 45:562-7.
14. Siddoway LA, Thompson KA, McAllister CB et al. Polymorphism of propafenone metabolism and disposition in man: clinical and pharmacokinetic consequences. Circulation 1987; 75:785-91.
15. Reymer PW, Gagne E, Groenemeyer BE et al. A lipoprotein lipase mutation (Asn291Ser) is associated with reduced HDL cholesterol levels in premature atherosclerosis. Nat.Genet. 1995; 10:28-34.
16. Groenemeijer BE, Hallman MD, Reymer PW et al. Genetic variant showing a positive interaction with beta-blocking agents with a beneficial influence on lipoprotein lipase activity, HDL cholesterol, and triglyceride levels in coronary artery disease patients. The Ser447-stop substitution in the lipoprotein lipase gene. REGRESS Study Group. Circulation 1997; 95:2628-35.
17. Wittrup HH, Tybjaerg-Hansen A, Nordestgaard BG. Lipoprotein lipase mutations, plasma lipids and lipoproteins, and risk of ischemic heart disease. A meta-analysis. Circulation 1999; 99:2901-7.
18. Mailly F, Tugrul Y, Reymer PW et al. A common variant in the gene for lipoprotein lipase (Asp9-->Asn). Functional implications and prevalence in normal and hyperlipidemic subjects. Arterioscler.Thromb.Vasc.Biol. 1995; 15:468-78.
19. Jukema JW, van Boven AJ, Groenemeijer B et al. The Asp9 Asn mutation in the lipoprotein lipase gene is associated with increased progression of coronary atherosclerosis. REGRESS

Study Group, Interuniversity Cardiology Institute, Utrecht, The Netherlands. Regression Growth Evaluation Statin Study. Circulation 1996; 94:1913-8.
20. Kuivenhoven JA, Jukema JW, Zwinderman AH et al. The role of a common variant of the cholesteryl ester transfer protein gene in the progression of coronary atherosclerosis. The Regression Growth Evaluation Statin Study Group. N.Engl.J.Med. 1998; 338:86-93.
21. Ordovas JM, Cupples LA, Corella D et al. Association of Cholesteryl Ester Transfer Protein-TaqIB Polymorphism With Variations in Lipoprotein Subclasses and Coronary Heart Disease Risk : The Framingham Study. Arteriosclerosis, Thrombosis, and Vascular Biology 2000; 20:1323-9.
22. Cambien F, Poirier O, Lecerf L et al. Deletion polymorphism in the gene for angiotensin-converting enzyme is a potent risk factor for myocardial infarction. Nature 1992; 359:641-4.
23. Agerholm-Larsen B, Nordestgaard BG, Tybjaerg-Hansen A. ACE gene polymorphism in cardiovascular disease: meta-analyses of small and large studies in whites. Arteriosclerosis, Thrombosis, and Vascular Biology 2000; 20:484-92.
24. Rieder MJ, Taylor SL, Clark AG, Nickerson DA. Sequence variation in the human angiotensin converting enzyme. Nat.Genet. 1999; 22:59-62.
25. Okamura A, Ohishi M, Rakugi H et al. Pharmacogenetic analysis of the effect of angiotensin-converting enzyme inhibitor on restenosis after percutaneous transluminal coronary angioplasty. Angiology 1999; 50:811-22.
26. Roses AD. Pharmacogenetics and the practice of medicine. Nature 2000; 405:857-65.
27. Lander E, Kruglyak L. Genetic dissection of complex traits: guidelines for interpreting and reporting linkage results. Nat Genet 1995; 11:241-7.
28. Rosenthal N, Schwartz RS. In search of perverse polymorphisms. N Engl J Med 1998; 338:122-4.
29. Wang XL, Mahaney MC, Sim AS et al. Genetic contribution of the endothelial constitutive nitric oxide synthase gene to plasma nitric oxide levels. Arterioscler.Thromb.Vasc.Biol. 1997; 17:3147-53.
30. Jukema JW. Matching treatment to the genetic basis of (lipid) disorder in patients with coronary artery disease. Heart 1999; 82:126-7.
31. Young RA. Biomedical discovery with DNA arrays. Cell 2000; 102:9-15.

9. MOLECULAR DIAGNOSIS OF THE MARFAN SYNDROME

P.N. Robinson

Introduction

The Marfan syndrome (MFS) is a pleiotropic disorder of connective tissue with highly variable clinical manifestations including aortic dilatation and dissection, ectopia lentis, and skeletal abnormalities such as scoliosis, pectus deformities, arachnodactyly and dolichostenomelia. The primary cause of death in MFS is aortic dissection or rupture as a consequence of progressive dilatation of the aortic root. The MFS is estimated to have a prevalence of 2-3 per 10,000 individuals, which makes it one of the most common hereditary disorders of connective tissue [1]. The average life expectancy of individuals with MFS has risen significantly since 1972 [2], which is due mainly to improved management of the cardiovascular complications, including beta-adrenergic blockade [3] routine imaging of the aorta, and prophylactic replacement of the aortic root before the diameter exceeds 5.5 to 6.0 cm [4].

Despite recent advances in molecular mutation screening, the diagnosis of MFS is still made primarily on clinical grounds. Diagnostic evaluation generally involves interpretation of ophthalmological and cardiological data in addition to a general examination. Clinical diagnosis of the MFS may be challenging, since not all affected individuals display a classic habitus, and the MFS should be regarded as a spectrum of diverse and highly variable manifestations in various organs; many of the physical findings associated with the MFS also are encountered in the general population or associated with other disorders of connective tissue.

In 1986, the so-called Berlin nosology [5] introduced the first widely accepted clinical criteria for the diagnosis of MFS, requiring involvement of the skeleton and at least two other organ systems to make the diagnosis in the index case, or involvement of at least two organ systems in the presence of at least one unequivocally affected first-degree relative. With the advent of molecular diagnosis, it became apparent that the criteria of the Berlin nosology for first-degree relatives of an individual with unequivocal MFS were not stringent enough, which had led to misdiagnosis of MFS in relatives with minor anomalies of connective tissue [6]. The Ghent nosology [7] attempted to addressthese difficulties by defining major criteria with high diagnostic specificity and minor criteria with less specificity; to make the diagnosis, a constellation of findings

PA Doevendans and AA Wilde (eds.), Cardiovascular genetics, 101-110.

including major criteria in two organ systems and the involvement of a third organ system are required. More stringent requirements for the diagnosis of MFS in relatives of an unequivocally affected index case were introduced, and molecular evidence was included. Presence of a mutation in the fibrillin gene (FBN1) known to cause MFS or the presence of a haplotype around FBN1 (i.e., a particular constellation of polymorphic markers in the region around FBN1) associated with unequivocally diagnosed MFS in the family represent a major criterion. Importantly, the inability to detect a FBN1 mutation does not exclude MFS (table 1).

Clinicians also need to be aware of the age-dependent nature of most of the manifestations of MFS; for instance, in one study the average age of initial diagnosis was 11 years for aortic root dilatation and 10 years for scoliosis [8]. This means that the absence of specific manifestations such as aortic root dilatation cannot be used to rule out the diagnosis of MFS in a child with other features suggestive of MFS.

Fibrillin-1

The MFS is caused by mutations in the gene for fibrillin-1. Fibrillin-1 is a large (~320 kDa), multidomain glycoprotein comprised mainly of cysteine-rich structural repeats, the most common of which is a module with homology to the epidermal growth factor precursor (EGF). In all, fibrillin contains 47 EGF modules, 43 of which contain a consensus sequence for calcium binding and are termed calcium-binding EGF repeats (cbEGF): Stretches of up to 12 cbEGF repeats form rigid, rod-like structures that are interrupted by other types of modules including seven with homology to a motif also found in the latent transforming growth factor β1 binding protein (LTBP), and another motif ("Fib") that may represent a fusion between the cbEGF and the LTBP motifs [9]. Fibrillin-1 is the main component of a class of 10-12nm extracellular microfibrils found in a wide range of tissues both in association with elastin as elastic fibers and as elastin-free bundles. The microfibrils display a "beads on a string" structure and consist of several distinct proteins in addition to fibrillin, and are thought to be important for elastogenesis, elasticity, and homeostasis of elastic fibers [10].

The pathogenesis of MFS was initially hypothesized to be due to a dominant negative effect, whereby mutant defective fibrillin-1 monomers interfere with the polymerization of fibrillin and the assembly of mature microfibrils [11]. More recent work has suggested that fibrillin defects may lead to impaired tissue homeostasis [12] and cause increased susceptibility of fibrillin to proteolysis [13, 14].

FBN1 mutations in Marfan syndrome and other type-1 fibrillinopathies

At present, approximately 200 *FBN1* mutations have been published, most of which have been unique to one affected individual or family. An internet-based database for *FBN1* mutations [15] offers a summary of mutations and associated clinical features (http://www.umd.necker.fr). Mutations have been found in all regions of the gene, although there is a significant clustering of mutations in exons 24-32 [16].

Skeletal System
Major criterion: Presence of at least four of the following manifestations: 1) Pectus carinatum, 2) pectus excavatum requiring surgery, 3) reduced upper to lower segment ratio or increased arm-span to height ratio (>1.05), 4) positive wrist and thumb signs, 5) scoliosis (>20°) or spondylolithesis, 6) reduced extension of elbows (<170°), 7) medial displacement of medial malleolus causing pes planus, 8) protrusio acetabulae of any degree (ascertained on x-ray)
Minor criteria: 1) Pectus excavatum of moderate severity, 2) joint hypermobility, 3) highly arched palate with dental crowding, 4) Characteristic facial appearance (dolichocephaly, malar hypoplasia, enophthalmos, retrognathia, down-slanting palpebral fissures)
Involvement of the skeletal system: presence of at least two of the components comprising the major criterion, or one component of the major criterion plus two of the minor criteria
Ocular System
Major criterion: Bilateral Ectopia lentis
Minor criteria: 1) Abnormally flat cornea (as measured by keratometry), 2) increased axial length of globe (as measured by ultrasound), 3) hypoplastic iris or hypoplastic ciliary muscle causing a decreased miosis
Involvement of the ocular system: presence of at least two of the minor criteria
Cardiovascular System
Major criteria: 1) Dilatation of the ascending aorta with or without aortic regurgitation and involving at least the sinuses of Valsalva 2) dissection of the ascending aorta
Minor criteria: 1) Mitral valve prolapse with or without mitral valve regurgitation, 2) dilatation of main pulmonary artery, in absence of valvular or peripheral pulmonic stenosis or any other obvious cause, below the age of 40 years, 3) calcification of the mitral annulus below the age of 40 years, 4) dilatation or dissection of the descending thoracic or abdominal aorta below the age of 50 years
Involvement of the cardiovascular system: presence of at least one of the minor criteria
Pulmonary System
Major criteria: none
Minor criteria: 1) Spontaneous pneumothorax, 2) apical blebs (ascertained by chest radiography)
Involvement of the pulmonary system: presence of at least one minor criterion
Skin and Integument
Major criterion: Lumbosacral dural ectasia by CT or MRI
Minor criteria: 1) Striae atrophicae (stretch marks) not associated with marked weight changes, pregnancy or repetitive stress, 2) recurrent or incisional herniae
Involvement of the integumentary system: presence of at least one minor criterion
Family History
Major criteria: 1) Having a parent, child, or sibling who meets the diagnostic criteria listed below independently, 2) Presence of a mutation in *FBN1* known to cause the Marfan syndrome, 3) Presence of a haplotype around *FBN1*, inherited by descent, known to be associated with unequivocally diagnosed Marfan syndrome in the family
Minor criteria: none
For the family history to be contributory, one of the major criteria must be present

Table 1. "Ghent" Diagnostic Criteria for MFS. *For the index case, major criteria must be present in at least two different organ systems, and a third organ system must be involved as defined in the table. The diagnosis can be made in a family member if a major criterion is present in one organ system, a second organ system is involved, and if the family history is positive for a major criterion.*

The majority of mutations represent missense mutations, most of which affect cbEGF modules dispersed throughout the gene. Premature truncation codon (PTC) mutations and mutations at the transition between introns and exons, affecting splice consensus sequences are also relatively common [15].

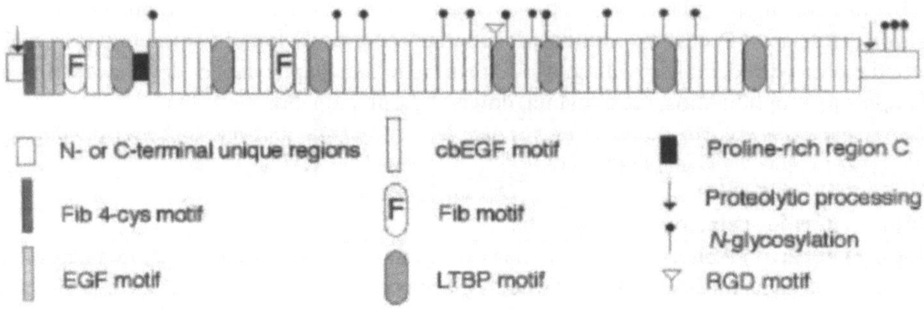

Figure 1. Domain structure of fibrillin-1

In addition to mutations found in individuals with classic MFS syndrome, *FBN1* mutations have been identified in a series of related disorders of connective tissue, termed type-1 fibrillinopathies [17]. The neonatal MFS (nMFS) represents the severest end of the Marfan clinical spectrum, and affected patients generally die in the first year of life. nMFS is characterized by a series of manifestations not found in classic MFS, including joint contractures, crumpled ears, and congestive heart failure due to mitral and tricuspid valve insufficiency in the first year or months of life. Mutations in nMFS cluster in exons 24-32 [18].

Patients carrying exon-skipping mutations tend to have severe phenotypes [19]. Additionally, point mutations associated with atypically severe phenotypes cluster in exons 24-32 [16]. Still other mutations in exons 24-32 have been associated with classic MFS, and at present there is no way of predicting which phenotype a novel mutation in these exons will be associated with [16].

The mild end of the clinical spectrum is represented by phenotypes lacking aortic dilatation and dissection. Since the identification of a *FBN1* mutation in a family with isolated ectopia lentis [20], a series of mutations in individuals with phenotypes characterized by various combinations of mainly ocular and skeletal abnormalities has been found, and such mutations have been shown to cluster in exons 59-65 [21].

In one study, a PTC mutation associated with an expression level of the mutant allele of 6% was identified in a patient with a clinically mild fibrillinopathy termed the MASS phenotype (Myopia, mitral valve prolapse, aortic root dilatation without dissection, skin abnormalities (striae) and skeletal involvement). In contrast, another patient with a somewhat higher level of mutant transcript (16%) had classic MFS. The authors postulated on the basis of these observations that severely reduced expression of the mutant allele due to PTC mutations leads to a preponderance of normal fibrillin monomers in the microfibrillar aggregates. Below a certain threshold of expression, there is mild disease. If an expression threshold is crossed (between 6% and 16% of wild type levels), sufficient mutant, truncated peptide is present to disturb the microfibrillar structure or assembly to such an extent that more severe disease occurs [11]. Subsequently, however, patients with classic MFS were shown to carry PTC mutations with expression levels of 7% [22] and 2% [23,24]. Therefore, the exact relationship between mutant transcript expression and clinical disease remains to be determined.

No.	Syndrome	Clinical features	Mutations	Category; Ref
1.	Marfan syndrome	See text, section 1	See text, section 10	B, E [15]
2.	Neonatal MFS (nMFS)	Severe manifestations (see text). Death usually in the first year of life due to congestive heart failure.	"Hotspot" in ex 24-27 and 31-32	B Reviewed in [18]
3.	Atypically severe MFS	atypically severe manifestations including aortic dissection before the age of 16 years	Clustering in exons 24-32	B [16]
4.	Mild Marfan-like Phenotypes	MFS-like phenotypes lacking aortic dissection	Clustering in exons 59-65	C(res.) [21]
5.	Shprintzen-Goldberg syndrome	craniosynostosis and marfanoid habitus	C1223Y (ex 29)	C(res.) [26]
6.	Familial arachnodactyly	arachnodactyly, dolichostenomelia, no cardiovascular manifestations	R1170H (ex 28)	C(res.) [27]
7.	Ectopia lentis	Bilateral ectopia lentis, in some cases scoliosis, no cardiovascular manifestations	E2447K (Ex 59)	C(res.) [20]
8.	Ascending aortic aneurysm and dissection without classical MFS	Ascending aortic aneurysm and dissection, no ectopia lentis, no specific skeletal findings	1) G1127S (ex 27) 2) D1155N (ex 27) 3) P1837S (ex 44)	C(res.) [28, 29]
9.	MASS-Phenotype	Mitral valve prolapse, aortic root dilatation without dissection, skeletal and skin abnormalities	5317insTTCA (ex 41)	C(res.) [11]
10.	New variant of the MFS	Skeletal features of MFS with joint contractures and knee joint effusions. Ectopia lentis. no cardiovascular manifestations	R122C (ex 4) (2x)	C(res.) [30, 31]
11.	Isolated skeletal features	High stature, scoliosis, pectus excavatum, arachnodactyly	R2726W (ex 64)	C(res.) [32]

Table 2. Type 1 fibrillinopathies. *FBN1 mutations have been associated not only with classic MFS, but also with a wide range of related phenotypes, termed "type 1 fibrillinopathies." The reader is referred to the original publications for details. C(res.): For entries 4 to 11, insufficient data are available at the present time to judge the full extent of clinical variability associated with these mutations. Although the phenotypes described appeared to "breed true" within affected families, it is still imperative to perform a full clinical evaluation including echocardiographic monitoring in all individuals in whom a fibrillin-1 gene mutation is identified.*

In addition to the above, a series of reports on individuals or families with variant fibrillinopathies has been published (table 2). Although these reports give an impression of the spectrum of disease associated with *FBN1* mutations, in most cases it is not yet possible to identify the molecular causes of this variation. It should also be noted that there is a striking intrafamilial variability in classic MFS, suggesting that the allelic mutation is not the only determinant of clinical severity. The clinical status of relatives carrying an identical *FBN1* mutation can vary widely with respect to onset of disease, organ-system involvement, and severity. Affected adults may not be aware of their status before being diagnosed following identification of an *FBN1* mutation [25].

Fibrillin-2 Mutations and Congenital Contractural Arachnodactyly

The fibrillin-2 gene (*FBN2*) is located on chromosome 5q23-31 and is closely related to fibrillin-1 (figure 1). The two fibrillins are differentially expressed and are likely to have different functional roles [33]. Mutations in *FBN2* cause a related disorder of connective tissue called congenital contractural arachnodactyly (CCA) characterized by a marfanoid habitus, arachnodactyly, crumpled ears, and mild contractures in the elbows, knees, and hips. To date, all identified *FBN2* mutations have been located between exons 24 and 34, analogous to the region involved in nMFS [34].

Mutation detection in Marfan syndrome

For reasons that are still not completely understood, *FBN1* mutation analysis has identified mutations in only a minority of patients analyzed to date. Initial attempts with cDNA-based screening methods display a sensitivity of 10-25% [35, 36]. In 1995, the first report on exonwise screening of all 65 *FBN1* exons was published [37]; a detection rate of 78% in a group of nine patients was achieved. However, subsequent studies could not reproduce this rate in larger patient groups; for instance, only 17 probable disease-causing mutations were identified in a group of 60 unrelated patients (28%) [38]. This suggests that clinical overdiagnosis of MFS may contribute to the overall low detection rate. Other factors such as the size of the gene (200kb, 65 exons) may also be partially responsible for the overall low detection rate. Also, mutation detection strategies have employed PCR-based methods that are not suitable for the detection of certain classes of mutation such as large deletions, when primer sites are lost (false negative results). There has been only one published report on Southern blotting analysis of samples from 20 MFS patients [39], in which no abnormalities were detected. Future efforts at mutation detection may therefore need to reassess Southern blotting and to analyze regions of the gene such as the promoter that have not been investigated for mutations to date.

The question of genetic heterogeneity in MFS has not yet been convincingly answered. On the one hand, there is a cumulative lod score of >150 for linkage between *FBN1* and classic MFS [40]. On the other hand, linkage to a yet to be cloned locus on chromosome 3p24.2-p25 has been shown in a large family with a Marfan-like phenotype for whom linkage to the fibrillins had been excluded (category E) [41]. Although the proportion of mutations at *FBN1* and at other loci remains to be determined, it is likely that no more than 25% ofcases of genuine MFS will be due to mutations at loci other than *FBN1* [42].

Conclusions: the role of *FBN1* mutation analysis in clinical practice

Accurate diagnosis or exclusion of MFS has important clinical implications regarding prophylactic medication with long-term β-adrenergic blockade [43, 44], surgery, and lifestyle modifications, and a false-negative diagnosis may have significant consequences. Despite recent advances in molecular analysis, MFS remains a clinical diagnosis. Optimally, the diagnosis and care of affected patients will be coordinated by a generalist who can coordinate care from a variety of specialties as appropriate. The clinician responsible for determining the diagnosis must evaluate a range of findings including data from the ophthalmologist and cardiologist [1].

At present, genetic testing for MFS can only be regarded as an adjunct to clinical evaluation. The identification of an *FBN1* mutation does not necessarily imply the diagnosis of MFS, because *FBN1* mutations have been found in individuals or families with variant type-1 fibrillinopathies who do not satisfy the diagnostic criteria for MFS. On the other hand, failure to find an *FBN1* mutation does not rule out the diagnosis of MFS, because current mutation detection techniques are not capable of finding *FBN1* mutations in all patients with unequivocal clinical MFS. Although suggestive data have been presented with respect to genotype-phenotype correlations, it is probably too early to incorporate such information into clinical decision making.

Molecular diagnosis is useful if the *FBN1* mutation is known in an individual with MFS; then, testing can be easily performed on relatives to determine whether individuals have inherited the same genetic predisposition to develop MFS (category B). Linkage analysis using intragenic polymorphisms [6] is available for families with a sufficient number of affected individuals (see above). Because of the difficulties in mutation detection and the extensive allelic heterogeneity in MFS, the role of mutation detection in sporadic cases or in making the initial diagnosis in a family is minor at the present time (category C). However, as knowledge concerning the full mutation spectrum associated with MFS and related disorders accumulates, and as mutation detection techniques become more efficient and economical, mutation detection is likely to become more important in the evaluation of affected individuals.

References

1. R. E. Pyeritz. The Marfan syndrome. Annu Rev Med 2000; 51: 481-510.
2. D. I. Silverman, K. J. Burton, J. Gray, M. S. Bosner, N. T. Kouchoukos, M. J. Roman, et al. Life expectancy in the Marfan syndrome. Am J Cardiol 1995; 75: 157-60.
3. J. Shores, K. R. Berger, E. A. Murphy and R. E. Pyeritz . Progression of aortic dilatation and the benefit of long-term β-adrenergic blockade in Marfan's syndrome. N Engl J Med 1994; 330: 1335-41.
4. V. L. Gott, P. S. Greene, D. E. Alejo, D. E. Cameron, D. C. Naftel, D. C. Miller, et al. Replacement of the aortic root in patients with Marfan's syndrome. N Engl J Med 1999; 340: 1307-13.
5. P. Beighton, A. de Paepe, D. Danks, G. Finidori, T. Gedde-Dahl, R. Goodman, et al. International Nosology of Heritable Disorders of Connective Tissue, Berlin, 1986. Am J Med Genet 1998; 29: 581-94.
6. L. Pereira, O. Levran, F. Ramirez, J. R. Lynch, B. Sykes, R. E. Pyeritz, et al. . A molecular approach to the stratification of cardiovascular risk in families with Marfan's syndrome. N Engl J Med 1994; 331: 148-53.
7. A. De Paepe, R. B. Devereux, H. C. Dietz, R. C. Hennekam and R. E. Pyeritz. Revised diagnostic criteria for the Marfan syndrome. Am J Med Genet 1996; 62: 417-26.
8. K. J. Lipscomb, J. Clayton-Smith and R. Harris. Evolving phenotype of Marfan's syndrome. Arch Dis Child 1997; 76: 41-6.
9. L. Pereira, M. D'Alessio, F. Ramirez, J. R. Lynch, B. Sykes, T. Pangilinan, et al. . Genomic organization of the sequence coding for fibrillin, the defective gene product in Marfan syndrome. Hum Mol Genet 1993; 2: 1762.
10. P. N. Robinson and M. Godfrey. The molecular genetics of Marfan syndrome and related microfibrillopathies. J Med Genet 2000, 37: 9-25.
11. H. C. Dietz, I. McIntosh, L. Y. Sakai, G. M. Corson, S. C. Chalberg, R. E. Pyeritz, et al.. Four novel FBN1 mutations: significance for mutant transcript level and EGF-like domain calcium binding in the pathogenesis of Marfan syndrome. Genomics 1993; 17: 468-75.
12. L. Pereira, S. Y. Lee, B. Gayraud, K. Andrikopoulos, S. D. Shapiro, T. Bunton, et al. . Pathogenetic sequence for aneurysm revealed in mice underexpressing fibrillin-1. Proc Natl Acad Sci U S A 1999; 96: 3819-23.
13. P. Booms, F. Tiecke, T. Rosenberg, C. Hagemeier and P. N. Robinson . Differential effect of FBN1 mutations on in vitro proteolysis of recombinant fibrillin-1 fragments. Hum Genet 2000; 107: 216-24.
14. D. P. Reinhardt, R. N. Ono, H. Notbohm, P. K. Muller, H. P. Bachinger and L. Y. Sakai. Mutations in calcium-binding epidermal growth factor modules render fibrillin-1 susceptible to proteolysis. A potential disease-causing mechanism in Marfan syndrome. J Biol Chem 2000; 275: 12339-45.
15. G. Collod-Béroud, C. Béroud, L. Ades, C. Black, M. Boxer, D. J. Brock, et al.. Marfan Database : new mutations and new routines for the software. Nucleic Acids Res 1998; 26: 229-3.
16. F. Tiecke, S. Katzke, P. Booms, P. Robinson, L. Neumann, M. Godfrey, et al. Classic, atypically severe and neonatal Marfan syndrome: twelve mutations and genotype-phenotype correlations in FBN1 exons 24-40. Eur J Hum Genetics 2001; 9: 13-21.
17. C. Hayward and D. J. Brock . Fibrillin-1 mutations in Marfan syndrome and other type-1 fibrillinopathies. Hum Mutat 1997; 10: 415-23.

18. P. Booms, J. Cisler, K. R. Mathews, M. Godfrey, F. Tiecke, U. C. Kaufmann, et al. Novel exon skipping mutation in the fibrillin-1 gene: two 'hot spots' for the neonatal Marfan syndrome. Clin Genet 1999; 55: 110-7.
19. W. Liu, C. Qian, K. Comeau, T. Brenn, H. Furthmayr and U. Francke . Mutant fibrillin-1 monomers lacking EGF-like domains disrupt microfibril assembly and cause severe Marfan syndrome. Hum Mol Genet 5: 1581-7.
20. L. Lönnqvist, A. Child, K. Kainulainen, R. Davidson, L. Puhakka and L. Peltonen. A novel mutation of the fibrillin gene causing ectopia lentis. Genomics 1994; 19: 573-6.
21. M. Palz, F. Tiecke, P. Booms, B. Göldner, T. Rosenberg, J. Fuchs, et al. Clustering of Mutations Associated with Mild Marfan-like Phenotypes in the 3' Region of FBN1 suggests a Potential Genotype-Phenotype Correlation. Am J Med Genet 2000; 91: 212-21.
22. R. A. Montgomery, M. T. Geraghty, E. Bull, B. D. Gelb, M. Johnson, I. McIntosh, et al. Multiple molecular mechanisms underlying subdiagnostic variants of Marfan syndrome. Am J Hum Genet 1998; 63: 1703-11.
23. D. Halliday, S. Hutchinson, S. Kettle, H. Firth, P. Wordsworth and P. A. Handford Molecular analysis of eight mutations in FBN1. Hum Genet 1999; 105: 587-97.
24. D. Hewett, J. Lynch, A. Child, H. Firth and B. Sykes. Differential allelic expression of a fibrillin gene (FBN1) in patients with Marfan syndrome. Am J Hum Genet 1994; 55: 447-52.
25. H. C. Dietz, R. E. Pyeritz, E. G. Puffenberger, R. J. Kendzior, Jr., G. M. Corson, C. L. Maslen, et al. Marfan phenotype variability in a family segregating a missense mutation in the epidermal growth factor-like motif of the fibrillin gene. J Clin Invest 1992; 89: 1674-80.
26. S. Sood, Z. A. Eldadah, W. L. Krause, I. McIntosh and H. C. Dietz . Mutation in fibrillin-1 and the Marfanoid-craniosynostosis (Shprintzen-Goldberg) syndrome. Nat Genet 1996; 12: 209-11.
27. C. Hayward, M. E. Porteous and D. J. Brock. A novel mutation in the fibrillin gene (FBN1) in familial arachnodactyly. Mol Cell Probes 1994; 8: 325-7.
28. U. Francke, M. A. Berg, K. Tynan, T. Brenn, W. Liu, T. Aoyama, et al. A Gly1127Ser mutation in an EGF-like domain of the fibrillin-1 gene is a risk factor for ascending aortic aneurysm and dissection. Am J Hum Genet 1995; 56: 1287-96.
29. D. M. Milewicz, K. Michael, N. Fisher, J. S. Coselli, T. Markello and A. Biddinger. Fibrillin-1 (FBN1) mutations in patients with thoracic aortic aneurysms. Circulation 1996; 94: 2708-11.
30. C. Ståhl-Hallengren, T. Ukkonen, K. Kainulainen, U. Kristofersson, T. Saxne, K. Tornqvist, et al. An extra cysteine in one of the non-calcium-binding epidermal growth factor-like motifs of the FBN1 polypeptide is connected to a novel variant of Marfan syndrome. J Clin Invest 1994; 94: 709-13.
31. C. Black, A. P. Withers, J. R. Gray, A. B. Bridges, A. Craig, D. U. Baty, et al. Correlation of a recurrent FBN1 mutation (R122C) with an atypical familial Marfan syndrome phenotype. Hum Mutat 1998; S198-200.
32. D. M. Milewicz, J. Grossfield, S. N. Cao, C. Kielty, W. Covitz and T. Jewett. A mutation in FBN1 disrupts profibrillin processing and results in isolated skeletal features of the Marfan syndrome. J Clin Invest 1995; 95: 2373-8.
33. H. Zhang, W. Hu and F. Ramirez. Developmental expression of fibrillin genes suggests heterogeneity of extracellular microfibrils. J Cell Biol 1995; 129: 1165-76.
34. E. S. Park, E. A. Putnam, D. Chitayat, A. Child and D. M. Milewicz. Clustering of FBN2 mutations in patients with congenital contractural arachnodactyly indicates an important role of the domains encoded by exons 24 through 34 during human development. Am J Med Genet 1998; 78: 350-5.
35. K. Tynan, K. Comeau, M. Pearson, P. Wilgenbus, D. Levitt, C. Gasner, et al. Mutation

screening of complete fibrillin-1 coding sequence: report of five new mutations, including two in 8-cysteine domains. Hum Mol Genet 1993; 2: 1813-21.
36. K. Kainulainen, L. Karttunen, L. Puhakka, L. Sakai and L. Peltonen. Mutations in the fibrillin gene responsible for dominant ectopia lentis and neonatal Marfan syndrome. Nat Genet 1994; 6: 64-9.
37. G. Nijbroek, S. Sood, I. McIntosh, C. A. Francomano, E. Bull, L. Pereira, et al. Fifteen novel FBN1 mutations causing Marfan syndrome detected by heteroduplex analysis of genomic amplicons. Am J Hum Genet 1995; 57: 8-21.
38. C. Hayward, M. E. Porteous and D. J. Brock . Mutation screening of all 65 exons of the fibrillin-1 gene in 60 patients with Marfan syndrome: report of 12 novel mutations. Hum Mutat 1997; 10: 280-9.
39. H. C. Dietz, G. R. Cutting, R. E. Pyeritz, C. L. Maslen, L. Y. Sakai, G. M. Corson, et al. Marfan syndrome caused by a rccurrent de novo missense mutation in the fibrillin gene. Nature 1991; 352: 337-339.
40. F. Ramirez. Fibrillin mutations in Marfan syndrome and related phenotypes. Curr Opin Genet Dev 1996; 6: 309-15.
41. G. Collod, M. C. Babron, G. Jondeau, M. Coulon, J. Weissenbach, O. Dubourg, et al. A second locus for Marfan syndrome maps to chromosome 3p24.2-p25. Nat Genet 1994; 8: 264-8.
42. W. O. Liu, P. J. Oefner, C. Qian, R. S. Odom and U. Francke . Denaturing HPLC-identified novel FBN1 mutations, polymorphisms, and sequence variants in Marfan syndrom and related connective tissue disorders. Genetic Testing 1998; 1: 237-42.
43. M. A. Salim, B. S. Alpert, J. C. Ward and R. E. Pyeritz. Effect of beta-adrenergic blockade on aortic root rate of dilation in the Marfan syndrome. Am J Cardiol 1994; 74: 629-33.
44. J. Shores, K. R. Berger, E. A. Murphy and R. E. Pyeritz. Progression of aortic dilatation and the benefit of long-term β-adrenergic blockade in Marfan's syndrome. N Engl J Med 1994; 330: 1335-41.

10. WILLIAMS-BEUREN SYNDROME AND SUPRAVALVULAR AORTIC STENOSIS

L. Pérez Jurado

Introduction

Supravalvular aortic stenosis (SVAS, Online Mendelian Inheritance in Man, [OMIM], #185500, search at http://www.ncbi.nlm.nih.gov/omim/) is an obstructive vascular lesion that involves the ascending aorta. It is often associated with stenoses of the pulmonary or other arteries. SVAS can occur sporadically, as an autosomal dominant condition with incomplete penetrance and variable expressivity, or associated with a more complex developmental disorder, Williams-Beuren syndrome (WBS, OMIM#194050). There was some controversy in the literature whether SVAS and WBS could be the same disorder [1,2]. The molecular basis of SVAS was discovered in 1993 when linkage studies of separate kindreds mapped the responsible locus to chromosome 7q [3,4] and a disruption of the elastin (ELN) gene (located at 7q11.23) was found in a family in which a translocation of chromosome 7 was cosegregating with SVAS [5]. Soon thereafter, hemizygosity at the ELN gene was found in all WBS cases studied [6] with deletions extending far outside the ELN locus. It became then clear that both entities, WBS and isolated SVAS, exist in a separate manner being allelic conditions. While SVAS is caused by mutations affecting only the elastin gene [7], WBS is a contiguous gene disorder due to a large deletion including both the elastin and additional genes [8]. Some forms of autosomal dominant cutis laxa (OMIM#123700) have been shown recently to be also allelic disorders caused by elastin mutations [9,10].

Williams-Beuren Syndrome

WBS is a developmental disorder with multisystem manifestations including distinctive facial features, mental disability with unique cognitive and personality profiles, vascular stenoses, short stature, occasional transient hypercalcemia of infancy, and connective tissue anomalies [11,12]. It occurs with an incidence of about 1/25,000 newborns with equal frequency in both sexes and all races, and without known predisposing factors [13]. While most cases are sporadic, a few instances of parent to child transmission confirming autosomal dominant inheritance have been reported [14,15]. WBS has also

PA Doevendansand AA Wilde (eds.), Cardiovascular genetics, 111-126.

been reported in concordant monozygotic twins and in discordant dizygotic twins. It was first reported under the name "Idiopathic Infantile Hypercalcemia" as a syndrome defined by hypercalcemia, characteristic face and failure to thrive [16]. It was then described independently by Williams and Beuren as a disorder involving characteristic face, SVAS and mental retardation [17,18]. Later on, multiple reports clearly demonstrated that the previously described clinical entities were one and the same, which might include a wider spectrum of abnormalities [11,19].

Clinical features

Cranio-Facial

Characteristic features that comprise the so called "elfin" face are bitemporal narrowing, periorbital fullness, malar flattening, full dropping cheeks, a bulbous nasal tip, a wide mouth with full lips and a small chin (figure 1).

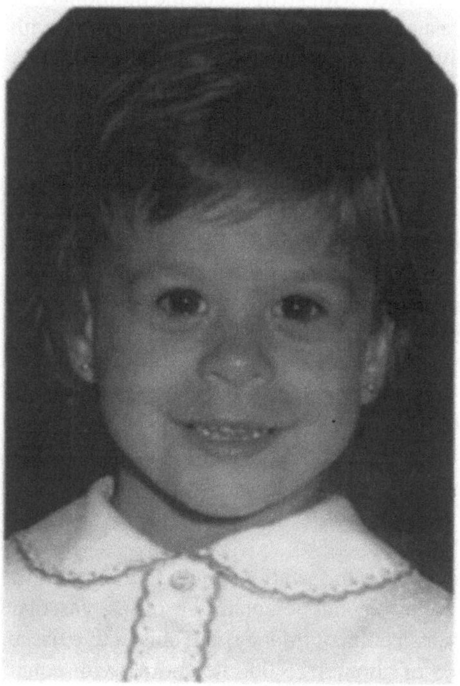

Figure 1*. A beautiful 2-year-old girl with WBS showing the typical facial features.*

Epicanthal folds may be present and the iris frequently has a stellate pattern [20]. Strabismus is a common finding that may be related to subnormal binocular vision [21]. Hyperopia and reduced stereoacuity have also been found [22]. Dental hypoplasia, absent or malformed teeth, and malocclusion are common.

Growth

Growth failure of prenatal onset is present in about one third of WBS patients. Failure to thrive often manifests in infancy and early childhood, in part related to feeding and gastrointestinal problems. Growth tends to be normal in childhood, but the pubertal growth spurt may be slightly premature and short. The final adult height is usually at the lower limit of normal, ≅10cm below the target [23]. The trunk may be relatively long for the extremities. Head circumference is slightly small but proportionate to height.

Skeletal and connective tissue abnormalities

Mild joint laxity is common in infancy but contractures may appear later in life [24]. Scoliosis, kyphosis and lordosis are common. Clinodactyly of the fifth finger, hallux valgus and radio-ulnar synostosis have also been reported. Manifestations of connective tissue weakness in other systems may include inguinal hernias, bladder diverticuli and intestinal diverticulosis. Skin is usually soft and finely wrinkled particularly on the hands, with decreased subcutaneous fat. Hair tends to be curly and may become prematurely grey, and nail hypoplasia is common. The voice is typically hoarse.

Cardiovascular manifestations

Cardiovascular involvement is detected in about 75% of patients during their lifetime [11]. SVAS is most common, with peripheral pulmonic stenosis next in frequency. Involvement of any other muscular arteries may occur, and vascular narrowing may be progressive. Increased carotid arterial wall thickness is a consistent ultrasonographic finding in all WBS patients [25]. There are cases of sudden death probably associated with primary or secondary occlusion of the coronary arteries [26]. Hypertension is relatively common and may be related to narrowing of the renal artery in some cases [27].

Neurobehavioral features

The neurobehavioral phenotype is characterized by a distinctive cognitive profile and an unusual personality profile [28,29]. WBS patients show mild to moderate mental retardation or learning disability with marked deficits in motor co-ordination and visual spatial abilities. The visual spatial processing dysfunction translates into markedly impaired visual learning abilities and may contribute to gait instability. In contrast, their language skills are relatively preserved with a loquacious speech rich in clichés, intonations and unusual aphorisms, although their command of grammar and comprehension is worse than it appears. In addition, a clear strength in auditory rote memory and face processing is evident in WBS individuals. Relative to overall level of adaptive behavior functioning, WBS individuals show clear strength in socialization skills and communication skills, and clear weakness in daily living skills and motor skills. Their personality involves overfriendliness and empathy, with an undercurrent of anxiety related to social situations and some features of obsessive-compulsive disorder. In adulthood, emotional and behavioral problems are common [30]. Hyperactive behavior and short attention span can occur, compounding the existing learning problems.

Mild muscle hypotonia is common and may be due to an actual myopathy [31]. However, hyperreflexia and hypertonia may also develop in late childhood; in these cases, symptomatic Chiari type I malformation should be ruled out [32]. Hyperacusis manifests in up to 85% of WBS patients. Musical ability is usually described in WBS and there are anecdotal reports of WBS syndrome individuals with exceptional musical talent or even "perfect pitch" [33]. However, contrasted and objective data are still lacking.

Brain morphology
A few differences have been found in WBS patients' brains by magnetic resonance imaging (MRI) [34]. Brain and brainstem sizes are globally decreased with relative preservation of the cerebellum and temporal gyrus. There is also some gross discrepancy in size between the larger frontal and temporal cerebral regions and the smaller parietal and occipital areas. The corpus callosum midline length is decreased, may be due to a decreased size of the splenium. There is a relative preservation of cerebral gray matter volume and disproportionate reduction in cerebral white matter volume. Assymetries have been noted in the occipital lobes and the planum temporale with a relative decrease of the gray matter volume on the right side. A consistent finding is a short central sulcus that does not become opercularized in the interhemispheric fissure, bringing attention to a possible developmental anomaly affecting the dorsal half of the hemispheres [35]. There is a correlation between frontal/temporal sparing and preservation of language and social skills relative to motor and visual abilities. Chiari type I malformation can also be found by MRI in subjects with WBS even in the absence of neurological signs [32]. The cortical cytoarchitecture is relatively normal in most brain areas, except for some regions that show increased cell size and decreased cell-packing density. Acquired pathology of microvascular origin likely related to underlying hypertension has been reported [35].

Brain electrophysiology
Event related potentials during two relatively spared cognitive functions, face processing and language processing, have shown very consistent differences between WBS patients and controls [36]. These data are suggestive of an abnormal cerebral specialization, using different pathways to accomplish those functions in WBS.

Hypercalcemia
Hypercalcemia is not often noted in WBS patients and, if found, tends to resolve by 2-4 years of age. The hypercalcemia reported in the initial description of the syndrome was probably triggered by the high-dose vitamin D supplements provided to infants for preventing rickets [19]. Calcium levels are usually found in the upper limit of normal. However, the presence of nephrocalcinosis as well as the history of irritability, feeding problems, and constipation might be related in part to undetected hypercalcemia. No consistent abnormality in the regulation of calcium metabolism has been found, except for a delayed renal clearance of calcium following exogenous overload [37,38].

Gastro-intestinal problems
Gastroesophageal reflux is relatively common and may be the cause of colic in infants [39]. Hiatal hernia and/or reflux may occur in adults as well. Chronic constipation is also a common problem and may lead to rectal prolapse in 15% of individuals with WBS. In case of chronic abdominal pain, the diagnosis of diverticulosis and diverticulitis should be considered.

Genitourinary complications
Renal anomalies have been described in about 18% of WBS patients screened by ultrasound [40,41], including nephrocalcinosis, diverticuli of the bladder and structural

anomalies (duplicated kidney, hypoplasia and ectopic placement). Urinary frequency and nocturnal enuresis are frequent complaints, and could be related to hypercalciuria and/or bladder dyssynergia.

Rare complications
Hypothyroidism and coeliac disease have been reported to occur in WBS individuals with higher frequency than in the population [42,43].

Follow-up
Medical care should be individualized for every child, adolescent or adult with WBS [39]. Periodic follow-up is required by a multidisciplinary team including a geneticist, a cardiologist, a physical therapist, and other specialists depending on the complications. It is very important an early and adequate psychological evaluation and follow-up to provide educational needs. There is no specific treatment except for the medical complications if they occur (hypertension, SVAS, symptomatic hypercalcemia, etc…). In general, there is no need to decrease dietary calcium although vitamin D or multi-vitamin supplementations should probably be avoided. To prevent or minimize constipation, a dietary regimen is recommended. In cases of attention deficit-hyperactivity disorder, environmental modifications should be implemented and psychostimulant medication may be beneficial. There are excellent guidelines for medical monitoring of patients with WBS written by a panel of experts on WBS and available through the web pages of the Williams Syndrome Association of the Unites States (http://www.williams-syndrome.org).

Molecular basis and mutational mechanism in WBS

WBS is a contiguous gene disorder caused by a heterozygous microdeletion at chromosome band 7q11.23. A common deleted interval was defined in the great majority of patients by deletion mapping with polymorphic markers, and confirmed by the detection of common junction fragments [44-46]. Physical mapping of the region has been difficult due to the presence of several repeat clusters recently characterized [46.47]. The WBS deleted region is flanked by a complex arrangement of large (~100kb) blocks of chromosome 7-specific segmental duplications, also called low copy repeats or duplicons (figure2) [47]. It has been shown that the majority of deletions arise from crossover events between both chromosome 7 homologues during meiosis, although intrachromosomal rearrangements have also been observed [48,49]. Fine mapping of deletion ends in patients, has shown that the chromosomal breakpoints cluster into narrowly defined physical regions at the centromeric and middle segmental duplications [46,47]. Therefore, it appears that there is a common mutational mechanism for the majority of 7q11.23 deletions causing WBS that somehow explains the high mutation rate ($\sim 0.5 \times 10^{-4}$ per gamete per generation): WBS deletions arise as a consequence of unequal crossing over between highly homologous sequences (segmental duplications in 7q11.23), which confer susceptibility to local chromosome rearrangements through misalignment during chromosome pairing.

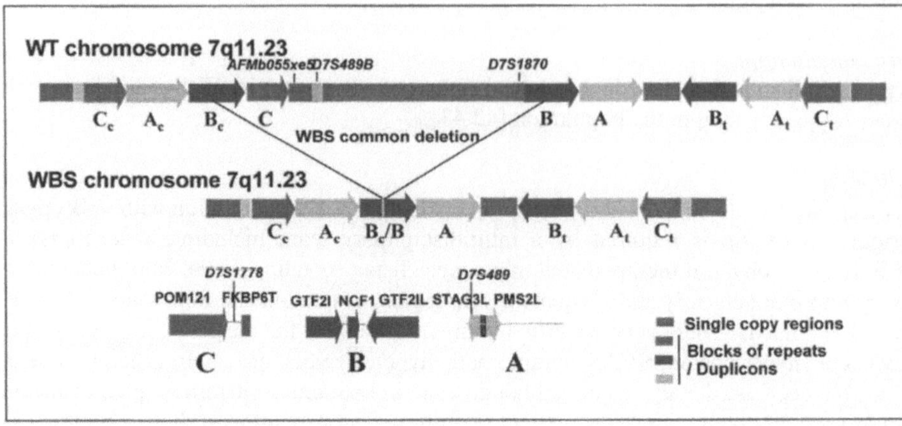

Figure 2. ***(see color section)*** *Schematic representation of the 7q11.23 genomic region. The single copy region that is commonly deleted in WBS patients (blue square from AFMb055xe5 to D7S1870 in the upper panel) contains 25-30 genes and is flanked by a complex arrangement of blocks of chromosome 7-specific low copy repeats or duplicons (called A, B and C) [47]. The arrow orientation from centromere to telomere of the middle duplicons is arbitrarily depicted as a reference for the relative orientation of the centromeric (A_c, B_c, C_c) and telomeric (A_t, B_t, C_t) blocks. The location of single copy polymorphic markers that internally limit the deleted interval (AFMb055xe5 and D7S1870) and two multiple copy polymorphic loci (D7S489 and D7S1778) within the duplicons are indicated. Most WBS chromosomes (middle panel) arise as a consequence of unequal recombination between the centromeric B_c and middle B duplicons. The lower panel shows the gene/pseudogene composition of each putatively ancestral duplicon. Block A contains sequences related to the PMS2 mismatch repair gene (PMS2L) and the stromal antigen 3 gene (STAG3L) that are also present in other chromosome 7 locations. Block B contains the GTF2I, NCF1 genes, and another gene related to GTF2I (GTF2IL). Block C comprises the POM121 gene and the four first exons of FKBP6.*

The order of the intradeletion genes is fully conserved in mouse although the deletion region is inverted relative to the human map, exactly at the flanking regions [47]. In addition, data indicative of similar duplicons or low-copy repeats have been found in other primates but not in mouse or other mammals [50,51]. Therefore, comparative mapping suggests that the human 7q11.23 chromosomal region has evolved through serial, evolutionarily recent, rearrangements leading to segmental genomic duplications.

The commonly deleted interval has been estimated to encompass ~1.6 Mb [46,52]. Up to date, 18-19 genes located within this deleted interval have been characterized [51,53-69], including genes that code for structural proteins, transcription factors, transmembrane receptors and other proteins involved in signal transduction and neuronal tasks (table) [reviewed in 8].

There are at least 8 additional incompletely characterized genes that lie within the commonly deleted interval, most of them located in a region that has not been completely sequenced as yet, between WBSCR14 and ELN.

Table. Genes commonly deleted in WBS ordered from centromere to telomere.

Gene	**Protein products**	**Putative function / functional clues** [70-82]	**Phenotypic contribution Other comments**
POM121	Pore membrane protein of the nuclear envelope	Biogenesis of nuclear envelope and cytoplasmatic annulate lamellae	Multiple copy gene, only one copy deleted (ancestral?)
FKBP6	FK-506 binding protein of 36kDa	Immunophilin family member	
FZD9	*Drosophila frizzled* homolog 9	Cell membrane receptor for wingless-related proteins	
WBSCR9/WSTF	*Drosophila Acf1* homolog	Transcription factor? Chromatin assembly	
BCL7B	Homolog of BCL7A disrupted by a leukemic translocation breakpoint	Atopy-related IgE autoantigen in atopic dermatitis	
TBL2/WS-ßTRP	Transducin ß-like 2	ß-transducin family member of unknown function	
WBSCR14/WS-bHLH	b-Helix-Loop-Helix protein	Transcription factor highly expressed in adult liver	
STX1A	Syntaxin 1A	Presynaptic vesicle protein brain-specific	
CLDN3 and CLND4	Claudin family members Clostridium perfringens enterotoxin receptors	Part of tight junction structures / paracellular barrier in epithelial tissues	
ELN	Elastin	Main component of the elastic fibers in the extracellular matrix	Happloinsufficiency causes the cardiovascular phenotype
LIMK1	LIM-kinase 1	Signal transduction in neuronal synapses regulating changes in cytoskeletal structure	Hemizygosity might contribute to impaired visuo-spacial contruction
EIF4H/WBSCR1	Eukaryotic initiation factor EIF4H	Positive regulator of translation initiation	
WBSCR15	Protein without known motifs	Unknown	
RFC2	Subunit 2 of the pentameric replication factor C	DNA elongation during replication	
CYLN2	Neuronal cytoplasmatic linker protein CLIP-115	Intracellular organelle transportation binds to microtubules	
GTF2IRD1/WBSCR11	GTF2I-related domain	Enhancer-binding protein and transcriptional regulator	
GTF2I	TFII-I/BAP135/SPIN	Transcription initiator factor involved in both basal and activated transcription	Multiple copy, the gene is deleted while two truncated pseudogenes are not
NCF1	Neutrophilic cytosolic factor 1, p47-phox	Phagocyte NADPH oxidase subunit. Antimicrobial activity	Multiple copy gene, only one copy (gene or pseudogene) deleted

Pathogenesis of the vascular disorder

Elastic fibers are found in the extracellular matrix of many tissues. They are extracellular matrix polymers, composed of at least 19 different proteins that comprise both the microfibrillar and the more abundant amorphous component (elastin). Elastin is produced as a precursor molecule, tropoelastin, that undergoes extensive post-translational modification by lysyl oxidase [74]. Elastin molecules are aligned on a network of fibrillin and other microfibril-associated proteins to form ordered elastic fibers, which are stabilized by the formation of intermolecular crosslinks known as desmosines. The hydrophobic regions of the chains, between the crosslinks, are highly mobile.

Pathological specimens from the aorta, skin and pulmonary arteries of WBS patients have demonstrated disorganized elastin deposition [83,84]. Hemizygosity at ELN leads to a reduced amount of elastin protein that would affect arterial compliance. In addition, compensatory increases in elastin lamellae and smooth muscle have been found in the arterial wall of WBS individuals. Progressive vascular narrowing might be triggered or accelerated by hemodynamic stress.

Further confirmation that ELN haploinsufficiency causes the cardiovascular phenotype of WBS comes from mouse models. Mice lacking elastin have been generated by homologous recombination [85]. Homozygous animals (ELN -/-) died of an obstructive arterial disease that resulted from subendothelial cell proliferation and reorganization of smooth muscle not associated with hemodynamic stress, as the disease still occurred in arteries isolated in organ culture without hemodynamic stress. Heterozygous animals (ELN +/-) showed a 50% reduction in ELN mRNA and protein levels, but arterial compliance at physiologic pressures was nearly normal. This discrepancy was explained by a paradoxical increase of 35% in the number of elastic lamellae and smooth muscle in ELN +/- arteries [86]. Thus, ELN hemizygosity in mice, like in humans, induces a compensatory increase in the number of rings of elastic lamellae and smooth muscle during arterial development. Humans appear to be more sensitive to reduced ELN expression, developing significant arterial thickening with increased risk of obstructive vascular disease.

The observed phenotypic variability of the cardiovascular features in WBS (25% non penetrance and diverse degrees of severity) is considered typical of phenotypes produced by haploinsufficiency, where genetic background is expected to have a major modifying effect. Likely, ELN gene happloinsuffiency may also be responsible at least in part for other connective tissue manifestations of the WBS phenotype, including the periorbital fullness and thick lips, inguinal hernias, skin and joint changes, and diverticuli of bladder and intestine.

Pathogenesis of other features and clinical molecular correlations

Happloinsufficiency for genes affected by the deletion must be the pathogenic mechanism for the neurobehavioral and metabolic disturbances. However, despite the number of known genes commonly deleted, the non-vascular features of WBS have not yet been clearly attributed to specific genes. Based on two families with deletions involving ELN and LIMK1, hemizygosity of LIMK1 was proposed as a contributing factor to impaired visuospatial constructive cognition in WBS [63]. However, this claim was not confirmed by clinical and molecular studies of three different patients with similar heterozygous LIMK1 deletions [87]. A phenotypic map for some clinical manifestations has been proposed based on a few atypical patients with smaller deletions and either a full phenotype (two patients with a deletion including ELN to GTF2I) [88] or partial phenotypes (several deletions surrounding ELN) [89]. Other genes close to ELN (including RFC2, EIFH4, STX1A) appear to be excluded from contributing significantly to the phenotype while the genes mainly responsible for abnormal cognition, map to the telomeric interval of the deletion, CYLN2, GTF2IRD1 and GTF2I [89]. Genes from POM121 to WBSCR14, at the centromeric edge of the deletion might contribute to other phenotypic aspects including mental retardation. However, these conclusions still lack strong supportive evidence and additional clinical and molecular studies are required.

On the other hand, while common phenotypic features can be defined, there is a wide range of clinical variability between patients. The molecular basis of this phenotypic variability, if any, remains unknown. Like in familial SVAS, where the variability within families is as great as that seen between families, environmental factors, genetic variants in the non-deleted allele, subtle imprinting effects and the genetic background may all contribute to the variable expression of the phenotype. Comparison of clinical data collected in a standardized quantifiable format with parental origin of the deletion revealed more severe growth retardation and microcephaly in the maternal deletion group and no correlation for other clinical features [44]. In other studies, however, no evidence for effects on stature by examining gender, ethnicity, cardiac status, or parental origin of the deletion was found [45,90].

Familial Isolated Supravalvular Aortic Stenosis

Familial SVAS is an autosomal dominant syndrome with the identical vascular phenotype of WBS, but without the associated mental or growth retardation and without hypercalcemia [1,91]. The term SVAS is not very appropriate since it refers to an extended arteriopathy, with multiple pulmonary and systemic arterial stenoses [91,92]. Some of the facial manifestations of WBS, mainly the configuration of the mouth, are also present in patients with islolated SVAS when compared with their unaffected relatives. Other connective tissue anomalies described in SVAS are an increased frequency of inguinal hernias and some premature aging of skin. Families with isolated SVAS also show marked variability of expression and incomplete penetrance [91] .

About 50 different mutations in heterozygosity at the ELN locus have been reported in familial and sporadic cases of isolated SVAS [93-96]. The mutation spectrum includes large and small gene deletions as well as a diversity of point mutations. All but four of the point mutations are predicted to cause either a complete absence of the gene product or a protein truncation (PTC) due to premature chain termination. Selective elimination of mutant transcripts by nonsense mediated mRNA decay has been demonstrated in skin fibroblasts of patients with PTC mutations and other frameshift mutations [95]. The consequences of missense mutations have not been analyzed yet, but they also could affect normal splicing resulting in decreased total mRNA. Therefore, most if not all ELN mutations lead to an overall decrease of the steady state levels of elastin mRNA resulting in reduced synthesis and secretion of tropoelastin. Functional haploinsufficiency seems to be the pathomechanism underlying most cases of nonsyndromic SVAS.

Cutis laxa congenital

Cutis laxa can be acquired as an autoimmune process but there are some congenital forms with either an autosomal recessive, X-linked, or autosomal dominant pattern of inheritance [97]. Congenital cutis laxa presents at birth with loose skin lacking elastic recoil, facial droping, floppy airway structures leading to fixed or collapsible upper airway obstruction, umbilical and inguinal hernias, and a hoarse voice. The cardiovascular phenotype may include mild dilatation of the proximal aorta and great vessels, tortuous, pulsatile external carotid arteries, multiple peripheral pulmonary stenoses, and redundant mitral or tricuspid valves. Patients have an aged appearance and may require cosmetic surgery for the skin problems. Histologically, dermal collagen fibers appear normal, but elastic fibers look fragmented with a paucity of amorphous elastin in the matrix [98].
Three different heterozygous mutations in the elastin gene have been described in patients with autosomal dominant cutis laxa [9,10] . All three mutations (in ELN exons 30 and 32) are predicted to cause a frameshift at the C terminus of the elastin protein, replacing a highly conserved sequence that contains the only two cysteines involved in crosslinking. The mutant transcript is expressed or even overrepresented compared to the normal transcript [99]. Electron microscopy of the skin sections of one patient showed abnormal branching and fragmentation in the amorphous elastin component with fewer microfibrils in the dermis, and reduced elastin deposition by immunocytochemistry [98]. These findings suggested that the mutant tropoelastin protein was synthesized, secreted, and incorporated into the elastic matrix, where it altered the architecture of elastic fibers. Interference with crosslinking would reduce elastic recoil in affected tissues and explain the cutis laxa phenotype. Therefore, a dominant negative effect of heterozygous ELN mutation is the most likely pathogenic mechanism for this condition.

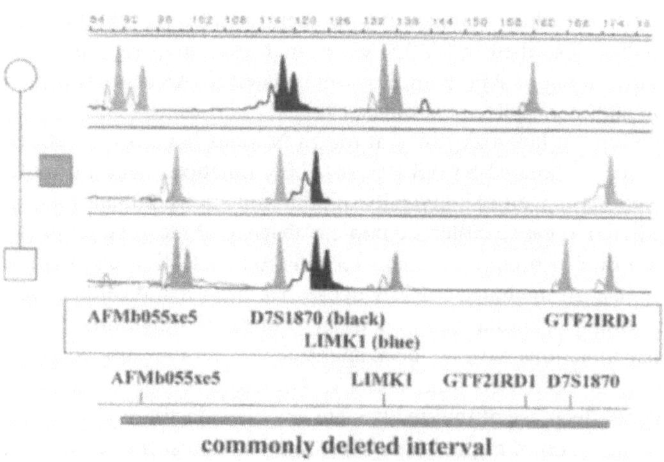

Figure 3. Results of a multiplex PCR for the diagnosis of WBS in a patient (middle panel), the mother (upper panel) and the father (lower panel). Lack of inheritance of maternal alleles is detected in the patient at all four informative polymorphic loci, indicating the presence of a *de novo* 7q11.23 deletion in the maternaly inherited chromosome. The location of the typed markers with respect to the commonly deleted interval is shown at the bottom.

Molecular Diagnostics: implications for treatment and counselling

The diagnosis of WBS can usually be made with high accuracy by expert clinicians. Molecular diagnostics is available and there is a great correlation between the presence of the deletion and the clinical phenotype. The most common method used is chromosomal fluorescence in situ hybridization (FISH) with a probe for the ELN locus, although alternative methods can be used such as typing intragenic polymorphic markers to detect failure of parental inheritance (figure 3). Molecular confirmation of the deletion is very relevant for follow-up as well as for genetic counseling (Category B). Obviously, detection of ELN hemizygosity implies a high risk for cardiovascular disease, different in patients with intact ELN. Recurrence risk in parents and other relatives of a WBS patient with a deletion is very low, <1% and probably not increased at all with respect to the general population. WBS indivuals may transmit the deletion, and then the disease, to 50% of their descendents (autosomal dominant). Exceptional patients without deletions may represent related syndromes or phenocopies. In these cases, clinical follow-up and genetic counseling must be different, done empirically if there is no alternative diagnosis.

A similar situation exist in SVAS families. SVAS shows variable penetrance within families but its potential progressive nature in some cases makes its presymptomatic diagnosis important. Therefore, the identification of the responsible mutation is important to identify all family members at risk (category B). That information facilitates appropriate clinical management, putative preventative treatments and genetic counseling. However, since the mutation may occur in different regions of the gene molecular diagnosis is not always straightforward.

Concluding remarks and future directions

Identification of the genes whose haploinsufficiency underlies the characteristic cognitive and personality profiles of WBS should provide new insight into the complex processes regulating the development and functioning of the central nervous system. However, the task of determining whether any of the deleted genes in WBS contributes to particular features of the phenotype is difficult. The identification of single gene defects in loci other than ELN in human patients with distinct features of the WBS phenotype would be very important. However, single gene defects may not be sufficient for a phenotypic effect, and additive effects of individual happloinsufficient loci may be necessary.

The identification of all the genes whose transcription may be affected by the deletion in typical and atypical patients is required to establish precise clinical-molecular correlations. Future studies should also focus on the functional characterization of the protein products of deleted genes, including the identification of their subcellular localization, interacting proteins, and pathways that might be affected by gene haploinsufficiency.

Finally, the answer to many of the remaining open questions about WBS, including the specific contribution of genes to the phenotype and the underlying pathophysiologic mechanisms of the disease, may rely on animal experimentation. Mice carrying identical deletion to humans as well as single gene knockouts should be generated. Recent progress in mouse and human genome projects has provided the framework required for these tasks [100-101].

References

1. Grimm T, Wesselhoeft H. The genetic aspects of Williams-Beuren syndrome and the isolated form of the supravalvular aortic stenosis: investigation of 128 families. Z Kardiol 1980; 69:168-72.
2. Garcia RE, Friedman WF, Kaback MM, Rowe RD. Idiopathic hypercalcemia and supravalvular aortic stenosis: documentation of a new syndrome. New Eng J Med. 1964; 271:117-20.
3. Ewart AK, Morris CA, Ensing GJ, et al. A human vascular disorder, supravalvular aortic stenosis, maps to chromosome 7. Proc Nat Acad Sci 1993; 90:3226-30.
4. Olson TM, Michels VV, Lindor NM, DJ, et al. Autosomal dominant supravalvular aortic stenosis: localization to chromosome 7. Hum Mol Genet 1993; 2: 869-73.
5. Curran ME, Atkinson DL, Ewart AK, et al. The elastin gene is disrupted by a translocation associated with supravalvular aortic stenosis. Cell 1993; 73:159-68.
6. Ewart AK, Morris CA, Atkinson D et al. Hemizygosity at the elastin locus in a developmental disorder, Williams syndrome. Nature Genet 1993; 5:11-6.
7. Chowdhury T, Reardon W. Elastin mutation and cardiac disease. Pediatr Cardiol 1999; 20:103-7.
8. Francke U. Williams syndrome: genes and mechanisms. Hum Mol Genet 1999; 8:1947-54.
9. Tassabehji M, Metcalfe K, Hurst J, et al. An elastin gene mutation producing abnormal tropoelastin and abnormal elastic fibres in a patient with autosomal dominant cutis laxa. Hum Mol Genet 1998; 7:1021-8.
10. Zhang, MC, He L, Giro M, et al. Cutis laxa arising from frameshift mutations in exon 30 of the elastin gene (ELN). J Biol Chem 1999; 274:981-6.
11. Morris CA, Demsey SA, Leonard CO, Dilts C, Blackburn BL. Natural history of Williams syndrome: physical characteristics. J Pediatr 1988; 113:318-26.
12. Burn J. Williams syndrome. J Med Genet 1986; 23:389-95.
13. Greenberg F. Williams syndrome professional symposium. Am J Med Genet 1990; 6 (suppl):85-8.
14. Morris CA, Thomas IT and Greenberg F. Williams syndrome: autosomal dominant inheritance. Am J Med Genet 1993; 47:478-81.
15. Sadler LS, Robinson LK, Verdaasdonk KR, Gingell R. The Williams syndrome: evidence for possible autosomal dominant inheritance. Am J Med Genet 1993; 47:468-70.
16. Fanconi VG, Giardet P, Schlesinger B, Butler N, Black J. Chronische hypercalcamie kambiniert mit osteosklerose, hyperazotamie, minderwuschs und kongenitalen missbildungen. Helv Paediatr Acta 1952; 7:314-49.
17. Williams JCP, Barratt-Boyes BG, Lowe JB. Supravalvular aortic stenosis. Circulation 1961; 24:1311-8.
18. Beuren AJ, Apitz J, Harmjanz D. Supravalvular aortic stenosis in association with mental retardation and a certain facial appearance. Circulation 1962; 26:1235-40.
19. Jones KL. Williams syndrome: an historical perspective of its evolution, natural history, and etiology. Am J Med Genet 1990; 6 (suppl):89-96.
20. Winter M, Pankau R, Amm M, Gosch A, Wessel A. The spectrum of ocular features in the Williams-Beuren syndrome. Clin Genet 1996; 49:28-31.
21. Olitsky SE, Sadler LS, Reynolds JD. Subnormal binocular vision in the Williams syndrome. J Pediatr Ophthalmol Strabismus 1997; 34:58-60.
22. Sadler LS, Olitsky SE, Reynolds JD. Reduced stereoacuity in Williams syndrome. Am J Med Genet 1996; 66:287-8.
23. Partsch CJ, Dreyer G, Gosch A, et al. Longitudinal evaluation of growth, puberty, and bone maturation in children with Williams syndrome. J Pediatr 1999; 134:82-9.
24. Kaplan P, Kirschner M, Watters G, Costa MT. Contractures in patients with Williams syndrome. Pediatrics 1989; 84:895-9.

25. Sadler LS, Gingell R, Martin DJ. Carotid ultrasound examination in Williams syndrome. J Pediatr 1998; 132:354-6.
26. Bird LM, Billman GF, Lacro RV, et al. Sudden death in Williams syndrome: report of ten cases. J Pediatr 1996; 129:926-31.
27. Broder K, Reinhardt E, Ahern J, et al. Elevated ambulatory blood pressure in 20 subjects with Williams syndrome. Am J Med Genet 1999; 83:356-60.
28. Bellugi U, Lichtenberger L, Jones W, Lai Z, St George M. The neurocognitive profile of Williams Syndrome: a complex pattern of strengths and weaknesses. J Cogn Neurosci. 2000; 12 (Suppl 1):7-29.
29. Mervis CB, Klein-Tasman BP. Williams syndrome: cognition, personality, and adaptive behavior. Ment Retard Dev Disabil Res Rev 2000; 6:148-58.
30. Udwin O. A survey of adults with Williams syndrome and idiopathic infantile hypercalcemia. Dev Med Child Neurol 1990; 32:129-41.
31. Voit T, Kramer H, Thomas C, et al. Myopathy in Williams-Beuren syndrome. Eur J Pediatr 1991; 150:521-6.
32. Mercuri E, Atkinson J, Braddick O, et al. Chiari I malformation in asymptomatic young children with Williams syndrome: clinical and MRI study. Europ J Paediatr Neurol 1997; 1:177-81.
33. Lenhoff HM, Wang PP, Greenberg F, Bellugi U. Williams syndrome and the brain. Scientific American 1997; 277:68-73.
34. Schmitt JE, Eliez S, Bellugi U, Reiss AL. Analysis of Cerebral Shape in Williams Syndrome. Arch Neurol 2001; 58:283-7.
35. Galaburda AM, Bellugi U. Multi-level analysis of cortical neuroanatomy in Williams syndrome. J Cogn Neurosci 2000;12(Suppl 1):74-88.
36. Mills DL, Alvarez TD, St George M, et al. Electrophysiological studies of face processing in Williams syndrome. J Cogn Neurosci 2000; 12(Suppl 1):47-64.
37. Forbes GB, Bryson MF, Manning J, Amirhakimi GH, Reina JC. Impaired calcium homeostasis in the infantile hypercalcemic syndrome. Acta Paediat Scand 1972; 61,305-9.
38. Kruse K, Pankau R, Gosch A, Wohlfahrt K. Calcium metabolism in Williams-Beuren syndrome. J. Pediatr 1992; 121:902-7.
39. Lashkari A, Smith AK, Graham JM. Williams-Beuren syndrome: an update and review for the primary physician. Clin Pediatr (Phila) 1999; 38:189-208.
40. Pankau R, Partsch CJ, Winter M, Gosch A, Wessel A. Incidence and spectrum of renal abnormalities in Williams-Beuren syndrome. Am J Med Genet 1996; 63:301-4.
41. Pober BR, Lacro RV, Rice C, Mandell V, Teele RL. Renal findings in 40 individuals with Williams syndrome Am J Med Genet 1993; 46:271-4.
42. Cammareri V, Vignati G, Nocera G, Beck-Peccoz P, Persani L. Thyroid hemiagenesis and elevated thyrotropin levels in a child with Williams syndrome. Am J Med Genet 1999; 85:491-4.Santer R, Pankau R, Schaub J, Burgin-Wolff A. Williams-Beuren syndrome and celiac disease. J Pediatr Gastroenterol Nutr 1996; 23:339-40.
43. Pérez Jurado LA, Peoples R, Wang Y-K et al. Molecular definition of the chromosome 7 deletion in Williams syndrome and parent-of-origin effects on growth. Am J Hum Genet 1996; 59: 618-25.
44. Wu YQ, Sutton VR, Nickerson E et al. Delineation of the common critical region in Williams syndrome and clinical correlation of growth, heart defects, ethnicity, and parental origin. Am J Med Genet 1998; 78: 82-9.
45. Peoples R, Franke Y, Wang YK, et al. A physical map, including a BAC/PAC clone contig, of the Williams-Beuren syndrome deletion region at 7q11.23. Am J Hum Genet 2000; 66:47-68.
46. Valero MC, de Luis O , Cruces J, Pérez Jurado LA. Fine-scale comparative mapping of the human 7q11.23 region and the orthologous regionon mouse chromosome 5G: the low-copy

repeats that flank the williams-beuren syndrome deletion arose at breakpoint sites of an evolutionary inversion(s). Genomics. 2000; 69:1-13.

47. Urbán Z, Helms C, Fekete G et al. 7q11.23 deletions in Williams syndrome arise as a consequence of unequal meiotic crossover. Am J Hum Genet 1996; 59:958-62.
48. Dutly F, Schinzel A. Unequal interchromosomal rearrangements may result in elastin gene deletions causing the Williams-Beuren syndrome. Hum Mol Genet 1996; 5:1893-98.
49. DeSilva U, Massa H, Trask BJ, Green ED. Comparative mapping of the region of human chromosome 7 deleted in Williams syndrome. Genome Res 1999; 9:428-36.
50. Pérez Jurado LA, Wang Y-K, Peoples R, et al. A duplicate gene in the breakpoint regions of the Williams-Beuren syndrome deletion encodes the initiator binding protein TFII-I and BAP-135, a phosphorylation target of BTK. Hum Mol Genet 1998; 7:325-34.
51. Hockenhull EL, Carette MJ, Metcalfe K, et al. A complete physical contig and partial transcript map of the Williams syndrome critical region. Genomics 1999; 58:138-45.
52. Meng X, Lu X, Morris CA, Keating MT. A novel human gene FKBP6 is deleted in Williams syndrome. Genomics 1998; 52:130-7.
53. Wang Y-K, Harryman-Samos C, Peoples R, et al. A novel human homologue of the Drosophila frizzled wnt receptor gene binds wingless protein and is in the Williams syndrome deletion at 7q11.23. Hum Mol Genet 1997; 6:465-72.
54. Lu X, Meng X, Morris CA, Keating MT. A novel human gene, WBSTF, is deleted in Williams syndrome. Genomics 1998; 54:241-9.
55. Peoples RJ, Cisco MJ, Kaplan P, Francke U. Identification of the WBSCR9 gene, encoding a novel transcrition regulator, in the Williams-Beuren syndrome deletion at 7q11.23. Cytogenet Cell Genet 1998; 82:238-46.
56. Jadayel DM, Osborne LR, Coignet LJA et al. The BCL7 gene family: deletion of BCL7B in Williams syndrome. Gene 1998 ; 224:35-44.
57. Meng X, Lu X, Li Z et al. Complete physical map of the common deletion region and characterization of three novel genes. Hum Genet 1998; 103:590-9.
58. Pérez Jurado LA, Wang Y-K, Francke U, Cruces J. TBL2, a novel transducin family member in the WBS deletion: characterization of the entire sequence, splice variants and the mouse ortholog. Cytogenet Cell Genet 1999; 86:277-84.
59. de Luis O, Valero MC, Jurado LA. WBSCR14, a putative transcription factor gene deleted in Williams-Beuren syndrome: complete characterisation of the human gene and the mouse ortholog. Eur J Hum Genet 2000; 8:215-22.
60. Osborne LR, Soder S, Shi XM, et al. Hemizygous deletion of the syntaxin 1A gene in individuals with Williams syndrome. Am J Hum Genet 1997; 61:449-52.
61. Paperna T, Peoples R, Wang Y-K, Kaplan P, Francke U. Genes for the CPE-receptor (CPETR1) and the human homolog of RVP (CPETR2) are localized within the Williams-Beuren syndrome deletion. Genomics 1998; 54:453-9.
62. Frangiskakis JM, Ewart AK, Morris CA et al. LIM-kinase 1 hemizygosity implicated in impaired visuospacial cognitive cognition. Cell 1996; 86:59-69.
63. Osborne L, Martindale D, Scherer SW, et al. Identification of genes from a 500 kb region that is commonly deleted in Williams syndrome. Genomics 1996; 36:328-36.
64. Doyle JL, DeSilva U, Miller W, Green ED. Divergent human and mouse orthologs of a novel gene (WBSCR15/Wbscr15) reside within the genomic interval commonly deleted in Williams syndrome. Cytogenet Cell Genet 2000; 90:285-90.
65. Peoples RJ, Pérez Jurado LA, Wang Y-K, Kaplan P, Francke U. The gene for the replication factor C subunit 2 (RFC2) is within the 7q11.23 Williams syndrome deletion. Am J Hum Genet 1996; 58:1370-3.
66. Hoogenraad CC, Eussen BHJ, Langeveld A et al. The murine CYLN2 gene: genomic organization, chromosome localization, and comparison to the human gene that is located within the 7q11.23 Williams syndrome critical region. Genomics 1998; 53:348-58.

67. Osborne LR, Campbell T, Daradich A, Scherer SW, Tsui LC. Identification of a putative transcription factor gene (WBSCR11) that is commonly deleted in Williams-Beuren syndrome. Genomics 1999; 57:279-84.
68. Franke Y, Peoples RJ, Francke U. Identification of GTF2IRD1, a putative transcription factor within the Williams-Beuren syndrome deletion at 7q11.23. Cytogenet Cell Genet 1999; 86:296-304.
69. Imreh G, Hallberg E. An integral membrane protein from the nuclear pore complex is also present in the annulate lamellae: implications for annulate lamella formation. Exp Cell Res 2000; 259:180-90.
70. Ito T, Levenstein ME, Fyodorov DV, et al. ACF consists of two subunits, Acf1 and ISWI, that function cooperatively in the ATP-dependent catalysis of chromatin assembly. Genes Dev 1999; 13:1529-39.
71. Natter S, Seiberler S, Hufnagl P, et al. Isolation of cDNA clones coding for IgE autoantigens with serum IgE from atopic dermatitis patients. FASEB J 1998; 14:1559-69.
72. Tsukita S, Furuse M. Pores in the wall: claudins constitute tight junction strands containing aqueous pores. J Cell Biol 2000; 149:13-6.
73. Rosenbloom J, Abrams WR, Mecham R. Extracellular matrix 4: the elastic fiber. FASEB J. 1993; 7:1208-18.
74. Stanyon CA, Bernard O. LIM-kinase1. Int J Biochem Cell Biol 1999; 31:389-94.
75. Reynolds N, Fantes PA, MacNeill SA. A key role for replication factor C in DNA replication checkpoint function in fission yeast. Nucleic Acids Res 1999; 27:462-9.
76. Richter NJ, Rogers GW, Hensold JO, Merrick WC. Further biochemical and kinetic characterization of human eukaryotic initiation factor 4H. J Biol Chem 1999; 274:35415-24.
77. Hoogenraad CC, Akhmanova A, Grosveld F, De Zeeuw CI, Galjart N. Functional analysis of CLIP-115 and its binding to microtubules. J Cell Sci 2000; 113:2285-97.
78. Bayarsaihan D, Ruddle FH. Isolation and characterization of BEN, a member of the TFII-I family of DNA-binding proteins containing distinct helix-loop-helix domains. Proc Natl Acad Sci U S A 2000; 97:7342-7.
79. O'Mahoney JV, Guven KL, Lin J, et al. Identification of a novel slow-muscle-fiber enhancer binding protein, MusTRD1. Mol Cell Biol 1998; 18:6641-52. .
80. Roy AL, Du H, Gregor PD, et al. Cloning of an inr- and E-box-binding protein, TFII-I, that interacts physically and functionally with USF1. EMBO J. 1997; 16:7091-104.
81. Nauseef WM. The NADPH-dependent oxidase of phagocytes. Proc Assoc Am Physicians. 1999;111:373-82.
82. Dridi SM, Ghomrasseni S, Bonnet D, et al. Skin elastic fibers in Williams syndrome. Am J Med Genet 1999; 87:134-8.
83. O'Connor WN, Davis JB, Geissler R, et al. Supravalvular aortic stenosis. Clinical and pathologic observations in six patients. Arch Pathol Lab Med 1985; 109:179-85.
84. Li DY, Brooke B, Davis EC, et al. Elastin is an essential determinant of arterial morphogenesis. Nature 1998; 393: 276-80.
85. Li DY, Faury G, Taylor DG, et al. Novel arterial pathology in mice and humans hemizygous for elastin. J Clin Invest 1998; 102:1783-7.
86. Tassabehji M, Metcalfe K, Karmiloff-Smith A et al. Williams syndrome: use of chromosomal microdeletions as a tool to dissect cognitive and physical phenotypes. Am J Hum Genet 1999; 64: 118-25.
87. Botta A, Novelli G, Mari A, et al. Detection of an atypical 7q11.23 deletion in Williams syndrome patients which does not include the STX1A and FZD3 genes. J Med Genet. 1999; 36:478-80.
88. Korenberg JR, Chen XN, Hirota H, et al. Genome structure and cognitive map of Williams syndrome. J Cogn Neurosci 2000; 12 (Suppl 1):89-107.

89. Wang MS, Schinzel A, Kotzot D, et al. Molecular and clinical correlation study of Williams-Beuren syndrome: No evidence of molecular factors in the deletion region or imprinting affecting clinical outcome. Am J Med Genet 1999; 86:34-43.
90. Stamm C, Friehs I, Ho SY, et al. Congenital supravalvar aortic stenosis: a simple lesion? Eur J Cardiothorac Surg 2001; 19:195-202.
91. McDonald AH, Gerlis LM, Sommerville J. Familial arteriopathy with associated pulmonary and systemic arterial stenosis. Brit. Heart J 1969; 31:375-85.
92. Tassabehji M, Metcalfe K, Donnai D, et al. Elastin: genomic structure and point mutations in patients with supravalvular aortic stenosis. Hum Mol Genet 1997; 6:1029-36.
93. Urban Z, Michels VV, Thibodeau SN, et al. Supravalvular aortic stenosis: a splice site mutation within the elastin gene results in reduced expression of two aberrantly spliced transcripts. Hum. Genet. 1999; 104: 135-142
94. Urban Z, Michels VV, Thibodeau SN, et al. Isolated supravalvular aortic stenosis: functional haploinsufficiency of the elastin gene as a result of nonsense-mediated decay. Hum Genet 2000; 106:577-88.
95. Metcalfe K, Rucka AK, Smoot L. Elastin: mutational spectrum in supravalvular aortic stenosis. Eur J Hum Genet 2000; 8:955-63.
96. Beighton PH. The dominant and recessive forms of cutis laxa. J Med Genet 1972; 9:216-21.
97. Sephel GC, Byers PH, Holbrook KA, Davidson JM. Heterogeneity of elastin expression in cutis laxa fibroblast strains. J Invest Derm 1989; 93:147-53.
98. Zhang MC, Giro M, Quaglino D, Davidson JM. Transforming growth factor-beta reverses a posttranscriptional defect in elastin synthesis in a cutis laxa skin fibroblast strain. J Clin Invest 1995; 95:986-94.
99. Nusbaum C, Slonim DK, Harris KL, et al. A YAC-based physical map of the mouse genome. Nat Genet 1999; 22:388-93.
100. Venter JC, Adams MD, Myers EW, et al. The Sequence of the Human Genome. Science. 2001; 291:1304-51.
101. International human genome sequencing consortium. Initial sequencing and analysis of the human genome. Nature 2001; 409:860-921.

11. MITOCHONDRIAL CARDIOMYOPATHY

R.J.E. Jongbloed , B.J.C. van den Bosch, I.F.M. de Coo, H.J.M. Smeets

Introduction

One of the important functions of mitochondria is the production of ATP by the process of oxidative phosphorylation (OXPHOS) [1]. OXPHOS defects become clinically manifest, if the ATP productions gets below a tissue specific threshold level. Based on energy consumption, the organs most likely to be affected are the central nervous system, skeletal and cardiac muscle, pancreas islets, liver and kidney. In case of the heart, OXPHOS defects may lead to hypertrophic (HCM), dilated (DCM) or hypertrophic dilated cardiomyopathy (HDCM), often as part of specific syndromes, but also as the sole expression of the defect [2]. Especially, when cardiomyopathies are identified by echocardiogram in infants, mitochondrial dysfunction has been reported and should be specifically evaluated [3]. Appropriate tests include oral glucose tolerance (high prevalence of diabetes) and lactate and creatine kinase levels in blood (often raised). Urine organic and amino acids may also be abnormal. Histochemical analysis of skeletal muscle biopsies may show subsarcolemmal accumulations of mitochondria (ragged red fibres) or cytochrome c oxidase deficiency. Studies of activities of the respiratory chain enzyme complexes involved in OXPHOS should also be performed. OXPHOS is generated by 5 enzyme complexes, which are located in the inner membrane of the mitochondria, and deficiencies of the OXPHOS complexes I, III and IV have frequently been reported in HCM and DCM [4]. Thirteen of the subunits of the enzyme complexes are encoded by the mtDNA, a small, circular DNA molecule of 16.6 kb (figure 1). It has a genetic code, which differs from the nuclear DNA, and codes also for 22 transfer RNAs and 2 ribosomal RNAs. The remaining subunits and all other proteins, involved in protein trafficking, unfolding and assembly or in mtDNA replication, transcription or translation are encoded by nuclear genes. Genetic defects causing mitochondrial disease, can therefore either be found in mitochondrial or nuclear genes.

Mitochondrial DNA and mutations

Defects in the mtDNA (figure 1) differ in a number of aspects from the defects in nuclear genes [5]. Firstly, the mtDNA and mtDNA diseases segregate maternally and

PA Doevendans and AA Wilde (eds.), Cardiovascular genetics, 127-137.

are transmitted through the cytoplasm of the oocyte to the offspring. Secondly, each cell contains several hundreds to thousands mitochondria, each with 2 to 10 copies mtDNA. Defects in mtDNA only become manifest, if the percentage mutated mitochondrial DNA (heteroplasmy), exceeds a tissue specific threshold level. Thirdly, mitochondria are randomly segregated to daughter cells during replication and changes in the percentage mutated mtDNA can occur among daughter cells and tissues. This somatic variation in family members, carrying the same mutations, can lead to different clinical manifestations of the same mutation. For example, the mtDNA 3243 mutation can either manifest as Mitochondrial Encephalopathy Lactic Acidosis and Stroke-like episodes (MELAS), deafness, HCM, renal failure or diabetes mellitus (figure 2). Extreme variations in mutation load occur during oogenesis, because the number of mtDNA molecules reduces drastically. The number of transmission units mentioned in literature varies between 1 and >100, which subsequently repopulate the oocyte and embryo [6,7]. Finally, the mutation rate of mtDNA is about 10-20 times higher than the nuclear DNA, because free radicals generated during OXPHOS are highly mutagenic and mitochondria have only limited repair mechanisms [8]. As the mtDNA lacks protecting histons and does not have large introns or intergenic regions, mutations often will have a pathogenic effect.

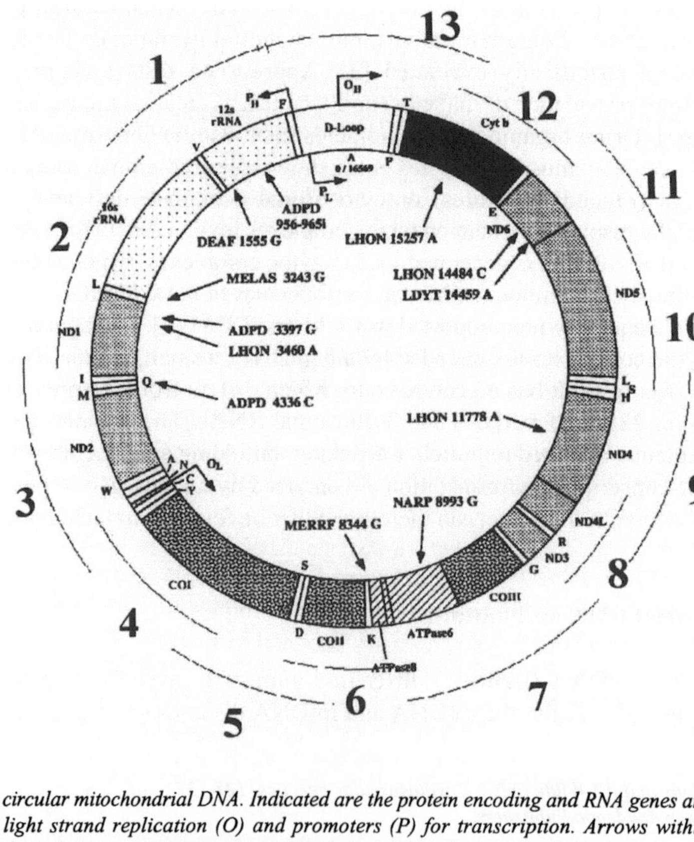

Figure 1. The circular mitochondrial DNA. Indicated are the protein encoding and RNA genes and the origin of heavy and light strand replication (O) and promoters (P) for transcription. Arrows within the circle indicate a number of common point mutations. Numbers 1-13 on the outside of the circle are the fragments generated for DHPLC analysis (figure 5).

The mode of inheritance of mitochondrial cardiomyopathy depends on the genetic defect involved. Single large deletions in the mtDNA are sporadic and are rarely, if ever, transmitted to the offspring. Point mutations in the RNA or protein encoding genes of the mtDNA show a maternal segregation pattern [9] (figure 2). Although mutations in the mtDNA can be the sole DNA defect involved, it is also possible that the mutated mtDNA is a risk factor, contributing to the development of HCM or DCM by exaggerating the effect of nuclear gene mutations [10]. In this respect, it is noteworthy that the high mutation rate in the mtDNA may lead to somatic OXPHOS impairment and may contribute to ageing and related diseases. Mutations in nuclear genes with a mitochondrial function or causing a mtDNA defect (multiple deletions in or reduced number [depletions] of mtDNA molecules) can either be autosomal dominant or recessive, or X-linked [11].

Mitochondrial DNA mutations in cardiomyopathies

Most mtDNA mutations associated with cardiomyopathy have been identified in tRNA genes. tRNA molecules have a tripletRNA code on one site complementary to mRNA, and carry an aminoacid in a different domain. After amino acid delivery to a growing peptide, the transfer RNA will pick up a new free amino acid. Therefore, the tRNAs are crucial components in the translation process and a mutation in one of the tRNA genes may impair the dynamics of translation in general. Mutations have been identified in a number of tRNA genes, some of which are described in more detail below, including the genes for tRNA-Leucine (UUR) (A3243G [12], A3260G [13], C3303T [14]), tRNA-Isoleucine (A4269G [15], A4295G [16], A4300G [17]), tRNA-Lysine (A8344G [18], G8363A [19]) and tRNA-Glycine (T9997C [20]). Mutations have also been described in the mtDNA rRNA genes (A1555G [21]) and protein encoding genes, for example as a rare association of Leigh disease (T8993G in the ATPase 6 gene [22]) or Parkinsonism/MELAS overlap syndrome (4 bp deletion cytochrome b gene [23]).

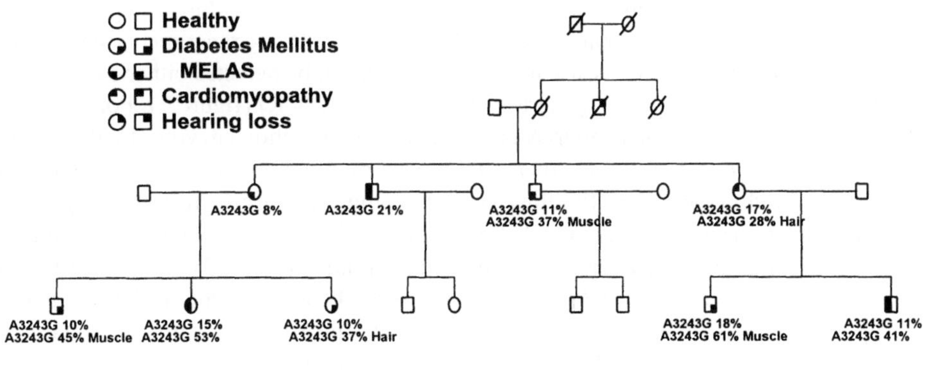

Figure 2. *Fictitious family with the MELAS A3243G mutation, based on own and literature data. The disease segregates solely through the maternal lineage and the clinical manifestations and percentage of the mutation vary broadly. Clinicians should be aware that these clinical features are caused by the same genetic defect.*

The A3243G mutation in the tRNA for leucine, is commonly associated with MELAS syndrome [12]. Cardiac involvement occurs in 20-30% of the patients with the full-blown MELAS syndrome, usually in the form of HCM, but also sometimes the Wolf-Parkinson-White syndrome is present. The A3243G mutation has also been described in a large pedigree with maternally inherited diabetes mellitus, sensorineural deafness, HCM and renal failure. Rarely, HCM is the predominant manifestation of this mutation. The C3303T mutation was described in a family with severe infantile cardiomyopathy, but presentation can range to moderate severe cardiomyopathy and isolated skeletal myopathy [14]. The A4300G mutation was described in a large Italian family with the heart as the only affected organ [17]. The A8344G mutation is associated with MERRF syndrome, so called because of the presenting symptoms (Myoclonic Epilepsy with Ragged Red Fibers) [18]. A review of 62 patients showed that 33% had cardiac problems. The A1555G mutation in the 12S rRNA gene is usually associated with maternally inherited deafness, but has been found in a family with maternally inherited restrictive cardiomyopathy [21].
Single large mtDNA rearrangements (deletion/duplication) are found in Kearns-Sayre syndrome patients, 20% of whom have cardiac involvement, typically consisting of conduction defects and DCM [24]. The clinical appearance of the Kearns-Sayre syndrome includes myopathy, ptosis, progressive external ophtalmoplegia and abnormal retinal pigmentation. A comprehensive database for the human mitochondrial DNA (mtDNA) is MITOMAP (www.gen.emory.edu/cgi-bin/MITOMAP). The database uses the mtDNA sequence as the unifying element for bringing together information on mitochondrial genome structure and function, pathogenic mutations and their clinical characteristics, population associated variation, and gene-gene interactions.

Detection of known mitochondrial DNA mutations

Large deletions and duplications usually occur in the mtDNA in patients with specific syndromes, like Chronic-Progressive External Ophthalmoplegia (CPEO), Kearns-Sayre syndrome, Pearson syndrome and diabetes mellitus with deafness. Duplications have also been found in patients with Pearson syndrome and Kearns-Sayre syndrome and deletions and duplications can co-exist. More than 100 rearrangements have been described in mitochondrial disease in general, which can be detected either by Southern blot analysis or long range polymerase chain reaction (PCR) (figure 3). For Southern blotting the 16.6 kb circular mtDNA is digested by a restriction enzyme (PvuII), which only cleaves once and linearizes the mtDNA. Size fractionation by gel electrophoresis, transfer to a nylon membrane (blotting) and screening with specific mtDNA probes will reveal if deletions are present and what part of the mtDNA is deleted. Long range PCR [25] has recently become a rapid and sensitive alternative (figure 3). The entire 16.6kb mtDNA molecule is amplified and the length of the PCR fragments is determined on an agarose gel. As PCR preferentially amplifies shorter fragments, it is not reliable to determine the mutation load from this assay and Southern blot analysis has to be performed to quantify the amount of deleted mtDNA. Also, discrimination between deletions and duplications can only be determined by Southern blot analysis. Sometimes multiple deletions can be observed, especially in CPEO, which are caused by nuclear gene defects [11].

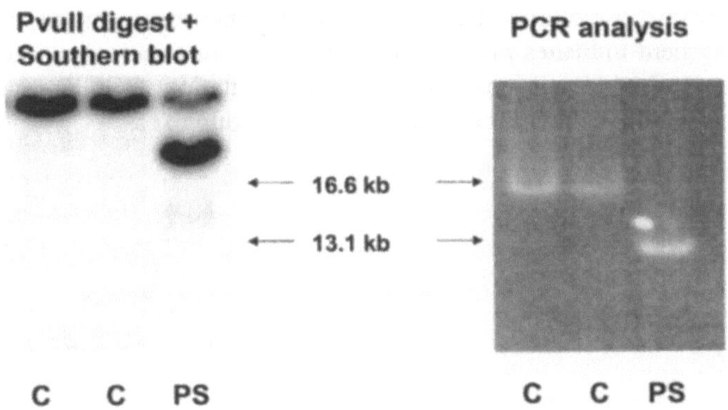

***Figure 3**. Detection of deletions in the mtDNA. The 16.6kb circular mtDNA can either be tested by Southern blot analysis of PvuII-digested DNA or long range PCR and agarose gel electrophoresis. A deletion of 3.4 kb is visible in the patient with Pearson syndrome (PS) and not in the controls (C). No normal mtDNA is visible after PCR, although the Southern blot analysis shows that it is present in substantial amount.*

Over 100 different point mutations in mtDNA, affecting protein encoding, tRNA and rRNA genes, have been described in patients with various manifestations of mitochondrial disease, about 20% involving cardiomyopathies. As the number of mutations increased, protocols were developed to determine which specific mutation should be tested in which case. The information used, includes clinical presentation, metabolic measurements, OXPHOS function and mitochondrial morphology. A broad variety of technologies exists to test with high sensitivity for known mutations. Mutation specific restriction digestion can be applied (figure 4). If the mutation does not change a restriction site, this can be accomplished by introducing an artificial restriction site by modifying the PCR primer. Alternative techniques are allele-specific primer extension, allele-specific oligonucleotide (see Chapter 1). In general mutation percentages of less than 1% are detectable allowing a reliable pre-screening in blood of patients, eliminating the necessity to start with muscle biopsy specimens.

Detection of unknown mtDNA mutations

Many methods can be used to screen for unknown heteroplasmic mutations. Two methods: 1. denaturing high-performance liquid chromatography (DHPLC) and 2. denaturing gradient gel electrophoresis (DGGE) detect specifically heteroduplexes (DNA strands composed of wild type and mutant DNA, carrying a mismatch at the site of the mutation), generated by heteroplasmic mutations. The advantage is that the large number of homoplasmic polymorphisms are not detected. A protocol was developed in which the entire mitochondrial DNA was amplified in 13 fragments [26]. Each fragment is cleaved by restriction enzymes, denatured and renatured. The fragments are loaded on the DHPLC column (Transgenomic Inc, San Jose, CA). Elution is performed at temperatures just below the melting temperature of the fragments and a denaturing acetonitrile gradient is applied. Heteroduplexes are less stable than homoduplexes and elute earlier from the column (figure 5). The presence of a single peak for each restriction fragment indicates no heteroduplexes, the presence of an additional peak indicates a heteroduplex and thus a heteroplasmic mutation. DGGE is also based on differences in melting behaviour of homo- and heteroduplexes.

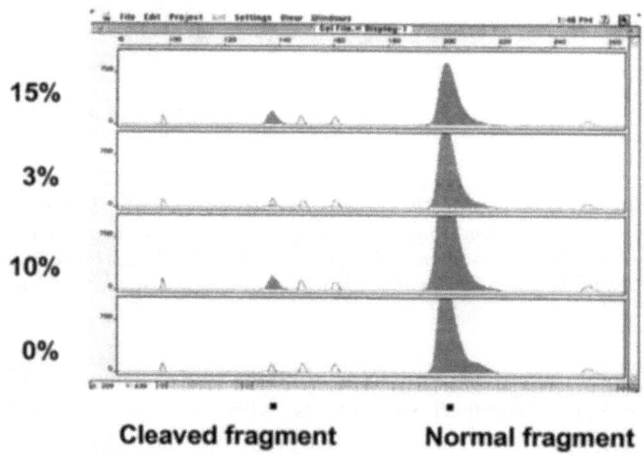

***Figure 4**. Mutation specific restriction digestion of the A3243G mutation. The mutation creates a restriction site and when the mutation is present the PCR fragment will be cleaved in two smaller fragments. One of the PCR primers is labelled and the digested PCR fragments are resolved on an ABI3100 automated sequencer. The electropherograms show the intact normal PCR fragment (N=normal) and one of the digestion products (Cleaved fragment). The ratio of the peaks gives the amount of mutated mtDNA in relation to the wild type. The negative control (0%) does not carry the mutation.*

Fragments are resolved by electrophoresis through a denaturing gradient of formamide and urea. Heteroduplexes melt at lower concentrations of denaturing agents than homoduplexes. Following melting the fragments get stuck in the agarose gel and the presence of 2 fragments with a different mobility is indicative of a mutation. Most other pre-screening methods do not discriminate between homoplasmic and heteroplasmic mutations.

Sequence analysis lacks the sensitivity to detect low amounts of heteroplasmic mutations. However, homoplasmic mutations can be detected best by sequence analysis or, in future, by DNA chips. Any pre-screening method will detect many sequence alterations, which have to be characterized by sequence analysis subsequenly. It is often difficult in case of homoplasmic mutations to discriminate genetically between neutral variants and pathogenic mutations. Functional tests of the mutations or model experiments need to be performed.

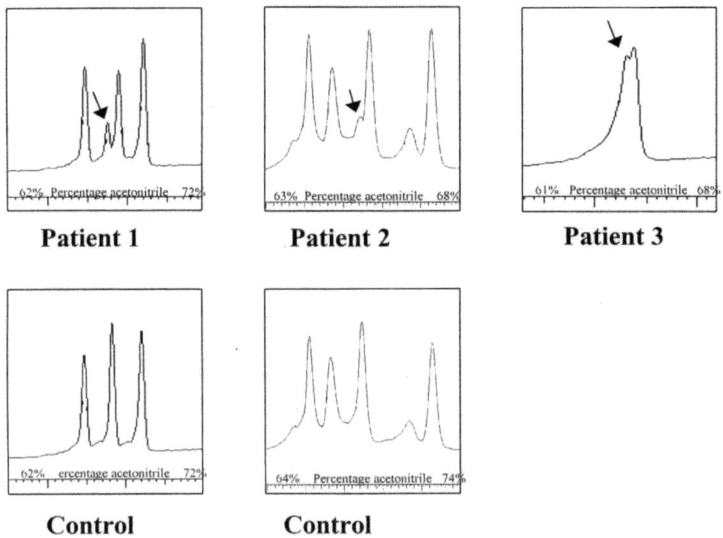

Figure 5. *DHPLC analysis of the mtDNA for heteroplasmic mutations. The circular mtDNA is shown in figure 1. The mtDNA is amplified in 13 fragments (numbered 1-13), which are digested in multiple fragments by restriction enzymes. The DHPLC patterns of 3 patients and their respective controls are shown. No control was available for the fragment of patient 3. The arrows indicate the heteroduplex peaks. Sequence analysis revealed that patient 1 carried the A3302G mutation (70%), patient 2 the T3271C mutation (80%) and patient 3 the T9176C mutation (93%).*

Mutations in nuclear genes with a mitochondrial function

Defects in the mtDNA can be caused by nuclear gene mutations. Alterations in genes affecting functions, such as replication of the mtDNA, may cause multiple deletions in the mtDNA [25]. Families have been described with an autosomal dominant inheritance pattern of chronic progressive external ophthalmoplegia (CPEO) and DCM and HCM. In 12 families with multiple deletions, more than 1/3 of the patients had cardiac abnormalities. Mutations in similar genes may cause the mtDNA depletion syndrome, which is characterized by a reduced level of the mtDNA in infancy [27]. This disease can be fatal within the first year of life and HCM has been found in some patients. Other nuclear genes with a mitochondrial function and defects can be associated with cardiomyopathy, like Friedreich ataxia (chapter 12). The technology to screen nuclear genes for mutations is described in the first chapter. A mouse model, in which the Adenine nucleotide translocator I gene was knocked out, developed classical hypertrophic cardiomyopathy followed by dilated cardiomyopathy [28]. Another model with a disruption of the mitochondrial transcription factor A gene developed features similar to Kearns Sayre syndrome, including dilated cardiomyopathy [29]. These genes are straightforward candidates for mitochondrial cardiomyopathies and it can be expected that many more genes will follow.

Investigational scheme for mitochondrial disease [30]

Clinical investigations	Blood: Creatine kinase, lactate, glucose
	Urine: Organic and amino acids
	CSF: Protein and lactate
	CXR, ECG +/- ECHO
	EEG/EMG
	CT/MRI
Specific syndromes	MELAS, MERRF, LHON, Leigh syndrome
Family investigations	Maternal inheritance of disease (manifestations may differ among affected family members!)
Histochemistry muscle	Ragged Red Fibres, COX deficiency
Biochemistry	OXPHOS complex enzyme deficiencies

DNA-investigations fall apart in 4 categories:

1. Analysis of specific mutations in the mtDNA
2. Screening for mtDNA deletions
3. Screening the entire mtDNA for point mutations
4. Analysis of nuclear genes, if mtDNA excluded

Investigations 1 and 2 yield results rapidly, as only a limited number of specific DNA mutations are being analyzed. A negative result does not exclude mtDNA involvement. Investigation 3 is quite laborious and takes considerable time. Investigation 4 can be rapid if a good candidate gene is available, but may last several years or may even remain unresolved, if this is not the case.

Management of patients:

No cure is available for patients with mitochondrial cardiomyopathy due to mtDNA defects. Management can be divided in counselling, supportive therapy (pacemaker) and pharmacological therapy (vitamins and co-factors). Counselling for prognosis, presymptomatic testing and inheritance is complex, because of the extreme clinical and genetic variability. Prenatal diagnosis is only a limited option for specific mutations.

Conclusion

Although frequently and increasingly reported, it is at this point unclear whether OXPHOS or mtDNA defects are a common cause of primary cardiomyopathies. In a study of 601 endomyocardial biopsy specimens of patients with DCM, 14% showed ultrastructurally abnormal mitochondria and 3% harbored likely pathogenic mtDNA mutations and defects in OXPHOS complexes I and IV [30]. As idiopathic DCM is supposed to be inherited in about 20% of the cases, a careful search for all potentially affected genes is important, including the mtDNA and nuclear genes involved mitochondrial functioning. This is especially the case if the cardiomyopathy is already present in the neonate or infant and the involvement of the mitochondria is supported by additional clinical and laboratory investigations or by maternal inheritance. In case of heteroplasmic or homoplasmic mtDNA mutations it can be difficult to judge the pathogenic effect, which may vary from contributing risk factor to primary cause. Insight in this may become especially important as mutations in the mtDNA were more frequently found in heart or muscle of patients with DCM than in control subjects, suggesting a possibly age-related, cumulative negative effect on heart function.

References

1. Lightowlers RN, Chinnery PF, Turnbull DM, Howell N. Mammalian mitochondrial genetics: heredity, heteroplasmy and disease. Trends Genet 1997; 13:450-55.
2. Santorelli FM, Tessa A, d'Amati G, Casali C. the emerging concept of mitochondrial cardiomyopathies. Am Heart J 2001; 141:e1.
3. Marin-Garcia J, Ananthakrishnan R, Goldenthal MJ, Filiano J, Perez-Atayde A. Mitochondrial dysfunction in skeletal muscle of children with cardiomyopathies. Pediatrics 1999; 103:456-59.
4. Towbin JA, Lipshultz SE. Genetics of neonatal cardiomyopathy. Curr Opin Cardiol 1999; 14:250-62.
5. Chinnery PF, Turnbull DM. Mitochondrial DNA and disease. Lancet 1999; 354:17-21.
6. Janssen RPS, De Boer K. The bottleneck: mitochondrial imperatives in oogenesis an ovarian follicular rate. Mol Cell Endocrinol 1998; 145:81-88.
7. Marchington DR, Hartshorne GM, Barlow D, Poulton J. Homoplasmic tract heteroplasmy in mtDNA from tissues and single oocytes: support for a genetic bottleneck. Am J Hum Genet 1997; 60:408-16.
8. Wallace DC. Mitochondrial diseases in man and mouse. Science 1999; 283:1482-8.
9. Chinnery PF, Turnbull DM. Mitochondrial DNA mutations in the pathogenesis of human disease. Molec Med Tod 2000; 6:425-32.
10. Arbustini E, Fasani R, Morbini P, et al. Coexistence of mitochondrial DNA and β myosin heavy chain mutations in hypertrophic cardiomyopathy with late congestive heart failure. Heart 1998; 80:548-58.
11. Zeviani M, Petruzzella V, Carrozzo R. Disorders of nuclear-mitochondrial intergenomic signalling. J Bioenerg Biomembr 1997; 29:121-30.
12. Hirano M, Pavlakis S. Mitochondrial myopathy, encephalopathy, lactic acidosis, and stroke-like episodes (MELAS): current concepts. J Child Neurol 1994; 9:4-13.
13. Zeviani M, Gellera C, Antozzi C et al. Maternally inherited myopathy and cardiomyopathy: association with mutation in mitochondrial DNA tRNA [LeuUUR] . Lancet 1991; 338:143-7.
14. Bruno C, Kirby DM, Koga Y, et al. The mitochondrial DNA C3303T mutation can cause cardiomyopathy and/or skeletal myopathy. J Pediatr 1999; 135:197-202.
15. Taniike M, Fukushima H, Yanagihara I, et al. Mitochondrial tRNA[Ile] mutation in fatal cardiomyopathy. Bichem Biophys Res Commun 1992; 186:47-53.
16. Merante F, Myint T, Tein I, et al. An additional mitochondrial tRNA [Ile] point mutation (A to G at nucleotide 4295) causing hypertrophic cardiomyopathy. Hum Mutat 1996; 8:216-22.
17. Casali C, Santorelli FM, d'Amati G, et al. A novel mtDNA mutation in maternally inherited cardiomyopathy. Biochem Biophys Res Commun 1995; 213:588-93.
18. Shoffner JM, Lott MT, Lezza AM, et al. Myoclonic epilepsy and ragged-red fiber disease (MERRF) is associated with a mitochondrial DNA tRNA[Lys] mutation. Cell 1990; 61:931-7.
19. Santorelli FM, Mak S-C, El-Schahawi M, et al. maternally inherited cardiomyopathy and hearing loss associated with a novel mutation in the mitochondrial DNA tRNALys gene (G8363A). Am j Hum Genet 1996; 58:933-9.
20. Merante F, Tein I, Benson L, et al. maternally inherited mitochondrial hypertrophic cardiomyopathy due to a novel T-to-C transition at nucleotide 9997 in the mitochondrial tRNA(gly) gene. Am J Hum Genet 1994; 55:437-46.
21. Santorelli FM, Tanji K, Manta P, et al. maternally inherited cardiomyopathy: an atypical presentation of the mtDNA 12S rRNA gene A1555G mutation. Am J Hum Genet 1999; 64:295-300.
22. Marin-Garcia J, Ananthakrishnan R, Korson M, et al. Cardiac mitochondrial dysfunction in Leigh syndrome. Pediatr Cardiol 1996; 17:387-9.
23. De Coo IF, Van Oost, BA, Renier WO, Ruitenbeek W, et al. A 4-base pair deletion in the mitochondrial cytochrome b gene associated with parkinsonism/MELAS overlap syndrome.

Ann Neurol 1999; 45:130-3.
24. Zeviani M, Moraes CT, DiMauro, et al. Deletions of mitochondrial DNA in Kearns-Sayre syndrome. Neurology 1998; 38:1339-46.
25. DeCoo IF, Gussinklo T, Arts PJ, Van Oost BA, Smeets HJM. A PCR test for progressive external ophthalmoplegia and Kearns-Sayre syndrome on DNA from blood samples. J Neurol Sci 1997; 149:37-40.
26. Van den Bosch BJ, De Coo RF, Scholte HR, et al. Mutation analysis of the entire mitochondrial genome using denaturing high performance liquid chromatography. Nucleic Acids Res 2000; 28:E89.
27. Marin-Garcia J, Ananthakrishnan R, Goldenthal MJ. Hypertrophic cardiomyopathy with mitochondrial DNA depletion and respiratory enzyme defects. Pediatr Cardiol 1998; 19:266-8.
28. Graham BH, Waymire KG, Cottrell, Trounce IA, MacGregor GR, Wallace DC. A mouse model for mitochondrial myopathy and cardiomyopathy resulting from a deficiency in heart/muscle isoform of the adenine nucleotide translocator. Nat genet 1997; 16:226-34.
29. Wang J, Wilhelmsson H, Graff C, et al. Dilated cardiomyopathy and atrioventricular conduction blocks induced by heart-specific inactivation of mitochondrial DNA gene expression. Nat Genet 1999; 21:133-137.
30. Arbustini E, Diegoli M, Fasani R, et al. Mitochondrial DNA mutations and mitochondrial abnormalities in dilated cardiomyopathy. Am J Pathol 1998; 153:1501-10.

12. HYPERTROPHIC CARDIOMYOPATHY

L. Carrier, R.J.E. Jongbloed, H.J.M. Smeets, P.A. Doevendans

Introduction

Up till a decade ago, diagnostic identification of acquired or hereditary cardiac diseases was based upon clinical observations and pedigree analysis and supported by instrumental and biochemical diagnostic tests. The molecular basis of the majority of these disorders was grossly unknown or speculative. In the last ten years, rapidly evolving and innovative strategies in molecular biology and genetics have completely changed this scenario. Families with well-documented hereditary disorders, sometimes known for several decades, appeared very attractive to start the search for the causative molecular defect. Using linkage analysis with DNA markers (DNA variants scattered along the genome), it became possible to search for linkage of particular markers and the disease-causing locus in a given family. Once the risk locus was identified, several strategies to identify the gene defect could be applied. By comparing families with identical genetic defects and by an inventory on the clinical features of all affected individuals it may be possible to establish genotype-phenotype correlations, which in turn can lead to an exact diagnosis.

In this chapter we discuss clinical and genetic guidelines to identify the familial form of primary HCM. HCM includes a group of primary myocardial disorders of previously undefined etiology, which are characterized by a high incidence of morbidity and mortality. Observations of myocardial diseases that can reasonably be interpreted as HCM were made in the middle of the last century at the Hospital La Salpêtrière in Paris by A. Vulpian, who called what he saw at the macroscopic level a "rétrécissement de l'orifice ventriculo-aortique" or « sub-aortic stricture » [1]. It was however only in the late 1950s that the unique clinical features of HCM were systematically described [2,3]. Hypertrophy can occur in either ventricle although usually there is involvement of the interventricular septum, with or without involvement of either the anterior wall or the posterior wall in continuity. A particular form of regional involvement affects the apex but spares the upper portion of the septum (apical hypertrophy) [4]. Typically, the left ventricular volume is normal or reduced. Systolic gradients are common. Typical morphological changes include myocyte hypertrophy and disarray surrounding the areas of increased loose connective tissue. Arrhythmias and premature sudden death are common [5]. Sudden death accounts for about 50% of the mortality in HCM. It may be

PA Doevendans and AA Wilde (eds.), Cardiovascular genetics, 139-154.

the first clinical manifestation in some affected individuals. Previous reports estimated its incidence to 2 to 4% annually in adults and 4 to 6% in children and adolescents [6-8] but these numbers are certainly overestimated because they are based on referral populations. Annual mortality rate in unselected patients has been reported to be 0.5 to 1.5% [9]. HCM is the most common cause of sudden death in young athletes, accounting for 36% of cases. Although HCM has been regarded largely as a relatively uncommon cardiac disease, the prevalence of echocardiographically defined HCM in a large cohort of apparently healthy young adults selected from a community-based general population was reported to be as high as 0.2% [10].

Familial hypertrophic cardiomyopathy (FHC)

Familial disease with autosomal dominant inheritance predominates, and the first large pedigree of familial hypertrophic cardiomyopathy (FHC) was reported in 1960 [11]. None of the previous hypotheses on the pathophysiological mechanisms would have predicted that defects in sarcomeric genes could be a possible molecular basis for the disease. The results of molecular genetic studies have nevertheless shown that all mutations found thus far concern nine different sarcomeric proteins (figure 1, Table 1): three myofilament proteins, the β–myosin heavy chain (β-MyHC), the ventricular myosin essential light chain (MLC-1s/v) and the ventricular myosin regulatory light chain (MLC-2s/v); four thin filament proteins, α–cardiac actin (α-cAct), cardiac troponin T (cTnT), cardiac troponin I (cTnI), and α-tropomyosin (α-TM); one myosin-binding protein, the cardiac myosin binding protein C (cMyBP-C), and finally the third filament protein, titin (TTN).
These genes certainly do not represent the whole spectrum of FHC disease genes since an additional locus was reported on chromosome 7q3 [12]. In these patients FHC was associated with the Wolff-Parkinson White Syndrome. One might reasonably hypothesize that disease genes yet to be identified include additional components of the sarcomere. Indeed, very recently, was reported as an abstract a mutation in *MYH6*, the strongly *MYH7* homologous gene encoding the α-MyHC in a FHC proband [13]. So, FHC is caused by a structural and/or functional impairment of the sarcomere, which is the contractile unit of striated muscle (figure 1). Sarcomeric gene mutations may also be associated to either the transition between hypertrophic and dilated cardiomyopathy [14] or to primary dilated cardiomyopathy [15,16]. This finding suggests that the position of the mutated amino acid triggers the development of either hypertrophic or dilated cardiomyopathy by impaired force generation versus impaired force transmission, respectively. The molecular mechanism by which the mutations lead to FHC and the basis for the diversity of the phenotypes is not completely elucidated. It has been generally accepted that cardiac hypertrophy is influenced by a dominant-negative mechanism, which can be explained by either production of a poison polypeptide or failing to incorporate a defective protein into the sarcomere leading to haploinsufficiency.

Table 1. Sarcomeric proteins and genes involved in FHC.

Protein	Gene	FHC Locus	Remarks
β–myosin heavy chain (β-MyHC)	*MYH7*	*CMH1* 14q11-q12	mainly missense mutations
Ventricular essential myosin light chain (MLC-1s/v)	*MYL3*	*CMH5* 3p	mid left ventricular chamber thickening
Ventricular regulatory myosin light chain (MLC-2s/v)	*MYL2*	*CMH6* 12q23-q24.3	Missense mutations and splice donor mutation
α–cardiac actin (α-cAct)	*ACTC*	*CMH8* 15q14	Missense mutations
Cardiac troponin T (cTnT)	*TNNT2*	*CMH2* 1q32	Missense mutations, in frame deletions, splice donor mutations; Mutations are particularly associated with poor prognosis and with only mild hypertrophy; low disease penetrance ± 80%
Cardiac troponin I (cTnI)	*TNNI3*	*CMH7* 19p13.4	Missense mutations and in frame deletion
α–tropomyosin (α-TM)	*TPM1*	*CMH3* 15q22.1	Missense mutations; poor prognosis
Cardiac myosin binding protein C (cMyBP-C)	*MYBPC3*	*CMH4* 11p11.2	Missense mutations, deletions, insertions; mostly truncated proteins; low disease penetrance ± 60% late onset.
Titin	*TTN*	*CMH9* 2q24.3	one missense mutation

In 1999, 143 mutations had been entered in the FHC database (Table 2) [17]. The two major genes appear to be MYH7 and MYBPC3, but one should note that not obligatory all the genes were screened to find the mutation in previous reports. Most of the FHC mutations are missense mutations or deletions that do not disrupt the reading frame with the exception of MYBPC3 in which most are frame shift mutations.

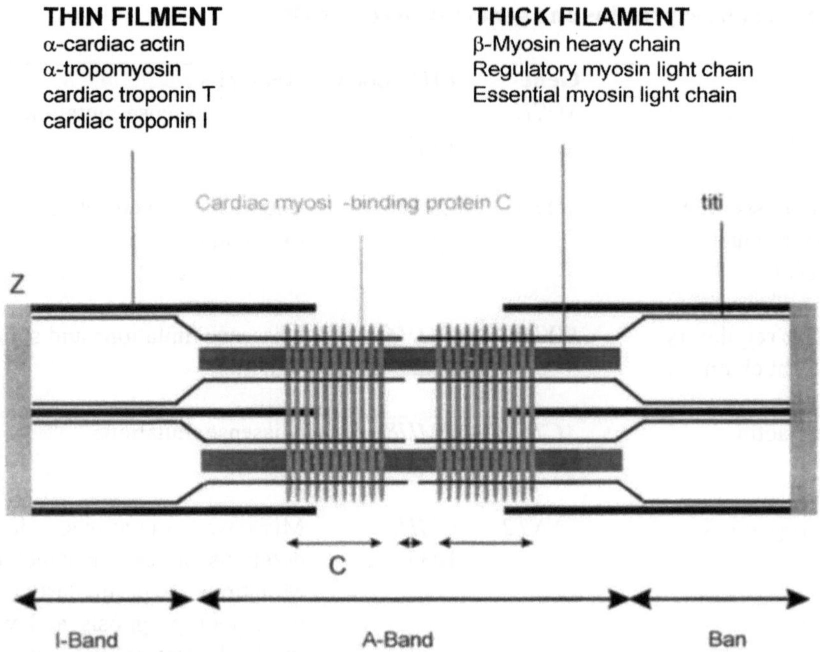

Figure 1. Schematic organization of the sarcomeric proteins associated with FHC (adapted from [18])

Table 2. Distribution of the FHC database mutations (from [18]).

Gene locus	# of mutations	# of missense mutations or deletions in frame	# of frameshift or nonsense mutations
MYH7	70	67	3
MYBP3	30	8	22
TNNT2	14	13	1
MYL2	8	7	1
TNNI3	8	8	-
ACTC	5	5	-
TPM1	5	5	-
MYL3	2	2	-
TTN	1	1	-

Mutations in the β-MyHC gene, MYH7 (CMH1 locus)

Jarcho *et al.* opened this field in 1989 by studying a large Canadian HCM family which had been previously reported by Pare *et al.* in 1961 [19,20]. Linkage analysis showed tight association of a disease locus with marker D14S26, and therefore identified the first locus for FHC, *CMH1*. Among the possible candidate genes involved in HCM, the closely linked cardiac α- and β-myosin heavy chain (MyHC) genes – *MYH6* and *MYH7*, respectively were suspected. Subsequently, a missense mutation was found in the *MYH7* gene [21]. Several other investigators have confirmed the linkage of HCM families to *CMH1* [22,23]. Likewise other groups excluded linkage of FHC families to *CMH1* indicating genetic heterogeneity [24,25]. The β-MyHC consists of 1,939 amino acids and is the major isoform in human ventricular cardiac myocytes and slow twitch skeletal muscles. It is composed of two parts, a globular amino-terminal part of 150 kDa, the heavy meromyosin (HMM) and the rod or tail of 70 kDa, the light meromyosin (LMM). HMM can be separated in two domains by papaïne digestion, the subfragments 1 and 2. Subfragment 2 contains the ATP- and actin-binding sites. More than seventy *MYH7* mutations were identified and most of them are located in HMM.

Mutations in the myosin light chain genes, MYL2 and MYL3 (CMH5 & CMH6 loci)
The muscle myosin proteins consist of two heavy chains and two pairs of light chains. The isoforms of light chains expressed in human ventricles are the ventricular essential myosin light chain (MLC-1s/v) and ventricular regulatory myosin light chain (MLC-2s/v). These two proteins are encoded by *MYL3* and *MYL2*, which are located on chromosome 3p and 12q23-q24.3, respectively [26]. Mutations in both genes were first described to be associated with a particular subtype of cardiac hypertrophy defined by mid left ventricular obstruction and skeletal myopathy [27]. However, it was later demonstrated that *MYL2* is also associated with classical forms of FHC [28].

Mutations in the α–cardiac actin gene, ACTC (CMH8 locus)
Actins are involved in various types of cell motility and they are ubiquitously expressed in all eukaryotic cells [29]. Actins are highly conserved proteins consisting of 377 amino acids. The polymerization of globular actin (g-actin) leads to a structural filament (f-actin) in the form of a two-stranded helix. In vertebrates, three main groups of actin isoforms, α, β and γ, have been identified. The α-actins are found in striated muscles and are a major component of the contractile apparatus. Two missense mutations were initially reported in the *ACTC* gene associated with a dilated form of cardiomyopathy [15]. Thereafter, Mogessen *et al.* reported *ACTC* mutations in families with FHC [30]. Recently three novel mutations (E99L, P164A and A331P) were identified in functionally distinct domains of α–cAct that were associated with an early onset and apical cardiac hypertrophy [31].

Mutations in the cardiac troponin T gene, TNNT2 (CMH2 locus)
Troponin T is the tropomyosin-binding subunit of troponin, which is required for thin filament regulation of contraction. It contains several putative functional domains: phosphorylation sites and protein-binding sites to α–tropomyosin, troponin I and troponin C. The gene *TNNT2* is composed of 17 exons spread over 17 kb and gives rise to multiple isoforms by the use of alternative exons and alternative acceptor sites [2]. Thierfelder *et al.* succeeded to map the *TNNT2* to chromosome 1q32 and presented three unrelated families with a missense mutation and one splicing site mutation in *TNNT2* causing cardiac hypertrophy in affected family members [33]. The splice site mutation was predicted to function as a null allele leading to haploinsufficiency and the authors

suggested that abnormal stoichiometry of sarcomeric proteins caused cardiac hypertrophy. Watkins *et al.* identified eight mutations in the *TNNT2* gene and estimated that mutations in this gene account for approximately 15% of familial HCM cases [34].

Mutations in the cardiac troponin 1 gene, TNN13 (CMH7 locus)
Because all the known FHC disease genes encoded major contractile elements in cardiac muscle, a Japanese group systematically screened cardiac sarcomere genes, including cardiac troponin I (*TNNI3*), and cardiac troponin C in a large group of unrelated patients with HCM. They found mutations in the *TNNI3* in several FHC patients [35]. Family studies showed that an R145G mutation was linked to HCM and a L206Q mutation had occurred 'de novo' strongly suggesting that *TNNI3* is the seventh FHC disease gene.

Mutations in the α– tropomyosin gene, TPM1 (CMH3 locus)
Tropomyosins are rigid rod-like ubiquitous proteins in the thin filament of the sarcomere. They associate with the actin filaments and contribute to the stability of the thin filament. The tissue-specific isoforms are generated by alternative splicing of the α-tropomyosin pre-mRNA. MacLeod and Gooding identified the sequence of the gene and Eyre *et al.* assigned the gene to chromosomal band 15q22 [36,37]. The tropomyosin gene gives rise to four isoforms. The α–tropomyosin gene, *TPM1,* has only 10 exons, which encode 284 amino acids. Four missense mutations have been described in *TPM1* previously [33,34]. Watkins *et al.* concluded that mutations in *TPM1* are a rare cause of HCM, accounting for approximately 3% of the cases. Recently, two novel *TPM1* mutations have been reported, the E180V mutation being associated to the transition between hypertrophic and dilated cardiomyopathy [14], and the V95A mutation showing unique features of mild cardiac hypertrophy with a high mortality rate [38].

Mutations in the cardiac myosin-binding protein C gene, MYBPC3 (CMH4 locus)
Cardiac myosin-binding protein C is located in the C-zone of the sarcomere A-bands and is tightly bound to myosin and titin. The *CMH4* locus was found in 1993 on chromosome 11p13-q13 [39]. Human *MYBPC3* was then localized by fluorescent *in situ* hybridization on chromosome 11p11.2 [40]. It was therefore anticipated that mutations in *MYBPC3* might cause FHC and indeed Bonne *et al.* and Watkins *et al.* simultaneously demonstrated splice mutations and a duplication in this gene in families with HCM [41,42]. Subsequently, several groups found *MYBPC3* mutations in FHC [43-48]. Most of the mutations produce a frame shift leading to a premature termination during translation, resulting in truncated proteins lacking at least the major myosin-binding site. *MYBPC3* is the most frequent mutated gene in French families with HCM (personal communication). The mechanism by which the truncation mutations lead to FHC is not fully understood, because neither the truncated protein nor a decrease of the normal protein was detected in the myocardial tissue of two patients with a *MYBPC3* mutation [44,48]. However, several *ex vivo* analyses and mouse models with *MYBPC3* mutations

Mutations in the titin gene, TTN (CMH9 locus)
Titin is a giant sarcomeric protein, extending from the M-band to the Z-disk of striated muscle sarcomere [54]. It's the third filament protein of the sarcomere. Titin is essential in the assembly of the highly ordered sarcomeres of striated muscles and responsible for the elasticity of relaxed striated muscle. Titin interacts with numerous sarcomeric proteins and provides a mechanical linkage. Only one missense mutation (R740L) has been reported in exon 14 [55]. The substitution occurred in a nonconservative domain located within the α–actinin binding site. The titin mutation may cause HCM in this patient *via* altered affinity to α-actinin.

Friedreich's s Ataxia

Friedreich's ataxia (FRDA) is the most common autosomal recessive ataxia, characterized by degeneration of the large sensory neurons and spinocerebellar tracts, cardiomyopathy and increased incidence of diabetes [56]. Initially, FRDA can be diagnosed with only an isolated HCM in young children even though additional features are not obvious, including ataxia, dysarthria and areflexia. The onset of the disease is before adolescence, most often between the age of 8 and 15 years, and is generally characterized by pyramidal weakness of the legs, dysarthria, nystagmus, diminished or absent tendon reflexes, Babinski sign, impairment of position and vibratory senses, scoliosis, pes cavus, and hammer toe. FRDA is caused by intronic GAA triplet repeat expansion in the frataxin gene [57], which is located on chromosome 9q13. The gene codes for a 18-kDa mitochondrial protein of unknown function. Frataxin has distant homology to *C. elegans* and yeast genes, where it is associated with the mitochondrial membrane, playing a role in regulating mitochondrial iron transport and in the stability of DNA structure. FRDA is caused by severely reduced levels of frataxin. This leads to mitochondrial iron accumulation and to a subsequent defect of respiratory chain and aconitase, probably due to cellular sensitivity to oxidative stress. In most patients FRDA is due to GAA-triplet repeat expansions in the first intron of the frataxin gene but in some cases the disease is due to mutations in the coding region. Most patients are homozygous for the expansions of a GAA triplet repeat within the frataxin gene but a few patients are compound heterozygotes with a point mutation and the GAA-repeat expansion. Recently, the first conditional mouse models for FRDA were generated by homologous recombination, and they exhibit important pathophysiological and biochemical features of the human disease [58]. These mice represent the first mammalian models to evaluate treatment strategies for the human disease.

Genetic analysis

For diagnostic DNA analysis of FHC it is crucial first of all that the diagnosis is unequivocally made without including any false-positives. This is one of the most important steps for the following genetic analyses. It is important that the clinician distinguishes a primary form (only cardiac symptoms) from a secondary form (associated with non-cardiac symptoms). Another important criterion is the age of onset. Primary

HCM is rarely symptomatic in infants and children while secondary HCM can disclose at any age. If HCM is diagnosed in infants and children, clinicians should always add biochemical evaluation and investigation of the neurologic system and skeletal musculature. Careful analysis of the family history and examination of the patient, and, if possible of relatives provides additional information. A sporadic case of HCM can be acquired (non-genetic) or can arise from a "*de novo*" mutation. In case of a positive family history the transmission mode can indicate whether the familial disease is inherited as an autosomal dominant, autosomal recessive or X-linked trait. An exclusively maternal transmission is suggestive for a mitochondrial defect.

Because FHC is very heterogeneous, linkage analysis is mainly the first option to initiate DNA analysis. A number of informative markers, closely linked to candidate genes, are used to investigate whether the disease gene co-segregates with a distinct locus. It should be emphasized that in FHC (with at least three affected and some unaffected relatives), it is much easier to establish the genetic etiology than in sporadic patients. Yet there are some limitations. Sometimes families are too small to perform adequate linkage analysis. In addition, a late clinical presentation of the disease (late-onset) or the presence of asymptomatic patients may obscure linkage analysis. In that case, the known disease genes are directly screened for mutations. For linkage analysis, it is very important to choose highly informative microsatellite markers with a high degree of heterozygosity. If linkage is obvious, a putative candidate gene can be located and a switch to the identification of the gene defect is made. DNA analysis is initiated by screening the complete coding sequence including intronic flanking regions. Depending on the strategy of DNA analysis and the laboratory equipment, identification of a mutation may take quite some time. Sometimes the large size of the gene hampers large routine screenings. If no linkage can be established a genome-wide screen is a next option to investigate whether a novel locus is involved. When a mutation is found in a proband, its disease –causing effect should be confirmed. Mutation should segregate in the family and should be absent in at least 200 normal control chromosomes to exclude low rates of polymorphisms.

Genotype-Phenotype relationships in familial hypertrophic cardiomyopathy

Before genetic analyses, it was well known that the pattern and extent of left ventricular hypertrophy varies greatly from one individual to another and even in first-degree relatives, and that a high incidence of sudden deaths occurs in some families [59]. Genetic studies have provided insight into the heterogeneity of FHC clinical features. However, the results must be seen as preliminary, because the available data relate to only a few hundred individuals, and it is obvious that although a given phenotype may be apparent in a small family, examining large or multiple families with the same mutation is required before drawing unambiguous conclusions. Several concepts nevertheless have emerged, at least for mutations in the *MYH7*, *TNNT2* and *MYBPC3* genes. For *MYH7*, it is clear that prognosis is very variable from one patient to the other (Category A) [60,61,8]. For example, the R403Q and R723G mutations appear to be associated with markedly reduced survival [60,62], whereas some others, such as the V606M, appear more benign [61]. The disease caused by *TNNT2* mutations is usually associated with a 20% incidence of non penetrance, a relatively mild and sometimes subclinical hypertrophy but a high incidence of sudden death which can occur even in the absence of significant clinical left ventricular hypertrophy (category A) [34,63,64]. In one family with a *TNNT2* mutation, however, penetrance is complete, echocardiographic data show a wide range of hypertrophy and there was no sudden cardiac death [65]. Mutations in *MYBPC3* seem to be characterized by specific clinical features with a mild phenotype in young subjects, a delayed age at the onset of symptoms and a favorable prognosis before the age of 40 [66,46]. Genetic studies have allowed the identification of patients with double mutations who develop a more severe form of the disease: compound heterozygotes for *MYH7* mutations [67], double heterozygotes for *MYH7* and *MYBPC3* mutations [68] and homozygotes for a *MYH7* mutation [69]. In addition, a detailed analysis of a "*de novo*" mutation in a French family with HCM allowed the description of the first case of germline mosaicism in FHC [70]. This mosaicism had been inherited from the mother but did not affect her somatic cells. Genetic studies have also revealed the presence of clinically healthy individuals carrying the mutant allele, which is associated in first-degree relatives with a typical phenotype of the disease. Several mechanisms could account for the large variability of the phenotypic expression of the mutations: the degree of functional impairment caused in the sarcomere by the mutation (that may vary markedly with the position of the mutation in the molecule and the type of protein involved), the role of environmental differences and acquired traits (e.g., differences in lifestyle, risk factors, and exercise) and finally the existence of modifier genes and/or polymorphisms that could modulate the phenotypic expression of the disease. The only significant results obtained so far concern the influence of the angiotensin I converting enzyme insertion/deletion (ACE I/D) polymorphism. Association studies showed that, compared to a control population, the D allele is more common in patients with HCM and in patients with a high incidence of sudden cardiac death [71-73]. It was also shown that the association between the D allele and hypertrophy is observed in patients with a *MYH7* R403 codon mutation, but not in *MYBPC3* mutation carriers [74], raising the concept of multiple genetic modifiers in FHC.The genetic status begins to be used as the criterion of reference to reassess diagnostic criteria and penetrance. The diagnosis of FHC is usually based on ECG and echocardiography, and it is generally accepted that echocardiography is a more accurate technique than ECG for the diagnosis in adults [5]. Analysis of a large genotyped population showed that, in fact, ECG and echocardiography have similar diagnostic values for FHC in adults, with an excellent specificity and a lower sensitivity [75]. As for penetrance, it was a much-debated issue. Before molecular genetics analyses, several studies have indicated either a full penetrance [76], or an incomplete one [77,78]. The penetrance of FHC has been re-assessed in a large French genotyped population, and it was found that it is incomplete, age-related and greater in males than in females [79]. This latter data has very important implications for genetic counseling especially for women under the age of fifty. One of the transgenic mouse models of FHC also shows a gender difference [80] and it provides now a good genetic model to look for a direct role of sexual hormones on myocardium and to study the role of putative modifier genes on sexual chromosomes.

Therapy in HCM

Two separate therapeutic approaches can be followed in HCM patients. One aimed at blocking the progression of hypertrophy and alleviating cardiac symptoms. The second target is prevention of arrhythmias [80]. There are three groups of individuals that should be distinguished: 1) Patients with complaints related to HCM, 2) Patients with hypertrophy, but no complaints, and 3) Carriers without disease characteristics and symptoms:

1) The need to treat patients with complaints is obvious, although the optimal treatment is not known. The wide range of therapeutic options going from pharmacological treatment, pacing, alcohol ablation, to surgical tissue resection in an attempt to improve cardiac function and reduce complaints is indicative for the confusion. All studies have different inclusion and assessment criteria, making comparisons between reports an arduous task. Different drugs have been tested, including Ca^{2+}-entry blockers, β-adrenoceptor blockers and ACE inhibitors. Early studies with Ca^{2+}-entry blockers indicate beneficial short-term effects on diastolic function, but only minor improvement after 6 months (considered to be long term in this study) [81]. Many studies focus on the reduction of the outflow tract obstruction, but it is questionable how important this is for symptoms and prognosis [81-84]. A retrospective study in the UK concluded improved survival in HCM children treated with high dose β-adrenoceptor blockers [83]. It has been shown that the outflow tract gradient can be reduced by left or biventricular pacing, septal alcohol injection or partial septal resection, with short term relieve of symptoms. These treatment modalities can be beneficial for the individual patient. With respect to arrhythmias, it is obvious that amiodarone has been drug of choice in this disease to relieve anginal complaints, prevent and treat atrial arrhythmias and prevent and control ventricular arrhythmias. There is little debate on the place of amiodarone in this patient group as shown by different studies, the question of course is whether implantable cardioverter defibrillators (ICD) are superior [85,86]. All patients with an outflow tract obstruction (including the asymptomatic patients) should receive endocarditis prophylaxis under the usual conditions.

2) Patients with the disease but without complaints will be less motivated to follow a strict drug regimen. How to attenuate the development of hypertrophy is again not well studied in this group. Rhythm control and sudden death prevention are important. Especially, in the setting of a family history with sudden death, or the identification of a mutation involved with a high incidence of sudden death (see above) would support prophylactic ICD placement. Again indicating the importance of the appropriate genetic diagnosis in this disease (Category A). The role of a preimplantation electrophysiological study is less obvious [85].

3) If you carry a mutation, does that make you a patient, in the absence of any signs of cardiac disease? For most individuals the answer is no. There are no reports on sudden death in gene carriers, without left ventricular disease. However, in the setting of troponin T mutations the situation is different as the signs of hypertrophy can be minor or absent, while a high incidence of sudden death has been reported [34,63,64]. Therefore, in these individuals, implantation of an ICD should be considered in the absence of any sign of disease.

Conclusions

It has become clear that the genetic basis of this group of cardiac disorders is extremely heterogeneous, thus complicating successful and fast identification of the causative molecular defect. During the differential diagnostic ways it is of crucial importance that the cardiologist establishes the type of cardiomyopathy and that the clinical geneticist adequately determines the mode of inheritance. In this respect it should be realized that cardiac tissue – paraffin-embedded or liquid nitrogen frozen, which is obtained from a deceased HCM patient is as suitable for genotyping as blood from alive subjects. The availability of this material can greatly accelerate adequate genotyping. Once the defect has been characterized it will be possible sometimes to offer patients or asymptomatic gene-carriers adequate therapeutic advice and suggest interventions to slow down further progress of the disease. Identification of the disease causing genes will be the basis for cell-biological studies, which may give insights into the pathogenesis of this group of cardiomyopathies. A fast method to screen multiple genes for pathologic mutations can be implemented in the new "microarray" technology. Soon, genotyping will be a mature and indispensable diagnostic tool to reveal the true nature of these cardiac disorders.

The aim for the near future is not only to identify new genes – major or modifiers - involved in HCM but also to better understand the molecular mechanisms by which the mutations lead to FHC. The analyses of human myocardial tissue, the *ex vivo* and *in vitro* studies, and the development of animal models by homologous recombination strategy will all help to investigate the pathogenesis of human FHC mutations.

References

1. Vulpian A, Contribution à l'étude des rétrécissements de l'orifice ventriculo-aortique. Archiv. Physiol., 1868;3:220-222.
2. Brock R, Functional obstruction of the left ventricle. Guys Hosp. Rep., 1957;106:221-238.
3. Teare D, Asymetrical hypertrophy of the heart in young adults. Br. Heart. J., 1958; 20:1-8.
4. Wigle ED, Sasson Z, Henderson MA, et al., Hypertrophic cardiomyopathy. The importance of the site and the extent of hypertrophy. A review. Prog. Cardiovasc. Dis., 1985; 28:1-83.
5. Maron BJ, Bonow RO, Cannon RO, et al., Hypertrophic cardiomyopathy: interrelations of clinical manifestations, pathophysiology, and therapy. N. Engl. J. Med., 1987; 316:780-789 and 844-852.
6. McKenna WJ and Camm AJ, Sudden death in hypertrophic cardiomyopathy: assessment of patients at high risk. Circulation, 1989;80:1489-1492.
7. Maron B, Hypertrophic cardiomyopathy. Lancet, 1997;350:127-133.
8. Spirito P, Seidman CE, Mckenna WJ, et al., The management of hypertrophic cardiomyopathy. New Engl. J. Med., 1997; 336:775-785.
9. Maron BJ, Olivotto I, Spirito P, et al., Epidemiology of hypertrophic cardiomyopathy-related death: revisited in a large non-referral-based patient population. Circulation, 2000;102:858-864.
10. Maron BJ, Gardin JM, Flack JM, et al., Prevalence of hypertrophic cardiomyopathy in a general population of young adults: echocardiographic analysis of 4111 subjects in the CARDIA study. Circulation, 1995; 92:785-789.
11. Hollman A, Goodwin JF, Teare D, et al., A family with obstructive cardiomyopathy (asymetrical hypertrophy). Br. Heart J., 1960;22:449-456.
12. MacRae CA, Ghaisas N, Kass S, et al., Familial hypertrophic cardiomyopathy with Wolff-Parkinson-White Syndrome maps to a locus on chromosome 7q3. J. Clin. Invest., 1995; 96:1216-1220.
13. Patton KK, Niimura H, Soults J, et al., Sarcomere protein gene mutations: a frequent cause of elderly-onset hypertrophic cardiomyopathy. Circulation, 2000;102 [Suppl.II]:178.
14. Regitz-Zagrosek V, Erdmann J, Wellnhofer E, et al., Novel Mutation in the -Tropomyosin Gene and Transition From Hypertrophic to Hypocontractile Dilated Cardiomyopathy. Circulation, 2000;102:e112-e116.
15. Olson TM, Michels VV, Thibodeau SN, et al., Actin mutations in dilated cardiomyopathy, a heritable form of heart failure. Science, 1998;280:750-752.
16. Kamisago M, Sharma SD, DePalma SR, et al., Mutations in Sarcomere Protein Genes as a Cause of Dilated Cardiomyopathy. N. Engl. J. Med., 2000; 343:1688-1696.
17. Fung DC, Yu B, Littlejohn T, et al., An online locus-specific mutation database for familial hypertrophic cardiomyopathy. Hum. Mutat., 1999;14:326-332.
18. Bonne G, Carrier L, Richard P, et al., Familial hypertrophic cardiomyopathy: from mutations to functional defects. Circ. Res., 1998; 83:579-593.
19. Paré JAP, Fraser RG, Pirozynski WJ, et al., Hereditary cardiovascular dysplasia: a form of familial cardiomyoapthy. Am. J. Med., 1961;31:37-62.
20. Jarcho JA, McKenna W, Pare JAP, et al., Mapping a gene for familial hypertrophic cardiomyopathy to chromosome 14ql. N. Engl. J. Med., 1989;321:1372-1378.
21. Geisterfer-Lowrance AAT, Kass S, Tanigawa G, et al., A molecular basis for familial hypertrophic cardiomyopathy: a β cardiac myosin heavy chain gene missense mutation. Cell, 1990; 62:999-1006.
22. Epstein N, Lin H, and Fananapazir L, Genetic evidence of dissociation (generational skips) of electrical from morphologic forms of hypertrophic cardiomyopathy. Am. J. Cardiol.,

1990; 66:627-631.

23. Hejtmancik JF, Brink PA, Hill R, et al., Localization of gene for familial hypertrophic cardiomyopathy to chromosome 14ql in a diverse US population. Circulation, 1991; 83:1592-1597.
24. Ko YL, Lien WP, Chen JJ, et al., No evidence for linkage of familial hypertrophic cadiomyopathy and chromosome 14ql locus D14S26 in a chinese family: evidence for genetic heterogeneity. Hum. Gen., 1992; 89:597-601.
25. Schwartz K, Dufour C, Fougerousse F, et al., Exclusion of myosin heavy chain and cardiac actin gene involvement in hypertrophic cardiomyopathies of several french families. Circ. Res., 1992; 71:3-8.
26. Macera MJ, Szabo P, Wadgaonkar R, et al., Localization of the gene encoding for ventricular myosin regulatory light chain (MYL2) to human chromosome 12q23q24.3. Genomics, 1992; 13:765-772.
27. Poetter K, Jiang H, Hassanzadeh S, et al., Mutation in either the essential or regulatory light chains of myosin are associated with a rare myopathy in human heart and skeletal muscle. Nature Genet., 1996; 13:63-69.
28. Flavigny J, Richard P, Isnard R, et al., Identification of two novel mutations in the ventricular regulatory myosin light chain gene (MYL2) associated with familial and classical forms of hypertrophic cardiomyopathy. J. Mol. Med., 1998; 76:208-214.
29. Kramer PL, Luty JA, and Litt M, Regional localization of the gene for cardiac muscle actin (ACTC) on chromosome 15g. Genomics, 1992;13:904-905.
30. Mogensen J, Klausen IC, Pedersen AK, et al., α-cardiac actin is a novel disease gene in familial hypertrophic cardiomyopathy. J. Clin. Invest., 1999; 103:R39-R43.
31. Olson TM, Doan TP, Kishimoto NY, et al., Inherited and de novo mutations in the cardiac actin gene cause hypertrophic cardiomyopathy. J. Mol. Cell. Cardiol., 2000; J. Mol. Cell. Cardiol.:1687-1694.
32. Farza H, Towsend P, Carrier L, et al., Genomic organization, alternative splicing and polymorphisms of the human cardiac troponin T gene. J. Mol. Cell. Cardiol., 1998; 30:1247-1253.
33. Thierfelder L, Watkins H, MacRae C, et al., α-tropomyosin and cardiac troponin T mutations cause familial hypertrophic cardiomyopathy: a disease of the sarcomere. Cell, 1994; 77:701-712.
34. Watkins H, McKenna WJ, Thierfelder L, et al., Mutations in the genes for cardiac troponin T and α-tropomyosin in hypertrophic cardiomyopathy. N. Engl. J. Med., 1995; 332:1058-1064.
35. Kimura A, Harada H, Park JE, et al., Mutations in the cardiac troponin I gene associated with hypertrophic cardiomyopathy. Nature Genet., 1997;16:379-382.
36. MacLeod AR and Gooding C, Human hTMα gene: expression in muscle and nonmuscle tissue. Mol. Cell. Biol., 1988; 8:433-440.
37. Eyre H, Akkari PA, Wilton SD, et al., Assignment of the human skeletal muscle alpha-tropomyosin gene (TPM1) to band 15q22 by fluorescence in situ hydridization. Cytogenet. Cell Genet., 1995; 69:15-17.
38. Karibe A, Tobacman LS, Strand J, et al., Hypertrophic cardiomyopathy caused by a novel α-tropomyosin mutation (V95A) is associated with mild cardiac phenotype, abnormal calcium binding to troponin, abnormal myosin cycling, and poor prognosis. Circulation, 2001; 103:65-71.
39. Carrier L, Hengstenberg C, Beckmann JS, et al., Mapping of a novel gene for familial hypertrophic cardiomyopathy to chromosome 11. Nature Genet., 1993; 4:311-313.
40. Gautel M, Zuffardi O, Freiburg A, et al., Phosphorylation switches specific for the cardiac isoform of myosin binding protein C: a modulator of cardiac contraction? EMBO J., 1995; 14:1952-1960.
41. Bonne G, Carrier L, Bercovici J, et al., Cardiac myosin binding protein-C gene splice

acceptor site mutation is associated with familial hypertrophic cardiomyopathy. Nature Genet., 1995; 11:438-440.
42. Watkins H, Conner D, Thierfelder L, et al., Mutations in the cardiac myosin binding protein-C gene on chromosome 11 cause familial hypertrophic cardiomyopathy. Nature Genet., 1995; 11:434-437.
43. Carrier L, Bonne G, Bährend E, et al., Organization and sequence of human cardiac myosin binding protein C gene (MYBPC3) and identification of mutations predicted to produce truncated proteins in familial hypertrophic cardiomyopathy. Circ. Res., 1997; 80:427-434.
44. Rottbauer W, Gautel M, Zehelein J, et al., Novel splice donor site mutation in the cardiac myosin-binding protein-C gene in familial hypertrophic cardiomyopathy. Characterization of cardiac transcript and protein. J. Clin. Invest., 1997; 100:475-482.
45. Moolman-Smook JC, Mayosi B, Brink P, et al., Identification of a new missense mutation in MyBP-C associated with hypertrophic cardiomyopathy. J. Med. Genet., 1998; 35:253-254.
46. Niimura H, Bachinski LL, Sangwatanaroj S, et al., Mutations in the gene for cardiac myosin-binding protein C and late-onset familial hypertrophic cardiomyopathy. N. Engl. J. Med., 1998; 338:1248-1257.
47. Yu B, French JA, Carrier L, et al., Molecular pathology of familial hypertrophic cardiomyopathy caused by mutations in the cardiac myosin binding protein C gene. J. Med. Genet., 1998; 35:205-210.
48. Moolman JA, Reith S, Uhl K, et al., A newly created splice donor site in exon 25 of the MyBP-C gene is responsible for inherited hypertrophic cardiomyopathy with incomplete disease penetrance. Circulation, 2000; 101:1396-1402.
49. Yang Q, Sanbe A, Osinska H, et al., A mouse model of myosin binding protein C human familial hypertrophic cardiomyopathy. J. Clin. Invest., 1998; 102:1292-1300.
50. Flavigny J, Souchet M, Sébillon P, et al., COOH-terminal truncated cardiac myosin-binding protein C mutants resulting from familial hypertrophic cardiomyopathy mutations exhibit altered expression and/or incorporation in fetal rat cardiomyocytes. J. Mol. Biol., 1999; 294:443-456.
51. McConnell BK, Jones KA, Fatkin D, et al., Dilated cardiomyopathy in homozygous myosin-binding protein-C mutant mice. J. Clin. Invest., 1999; 104:1235-1244.
52. Yang Q, Sanbe A, Osinska H, et al., In vivo modeling of myosin binding protein C familial hypertrophic cardiomyopathy. Circ. Res., 1999; 85:841-847.
53. Sébillon P, Bonne G, Flavigny J, et al., COOH-terminal truncated human cardiac MyBP-C alters myosin filament organization. C. R. Acad. Sci., 2001:In Press.
54. Labeit S and Kolmerer B, Titins: giant proteins in charge of muscle ultrastructure and elasticity. Science, 1995; 270:293-296.
55. Satoh M, Takahashi M, Sakamoto T, et al., Structural analysis of the titin gene in hypertrophic cardiomyopathy: identification of a novel disease gene. Biochem. Biophys. Res. Comm., 1999; 262:411-417.
56. Durr A, Cossee M, Agid Y, et al., Clinical and genetic abnormalities in patients with Friedreich's ataxia. N. Engl. J. Med., 1996; 335:1169-1175.
57. Campuzano V, Montermini L, Molto MD, et al., Friedreich's ataxia: autosomal recessive disease caused by an intronic GAA triplet repeat expansion. Science, 1996; 8:1423-1427.
58. Puccio H, Simon D, Cossée M, et al., Mouse models for friedreich ataxia exhibit cardiomyopathy, sensory nerve defect and Fe-S enzyme deficiency followed by intramitochondrial iron deposits. Nature genet., 2001; 27:181-186.
59. Klues HG, Schiffers A, and Maron BJ, Phenotypic spectrum and patterns of left ventricular hypertrophy in hypertrophic cardiomyopathy: morphologic observations and significance as assessed by two-dimensional echocardiography in 600 patients. J. Am. Coll. Cardiol., 1995; 26:1699-1708.
60. Watkins H, Rosenzweig T, Hwang DS, et al., Characteristic and prognostic implications

of myosin missense mutations in familial hypertrophic cardiomyopathy. N. Engl. J. Med., 1992; 326:1106-1114.

61. Fananapazir L and Epstein ND, Genotype-phenotype correlations in hypertrophic cardiomyopathy: Insights provided by comparisons of kindreds with distinct and identical β-myosin heavy chain mutations. Circulation, 1994; 89:22-32.
62. Enjuto M, Francino A, Navarro-Lopez F, et al., Malignant hypertrophic cardiomyopathy caused by the Arg723Gly mutation in β-myosin heavy chain gene. J. Mol. Cell. Cardiol., 2000; 32:2307-2313.
63. Moolman JC, Corfield VA, Posen B, et al., Sudden death due to troponin T mutations. J. Am. Coll. Cardiol., 1997; 29:549-555.
64. Nakajima-Taniguchi C, Matsui H, Fujio Y, et al., Novel missense mutation in cardiac troponin T gene found in japanese patient with hypertrophic cardiomyopathy. J. Mol. Cell. Cardiol., 1997; 29:839-843.
65. Forissier J-F, Carrier L, Farza H, et al., Codon 102 of the cardiac troponin T gene is a putative hot spot for mutations in familial hypertrophic cardiomyopathy. Circulation, 1996; 94:3069-3073.
66. Charron P, Dubourg O, Desnos M, et al., Clinical features and prognostic implications of familial hypertrophic cardiomyopathy related to cardiac myosin binding protein C gene. Circulation, 1998; 97:2230-2236.
67. Nishi H, Kimura A, Harada H, et al., A myosin missense mutation, not a null allele, causes familial hypertrophic cardiomyopathy. Circulation, 1995;91:2911-2915.
68. Richard P, Isnard R, Carrier L, et al., Double heterozygosity for mutations in the beta myosin heavy chain and in the cardiac myosin binding protein C genes in a family with hypertrophic cardiomyopathy. J. Med. Genet., 1999; 36:542-545.
69. Richard P, Charron P, Leclercq C, et al., Homozygotes for a R869G mutation in the beta-mysoin heavy chain gene have a severe form of familial hypertrophic cardiomyopathy. J. Mol. Cell. Cardiol., 2000; 32:1575-1583.
70. Forissier J-F, Richard P, Briault S, et al., First description of a germ line mosaicism in familial hypertrophic cardiomyopathy. J. Med. Genet., 2000; 37:132-134.
71. Marian AJ, Yu Q-T, Workman R, et al., Angiotensin-converting enzyme polymorphism in hypertrophic cardiomyopathy and sudden cardiac death. Lancet, 1993;342:1085-1086.
72. Lechin M, Quinones MA, Omran A, et al., Angiotensin-I converting enzyme genotypes and left ventricular hypertrophy in patients with hypertrophic cardiomyopathy. Circulation, 1995; 92:1802-1812.
73. Yonega K, Okamoto H, Machida M, et al., Angiotensin-converting enzyme gene polymorphism in japanese patients with hyeprtrophic cardiomyopathy. Am. Heart. J., 1995; 130:1089-1093.
74. Tesson F, Dufour C, Moolman JC, et al., The influence of the angiotensin I converting enzyme genotype in familial hypertrophic cardiomyopathy varies with the disease gene mutation. J. Mol. Cell. Cardiol., 1997; 29:831-838.
75. Charron P, Dubourg O, Desnos M, et al., Diagnostic value of electrocardiography and echocardiography for familial hypertrophic cardiomyopathy in a genotyped adult population. Circulation, 1997; 96:214-219.
76. Clark CE, Henry WL, and Epstein SE, Familial prevalence and genetic transmission of idiopathic subaortic stenosis. J. Engl. J. Med., 1973; 289:709-714.
77. Maron BJ, Nichols PF, Pickle LW, et al., Patterns of inheritance in hypertrophic cardiomopathy. Assessment by M-mode and two-dimensional echocardiography. Am. J. Cardiol., 1984; 53:1087-1094.
78. Greaves SC, Roche AHG, Neutze JM, et al., Inheritance of hypertrophic cardiomyopathy: a cross sectional and M mode echocardiographic study of 50 families. Br. Heart J., 1987; 58:259-266.
79. Charron P, Carrier L, Dubourg O, et al., Penetrance of familial hypertrophic

cardiomyopathy. Genetic counseling, 1997; 8:107-114.
80. Vikstrom KL, Factor SM, and Leinwand LA, Mice expressing mutant myosin heavy chains are a model for familial hypertrophic cardiomyopathy. Mol. Med., 1996; 2:556-567.
81. Tokushima T, Utsunomiya T, Ogawa T, et al., Short- and long-term effects of nisoldipine on cardiac function and exercise tolerance in patients with hypertrophic cardiomyopathy. Basic. Res. Cardiol., 1996; 91:329-336.
82. Sherrid MV, Pearle G, and Gunsburg DZ, Mechanism of benefit of negative inotropes in obstructive hypertrophic cardiomyopathy. Circulation, 1998; 97:41-47.
83. Ostman-Smith I, Wettrell G, and Riesenfeld T, A cohort study of childhood hypertrophic cardiomyopathy: improved survival following high-dose beta-adrenoceptor antagonist treatment. J. Am. Coll. Cardiol., 1999; 15:1813-1822.
84. Sherrid MV, Gunsburg D, and Sharma A, Medical treatment of hypertrophic cardiomyopathy. Curr. Cardiol., 2000; 2:148-153.
85. Zhu DW, Sun H, Hill R, et al., The value of electrophysiology study and prophylactic implantation of cardioverter defibrillator in patients with hypertrophic cardiomyopathy. Pacing Clin. Electrophysiol., 1998; 21(1 Pt 2):299-302.
86. Elliott PM, The Role of Pharmacologic Treatment to Prevent Sudden Death in the Implantable Cardioverter Defibrillator Era. Curr. Cardiol. Rep., 2001; 3:167-172.

13. DILATED CARDIOMYOPATHY

C. Marcelis, P.A. Doevendans, G. Bonne

Introduction

Dilated cardiomyopathy (DCM) is a primary heart muscle disease characterised by left ventricular dilatation with impaired contraction of the left ventricle and occasionally right ventricular disease. DCM has an incidence of 4/100.00 per year. It is a leading cause for heart failure and an important indication for cardiac transplantation. The disease is associated with a high risk of sudden death due to ventricular arrhythmias and a high mortality rate of 15-50% within 5 years.
A large number of primary cardiac and systemic diseases can cause systolic impairment and left ventricular dilatation, but in the majority of patients no identifiable cause is found (Idiopathic Dilated cardiomyopathy, IDC). In the past few years it has become increasingly clear that in at least 25% of the patients DCM has a genetic basis [1,2]. Familial DCM is a heterogeneous disorder with different inheritance patterns. Autosomal dominant inheritance is the most common, but autosomal recessive, X-linked and mitochondrial inheritance have also been recognized. In the last couple of years important progress has been made in unraveling familial DCM. Multiple genetic loci and several genes have been identified in familial DCM.
In this chapter we will outline how to recognise the disease and indicate the importance of genetic diagnostics. Thus far no mutation-based therapy is available, but clearly recognition of the disease and identification of the mutations will guide genetic counselling of patients and their relatives.

Clinical manifestations and diagnosis

Typically DCM presents with signs resulting from pulmonary congestion and low cardiac output (dyspnoe on exertion, fatigue). A wide variety of other symptoms can be attributed to the disease. In some patients arrhythmia, sudden cardiac death or systemic embolism may be the presenting symptom. Increasingly the diagnosis is made in asymptomatic individuals on routine medical screening or during family screening. For the diagnosis of DCM an echocardiogram is essential. The criteria are based on the Henry formulae and take into account sex and body size (see table 1). A left ventricular diameter of >112% represents 2 standard deviations of the predicted normal value.

PA Doevendans and AA Wilde (eds.), Cardiovascular genetics, 155-167.

Mestroni et al. (1999)[3] suggest a cut off value of 117%. This cut off value can be used in order to increase specificity for family studies. Before making the diagnosis of idiopathic dilated cardiomyopathy (IDC) other known causes of DCM should be excluded. ECG abnormalities in DCM patients include isolated T-wave changes, septal Q waves, AV-conduction prolongation and bundle branch block. Sinus tachycardia and supraventricular arrhythmias are common (especially atrial fibrillation). In DCM patients the ECG may remain remarkably normal. Exercise testing is of particular value in assessing functional limitations. A variety of other tests can be used routinely in the screening of DCM patients. Some tests are only indicated when a specific aetiology is suspected. (See Table 2)

Familial idiopathic DCM

Familial DCM is a clinically heterogeneous disorder. When identifying and studying families a series of problems can arise. First, the presentation of the disease (phenotype) of affected family members shows a significant variety, both between and within families. This might make it difficult to identify affected subjects. Second, the penetrance of the disease is variable and age dependent. Family members, especially the young individuals who are originally described as normal (on the basis of physical and echocardiographic examination), might develop the disease at a later age. Third, most of the known families are small, including only few patients. Often many of the patients are already deceased when families are identified. Classical linkage analysis may be difficult, as no DNA is available of deceased patients. A fourth important problem has been the lack of consensus on diagnostic criteria. For this reason a group of European Collaborators worked to define criteria for familial IDC [3].

Molecular basis of DCM

Familial DCM is not only clinically but also genetically heterogeneous. Autosomal dominant DCM with or without associated features (skeletal-muscle disease, conduction system disease, and deafness) is the most frequent. Autosomal recessive, X-linked and mitochondrial (matrilineal) inheritance patterns are described. In the past several years important progress has been made in unravelling the molecular background of familial DCM. Multiple genetic loci and at least 8 genes have been identified (see table 3). All presently identified genes are encoding proteins that are part of the cytoskeletal/ sarcolemmal structural support system. Mutations affect elements of the cell cytoarchitecture (cytoskeleton, sarcolemma) and elements that interact with the cytoskeleton.

Autosomal dominant DCM

At present 5 genes have been implied in familial 'pure' DCM: desmin (DES, chr. 2q35), actin (ACTC, chr. 15q11-qter), δ-sarcoglycan (SGCD, chr. 5q33), β-myosin heavy chain (MYH7, chr. 14q11.2) and cardiac troponin T (TNNT2, chr. 1q32). In addition 4 more loci have been identified [4,5,6,7].

Table 1. Definition of clinical status of members of families with idiopathic dilated cardiomyopathy.

Major criteria:
1. Ejection fraction of the left ventricle <0.45 and/or fractional shortening of <25%.
2. Left ventricular end diastolic dimension of >117% of the predicted value corrected for age, sex and body size.

Minor criteria:
1. Unexplained supraventricular or ventricular arrhythmias, frequent or repetitive before the age of 50 years.
2. Left ventricular dilatation >112% of the predicted value.
3. Left ventricular dysfunction: ejection fraction <50% or fractional shortening <28%.
4. Unexplained conduction disease: II or III AV-conduction defect, complete left bundle branch block, sinus nodal dysfunction.
5. Unexplained sudden death or stroke before 50 years of age.
6. Segmental wall motion abnormalities in the absence of intraventricular conduction defect or ischaemic heart disease.

Exclusion criteria:
1. Systemic arterial hypertension (>160/100 mmHg).
1. Coronary artery disease (obstruction >50% in a major branch.
2. History of chronic alcohol abuse with remission of DCM after 6 months abstinence.
3. Systemic disease known to cause DCM.
4. Pericardial disease.
5. Congenital heart disease.
6. Cor pulmonale.

Modified from Mestroni et al. 1999 [3]

Major and minor criteria are distinguished and exclusion criteria are added. A first-degree relative will be identified as 'affected' in the presence of:
- One major criterion.
- Or left ventricular dilatation with one minor criterion.
- Or three minor criteria.

When only one or two minor criteria are fulfilled the status would be identified as 'unknown'. The diagnosis of familial DCM is made in the presence of two or more affected individuals in a single family or in the presence of a first-degree relative of a DCM patient, with well-documented unexplained sudden death at <35 years of age.

Table 2. Baseline and additional evaluation of DCM patients. (from Mestroni et al., 1999, modified) [3]

Basic evaluation:

- 3 generation pedigree construction.
- Physical examination, incl. neuromuscular evaluation.
- Standard and ambulatory ECG.
- Echocardiography.
- Exercise testing.
- Chest X-ray.
- Laboratory examinations:

1. Full blood count.
2. Glucose.
3. Creatinine/ ureum/ elecrolytes.
4. Liver function tests (ALT, AST, GT, Bilirubine).
5. Cholesterol/ Triglycerides.
6. CK
7. TSH,T4

Proposed additional investigations:

• Angiography (coronary, ventriculographic)	
• Endomyocardial biopsy	For histologic and immunocytochemical studies.
• Skeletal muscle biopsy	If neuromuscular weakness is suspected.
• Sedimentation rate/ CRP	In children with suspect inflammation.
• Serum lactate/ pyruvate	If mitochondrial disease is suspected.
• Study of viral persistence	
• Metabolic studies	In pediatric DCM (for review see Schwartz et (al., 1996) 28)
• Ophthalmological examination	If mitochondrial disease is suspected or multiorgan disease.

The first gene identified in familial DCM was cardiac actin [8]. Actin is a member of the thin filament of the sarcomere unit. When a mutation is found near the dystrophin-binding site, there will be a DCM phenotype. In contrast mutations near the sarcomeric ends of Actin result in hypertrophic cardiomyopathy. Mutations near the dystrophin-binding site probably disrupt the link between actin and dystrophin (figure).

This way the actin cytoskeleton disassociates from the muscle membrane and extracellular matrix, leading to cell degeneration and necrosis. Since the identification of actin mutations in familial DCM several larger studies have been performed to look for additional actin mutations in DCM families [9,10,11]. Thus far no additional mutations have been identified. This implies that actin mutations are probably rare in familial DCM.

Desmin is a muscle-specific 53-kDa subunit of the class III intermediate filament. It is a part of the cytoskeleton of cardiac muscle, as well as skeletal and smooth muscle, and forms connections between the muscular and plasma domains. It is believed to play a role in the attachment or stabilisation of the sarcomere.

Table 3. Genes and loci in familial dilated cardiomyopathy

Inheritance	**Phenotype**	*Loci*	**Gene**	**Cat + Ref.**
AD pure	DCM pure	9q12-q13	?	D [4]
	DCM pure	1q32	?	D [5]
	DCM pure	2q24.3-q31	?	D [6]
	DCM pure	6q12-q16	?	D [7]
	DCM pure	2q35	*DES*: desmin	B [11,12]
	DCM pure	5q33	*SGCD*: δ-sarcoglycan	B [14]
	DCM pure	15q11-qter	*ACTC*: actin	B [8]
	DCM pure, early onset	14q11.2	*MYH7*: β-myosin	B [15]
	DCM pure, early onset	1q32	*TNNT2*: cardiac troponin T	B [15]
AD plus	DCM + CD	1q21	*LMNA*: lamin A/C	B [21,22]
	DCM + CD	2q14-q22	?	D [17]
	DCM + CD+ SN dysfunction	3p22-p25	?	D [18]
	DCM + mitral valve prolaps	10q21-q23	?	D [19]
	DCM + hearing loss	6q23-q24	?	D [20]
	DCM + CD + LGMD	6q22-q23	?	D [21]
	DCM + CD + MD = AD-EDMD	1q21	*LMNA*: lamin A/C	B [24]
	DCM + CD + LGMD = LGMD1B	1q21	*LMNA*: lamin A/C	B [25]
AR	LGMD +/- cardiomyopathy	17q21	*SGCA*: α-sarcoglycan	B [29]
	LGMD + severe cardiomyopathy	4q12	*SGCB*: β-sarcoglycan	B [30]
	LGMD + cardiomyopathy (Brazil)	5q33	*SGCD*: δ-sarcoglycan	B [13]
X-linked	DCM pure	Xp21.3	*DYS*: dystrophin	B [32]
	DCM lethal in infancy	Xq28	*TAZ*: tafazzin	B [40, 41]
	DCM + Myopathy = Barth syndrome	Xq28	*TAZ*: tafazzin	B [40,41]
	DCM + CD + MD = XL-EDMD	Xq28	*EMD*: emerin	B [42]

AD: autosomal dominant, AR: autosomal recessive, DCM: dilated cardiomyopathy, CD: conduction defect, SN: sinus node, LGMD: limb girdle muscular dystrophy, MD: muscular dystrophy, EDMD: Emery-Dreifuss muscular dystrophy.

Desmin mutations were first identified in families with a skeletal myopathy with cardiac involvement, predominantly conduction disorders and restrictive cardiomyopathy [12]. Later it was described in a family with pure DCM [13]. In the latter family the mutation was located in the carboxy tail domain of Desmin, while in the families with skeletal myopathy the mutations were found in the rod domain. This suggests a binding site-specific phenotype for the distinct mutations. Thus far no further desmin mutations have been described in 'pure' familial DCM [11,13].

δ-sarcoglycan is a member of the dystrophin-associated glycoprotein complex (DAG; i.e. the sarcoglycans and dystroglycans). Mutations in this gene have been first identified in autosomal recessive limb-girdle muscular dystrophy (LGMD2F)[14]. LGMD is a disorder with mild to severe skeletal muscle disease. Cardiac involvement has been documented in a subgroup of patients with this disease. Recently, mutations in this gene have been described in familial autosomal dominant late-onset DCM [15]. The mutations found in DCM are similar to those found in LGMD2F, except that they are heterozygous instead of homozygous. This might suggest that heterozygous mutation carriers within LGMD2F families might be at risk to develop DCM later in life.

Most recently mutations in sarcomere protein genes (β-myosin heavy chain, troponin T) have been identified in familial DCM [16]. Mutations in these genes were found in families with early-onset DCM with a severe phenotype. For some time mutations in these genes have been known to cause familial hypertrophic cardiomyopathy (FHC, see Chapter 12). In DCM a cardiac phenotype with increased ventricular volumes and ventricular wall thinning without specific histopathological changes is found. In FHC the phenotype is almost the opposite with marked thickening of the ventricular wall with important (asymmetric) thickening of the interventricular septum. In FHC histologically distinctive myocyte disarray with interstitial fibrosis is found. While in FHC contractile function is hyperdynamic, in DCM contraction is impaired. How do allelic mutations in sarcomeric proteins cause such distinct cardiac phenotypes? Biophysical evidence suggests that mutant sarcomeres in FHC exhibit increased actin-activated ATPase activity with greater force production and faster actin-filament sliding. This way the contractile function might be increased. The sarcomere mutations in DCM are located in domains that are involved in the generation of the power stroke of contraction. Mutations in these domains can be predicted to reduce the production of contractile force by the sarcomere, leading to the DCM-phenotype. The identification of sarcomere gene mutations in 10% of DCM families indicates that they are a major cause of DCM and might imply a role for other sarcomere proteins.

In addition to autosomal dominant DCM restricted to the heart there are also several AD disease phenotypes that include additional features, such as conduction system disease, mitral valve prolaps, sinus node dysfunction, muscle weakness and hearing loss [17-21]. Several loci for these diseases are identified (see table 3).

Mutations in the lamin A/C gene have been identified in families with autosomal dominant DCM with conduction system disease (DCM-CD)[22,23]. The most common conduction system abnormality in these families is atrioventricular heart block, which often precipitates left ventricular dilatation and impaired contractile function. Lamins A/C mutations were first described in autosomal dominant Emery-Dreyfuss muscular dystrophy (AD-EDMD)[24] and shortly after in an autosomal dominant form of limb-girdle muscular dystrophy (LGMD1B)[25]. These two muscle disorders are characterized by a skeletal involvement (proximal weakness +/- contractures) and a cardiac involvement that is similar to what is observed in DCM-CD. Mutations in the same gene have also been implied in a very distinct disease, familial partial lipodystrophy or Dunnigan-Kobberling syndrome (FPLD)[26,27]. This is an autosomal dominant condition characterised by abnormal fat distribution, caused by regional and progressive adipocyte degeneration, with insulin resistance and hyperlipidaemia.

Lamin A and C are highly conserved proteins that arise from one single gene by alternative splicing and are expressed in all differentiated cells. They are components of nuclear lamina, a nucleoskeletal structure associated with the nucleoplasmic surface of the inner nuclear membrane of the nuclear envelope. Lamins contribute to the structural integrity of the nuclear envelope and provide mechanical support for the nucleus. Mutations in Lamins A and C might destabilize the association of these lamins with the nuclear envelope. This would make the lamina less affective as a load-bearing structure, particularly in muscle [28]. Eventually this increased fragility would translate into physical damage leading to cell death and tissue damage. In cardiac muscle, loss

of individual cardiomyocytes will be cumulative and will eventually lead to conduction blocks. This accumulation of damaged nuclei as a result of a reduction in the load-bearing properties of the lamina can also take place in skeletal muscle.
In contrast to mutations in skeletal and cardiac disorders (EDMD, LGMD1B and DCM-CD) that are localized along the gene, mutations in familial partial lipodystrophy (FPLD) are restricted to a specific site. Ninety percent of the muations identified in FPLD patients are located on R482, the remaining muations being localized in the same region, within the globular domain of lamin A/C [29]. This suggests a specific function of this site in the adipocyte [26].

Autosomal recessive DCM

Autosomal recessive 'pure' DCM is probably rare and, to our knowledge, no loci have been identified. On the other hand DCM is a frequent feature in a number of autosomal recessive disorders, including several metabolic disorders in childhood. Schwartz et al. reviews the management of DCM in the pediatric population in detail [30].
In several of the AR limb-girdle muscular dystrophies the responsible gene defects have been identified (table 3). Mutations in α–, β- and δ-sarcoglycan have described in AR-LGMD families [14,31,32]. In these LGMD's dilated cardiomyopathy can be an important feature. This, together with the identification of δ-sarcoglycan mutations in AD-DCM [15], suggests an important role for the sarcoglycans in DCM.

X-linked DCM

X-linked inheritance of idiopathic DCM was first described by Berko et al. in 1987 [33]. Since then many families have been described. X-linked inheritance can be suspected in a pedigree where only males are affected, who inherit the disease from their non-expressing mother and no male-to-male transmission takes place. In 1993 Muntoni et al. [34] were the first to describe a defect in the dystrophin gene as a causal factor of X-linked dilated cardiomyopathy.
The dystrophin gene had been an important candidate because of the association of mutations in this gene with Duchenne muscular dystrophy (DMD) and Becker muscular dystrophy (BMD). Typically DMD-patients have mutations in the dystrophin gene that result in a total lack of expression of the sarcolemmal protein dystrophin. In BMD, patients have residual expression of a partially functional dystrophin in the muscle [35]. Cardiac involvement, and especially dilated cardiomyopathy, has been an integral part of these diseases [36,37]. Cardiac involvement can also be present in female carriers of DMD and BMD. Up to 8% of DMD carriers have dilated cardiomyopathy and an additional 18% have left ventricle dilatation even without muscle weakness [38,39]. DCM is probably rare in BMD carriers.
Unlike patients with typical DMD or BMD, patients with X-linked DCM do not have symptoms of skeletal muscle weakness. The only sign of neuromuscular involvement is usually an increased serum creatine kinase (CK). Ferlini et al. [40] reviewed the published dystrophin mutations in an attempt to find a genotype-phenotype correlation and speculated on possible pathogenic mechanisms underlying the disease. Some of the

mutations found in X-linked DCM are similar to those found in DMD and BMD, others seem to be DCM specific. Two main regions of the dystrophin gene are most commonly involved in X-linked DCM. Mutations in the 5' end region of the gene are associated with a more severe cardiac phenotype. These mutations are known to affect splicing. Because splicing is often tissue specific this might explain the cardiac specific phenotype. Mutations in the spectrin-like region (around exons 48-49) are associated with a less severe cardiac phenotype. The role of these mutations in the pathogenesis of the cardiac specific phenotype of these patients is not clear. It is suggested that introns in this region contain sequences that are involved in gene expression and thus might be involved in the cardiac specific phenotype. Franz et al. [41] reported a family with a nonsense mutation in exon 29. In contrast to other dystrophin mutations this mutation did not cause DCM by a diminished expression of dystrophin but it seemed to affect the sarcoglycan assembly in the heart muscle. Dystrophin interacts with actin and the sarcolemmal dystrophin-associated glycoprotein complex. Disruption of this interaction due to a mutation in the rod region of dystrophin will cause membrane instability and may lead to cardiomyopathy.

A second gene implicated in X-linked DCM is the gene G4.5 or taffazin. Mutations in this gene were first described in Barth syndrome, an X-linked cardioskeletal myopathy with neutropenia and abnormal mitochondria [42]. Mutations in the same gene were found in infantile fatal cardiomyopathy and isolated left ventricular compaction [43] The exact function of the gene is unknown.

A third X-linked disorder associated with DCM is X-linked Emery-Dreifuss muscular dystrophy which is associated with mutations in the gene emerin [44]. Emerin is an integral protein of the nuclear envelope and interacts with Lamin-A/C giving strength to the nucleus. Only two cases with emerin mutations and exclusively cardiac involvement, i.e. DCM-CD, are reported [45].

Mitochondrial DCM

When mitochondrial DNA-defects are associated with DCM the inheritance pattern will usually fit matrilineal inheritance in which the disease is only transmitted by (affected) females. Often a case clinically presents as sporadic. The presence of lactacidaemia suggests mitochondrial disease. The role of mitochondria in cardiac disease is extensively reviewed in chapter 11.

Future

Despite the increased knowledge on genetic involvement in DCM as described above, the role for genetic testing in (familial) DCM is still limited. The proportion of cases that can be explained by a mutation in one of the known genes is still small. An important problem at the moment is the lack of knowledge on genotype-phenotype correlations. No population-based studies reflecting the whole spectrum of gene mutations in DCM have been described. More knowledge on genotype-phenotype correlations is necessary for appropriate counselling of DCM patients and their relatives and will help to direct molecular diagnosis in individual families.

At present the availability of therapeutic options is still limited for the majority of cases. Identifying the molecular defects in DCM families and studying their role in the pathogenesis of DCM will help in understanding the development of heart failure. This understanding may in the future help to expand the therapeutic possibilities, and possibly gene specific treatment, for DCM-patients.

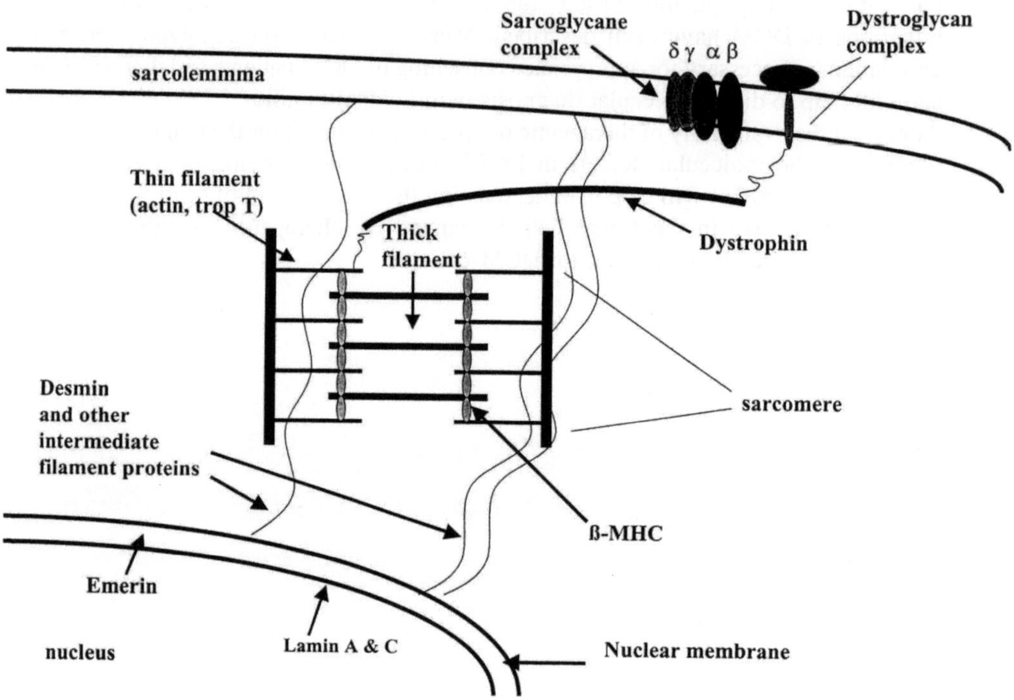

Figure 1. *Schematic drawing of cardiomyocyte indicating proteins that can cause dilated cardiomyopathy.*

References

1. Michels VV, Moll PP, Miller FA, Tajik AJ, Chu JS, Driscoll DJ, Burnett JC, Rodeheffer RJ, Chesbro JH, Tazelaar HD. The frequency of familial dilated cardiomyopathy in a series of patients with idiopathic dilated cardiomyopathy. N Engl J Med 1992; 326: 77-82.
2. Keeling PJ, Gang Y, Smith G, Seo H, Bent SE, Murday V, Caforio AL, McKenna WJ. Familial dilated cardiomyopathy in the United Kingdom. Br Heart J 1995; 73: 417-21.
3. Mestroni L, Maisch B, Mc Kenna WJ, Schwartz K, Charron P, Rocco C, Tesson F, Richter A, Wilke A, Komajda M. Guidelines for the study of familial dilated cardiomyopathy. Eur Heart J 1999; 20: 93-102.
4. Krajinovic M, Pinamonti B, Sinagra G, Vatta M, Severini GM, Milasin J, Falaschi A, Camerini F, Giacca M, Mestroni L. Linkage of familial dilated cardiomyopathy to chromosome 9. Heart Muscle Disease Study Group. Am J Hum Genet 1995; 57: 846-52.
5. Durand J-B, Bachinski LL, Bieling LC, Czernuszewicz GZ, Abchee AB, Yu QT, Tapscott T, Hill R, Ifegwu J, Marian AJ, Brugada R, Daiger S, Gregoritch JM, Anderson JL, Quinones M, Towbin JA, Roberts R. Localisation of a gene responsible for familial dilated cardiomyopathy to chromosome 1q32. Circulation 1995; 92: 3387-9.
6. Siu BL, Niimura H, Osborne JA, Fatkin D, MacRae C, Solomon S, Benson DW, Seidman JG, Seidman CE. Familial dilated cardiomyopathy locus maps to chromosome 2q31. Circulation 1999; 99: 1022-1026
7. Sylvius N, Tesson F, Gayet C, Charron, P, Benaiche A, Peuchmaurd M, Duboscq-Bidot L, Feingold J, Beckmann JS, Bouchier C, Komajda M. A new locus for autosomal dominant dilated cardiomyopathy identified on chromosome 6q12-q16. Am J Hum Genet 2001; 68: 241-6.
8. Olson TM, Michels VV, Thibodeau SN, Tai YS, Keating MT. Actin mutations in dilated cardiomyopathy, a heritable form of heart failure. Science 1998; 280: 750-2.
9. Takai E, Akita H, Shiga N, Kanazawa K, Yamada S, Terashima M, Matsuda Y, Iwai C, Kawai K, Yokota Y, Yokoyama M. Mutational analysis of the cardiac actin gene in familial and sporadic dilated cardiomyopathy. Am J Med Genet 1999; 86: 325-7.
10. Mayosi BM, Khogali S, Zhang B, Watkins H. Cardiac and skeletal actin gene mutations are not a common cause of dilated cardiomyopathy. J Med Genet 1999; 36: 796-7.
11. Tesson F, Sylvius, Pilotto A, Dubosq-Bidot L, Peuchmard M, Bouchier C, Benaiche A, Mangin L, Charron P, Gavazzi A, Tavazzi L, Arbustini E, Komajda M. Epidemiology of desmin and cardiac actin gene mutations in a European population of dilated cardiomyopathy. Eur Heart J 2000; 21: 1872-6.
12. Goldfarb LG, Park KY, Cervenakova L, Gorokhova S, Lee HS, Vasconcelos O, Nagle JW, Semino-Mora C, Sivakumar K, Dalakas MC. Missense mutations in desmin associated with familial cardiac and skeletal myopathy. Nat Genet 1998; 19: 402-3.
13. Li D, Tapscoft T, Gonzales O, Burch PE,Quinones MA, Zoghbi WA, Hill R, Bachinski LL, Mann DL, Roberts R. Desmin mutation responsible for idiopathic dilated cardiomyopathy. Circulation 1999; 100: 461-4.
14. Nigro V, de Sa Moreira E, Piluso G, Vainzof M, Belsito A, Politano L, Puca AA, Passos-Bueno MR, Zatz M. Autosomal recessive limb-girdle muscular dystrophy, LGMD2F, is caused by a mutation in the delta-sarcoglycan gene. Nat Genet 1996; 14: 195-8.
15. Tsubata S, Bowles KR, Vatta M, Zintz C, Titus J, Muhonen L, Bowles NE, Towbin JA. Mutations in the human delta-sarcoglycan gene in familial and sporadic dilated cardiomyopathy. J Clin Invest 2000; 106: 655-62.
16. Kamisago M, Sharma SD, DePalma SR, Solomon S, Sharma P, McDonough B, Smoot L, Mullen MP, Woolf PK, Wigle ED, Seidman JG, Seidman CE, Jarcho J, Shapiro LR. Mutations in Sarcomere Protein Genes as a Cause of Dilated Cardiomyopathy. N Engl J Med 2000; 343:

1688-96.
17. Jung M, Poepping I, Perrot A, Ellmer AE, Wienker TF, Dietz R, Reis A, Osterziel KJ. Investigation of a Family with Autosomal Dominant Dilated Cardiomyopathy Defines a Novel Locus on Chromosome 2q14-q22. Am J Hum Genet 1999; 65: 1068-1077.
18. Olson TM, Keating MT. Mapping a cardiomyopathy locus to chromosome 3p22-p25. J Clin Invest 1996; 97: 528-32.
19. Bowles KR, Gajarski R, Porter P, Goytia V, Bachinski L, Roberts R, Pignatelli R, Towbin JA. Gene mapping of familial autosomal dominant dilated cardiomyopathy to chromosome 10q21-23. J Clin Invest 1996; 98: 1355-60.
20. Schönberger J, Levy H, Grünig E, Sangwatanaroj S, Fatkin D, MacRae C, Stäcker H, Halpin C, Eavey R, Philbin EF, Katus H, Seidman JG, Seidman CE. Dilated cardiomyopathy and sensorineural hearing loss: a heritable syndrome that maps to 6q23-24. Circulation 2000; 101: 1812-8.
21. Messina DM, Speer MC, Pericak-Vance MA, McNally EM. Linkage of Familial Dilated Cardiomyopathy with Conduction Defect and Muscular Dystrophy to Chromosome 6q23. Am J Hum Genet 1997; 61: 906-17.
22. Fatkin D, MacRae C, Sasaki T, Wolff MR, Porcu M, Frenneaux M, Atherton J, Vidaillet HJ, Spudich S, De Girolami U, Seidman JG, Seidman CE, Muntoni F, Muehle G, Johnson W, McDonough B. Missense Mutations in the Rod Domain of the Lamin A/C Gene as Causes of Dilated Cardiomyopathy and Conduction-System Disease. N Engl J Med 1999; 341: 1715-24.
23. Becane HM, Bonne B, Varvous S, Muchir A, Ortega V, Hammouda EA, Urtizberea JA, Lavergne T, Fardeau M, Eymard B, Weber S, Schwartz K, Duboc D. High incidence of sudden death of conduction system and myocardial disease due to lamins A/C gene mutation. PACE 2000; 23: 1661-6.
24. Bonne G, Di Barletta MR, Varnous S, Becane H, Hammouda EH, Merlini L, Muntoni F, Greenberg CR, Gary F, Urtizberea JA, Duboc D, Fardeau M, Toniolo D, Schwartz K. Mutations in the gene encoding lamin A/C cause autosomal dominant Emery-Dreifuss muscular dystrophy. Nat Genet 1999; 21: 285-8.
25. Muchir A, Bonne G, van der Kooi AJ, van Meegen M, Baas F, Bolhuis PA, de Visser M, Schwartz K. Identification of mutations in the gene encoding lamins A/C in autosomal dominant limb girdle muscular dystrophy with atrioventricular conduction disturbances (LGMD1B). Hum Mol Genet 2000; 9: 1453-9.
26. Shackleton S, Lloyd DJ, Jackson SNJ, Evans R, Niermeijer MF, Singh BM, Schmidt H, Brabant G, Kumar S, Durrington PN, Gregory S, O'Rahilly S, Trembath RC. LMNA, encoding lamin A/C, is mutated in partial lipodystrophy. Nat Genet 2000; 24: 153-6.
27. Cao H, Hegele RA. Nuclear lamin A/C R482Q mutation in Canadian kindreds with Dunnigan-type familial partial lipodystrophy. Hum Mol Genet 2000; 9: 109-12.
28. Hutchison CJ, Alvarez-Reyes M, Vaughan OA. Lamins in disease: why do ubiquitously expressed nuclear envelope proteins give rise to tissue-specific disease phenotypes? J Cell Science 2000;114:9-19.
29. Vigouroux C, Magré J, Vantyghem MC, Bouruï C, Lascols O, Shackleton S, Lloyd DJ, Guerci B, Padova G, Valensi P, Grimaldi A, Piquemal R, Touraine P, Trembath RC, Capeau J. Lamin A/C gene: sex-determined expression of mutations in Dunnigan-type familial partial lipodystrophy and absence of coding mutations in congenital and acquired generalized lipoatrophy. Diabetes 2000; 49: 1958-62.
30. Schwartz ML, Cox GF, Lin AE, Korson S, Perez-Atayde A, Lacro RV, Lipschultz SE. Clinical approach to genetic cardiomyopathy in children. Circulation 1996; 94: 2021-38.
31. Piccolo F, Roberds SL, Jeanpierre M, Leturcq F, Azibi K, Beldjord C, Carrie A, Recan D, Chaouch M, Reghis A, El Kerch F, Sefiani A, Voit T, Merlini L, Collin H, Eymard B, Beckmann JS, Romero NB, Tome FMS, Fardeau M, Campbell KP, Kaplan J-C. Primary adhalinopathy: a common cause of autosomal recessive muscular dystrophy of variable severity. Nat Genet 1995; 10: 243-5.

32. Lim LE, Duclos F, Broux O, Bourg N, Sunada Y, Allamand V, Meyer J, Richard I, Moomaw C, Slaughter C, Tome FMS, Fardeau M, Jackson CE, Beckmann JS, Campbell KP. Beta-sarcoglycan: characterisation and role in limb-girdle muscular dystrophy linked to 4q12. Nat Genet 1995; 11: 257-65.
33. Berko BA, Swift M. X-linked dilated cardiomyopathy. N Engl J Med 1987; 316: 1186-91.
34. Muntoni F, Cau M, Ganau A, Congiu R, Arvedi G, Mateddu A, Marrosu MG, Cianchetti C, Realdi G, Cao A. Brief report: deletion of the dystrophin muscle-promoter region associated with X-linked dilated cardiomyopathy. N Engl J Med 1993; 329: 921-5.
35. Dubowitz V. Muscle disorders in childhood. 2nd edn. London: WB Saunders, 1995.
36. Perloff JK, de Leon AC, O'Doherty. The cardiomyopathy of progressive muscular dystrophy. Circulation 1966; 33: 625-48.
37. Nigro G, Comi L, Politano L, Bain R. The incidence and evolution of cardiomyopathy in Duchenne and Becker muscular dystrophy. Int J Cardiol 1990; 26: 271-7.
38. Hoogerwaard EM, van der Wouw PA, Wilde AAM, Bakker E, Ippel PF, Oosterwijk JC, Majoor-Krakauer DF, van Essen AJ, Leschot NJ, de Visser M. Cardiac involvement in carriers of Duchenne and Becker muscular dystrophy. Neuromusc Dis 1999; 9: 347-51.
39. Hoogerwaard EM, Bakker E, Ippel PF, Oosterwijk JC, Majoor-Krakauer DF, Leschot NJ, van Essen AJ, Brunner HG, van der Wouw PA, Wilde AAM, de Visser M. Signs and symptoms of Duchenne muscular dystrophy and Becker muscular dystrophy among carriers in the Netherlands: a cohort study. Lancet 1999; 353: 2116-9.
40. Ferlini A, Sewry C, Melis MA, Mateddu A, Muntoni F. X-linked dilated cardiomyopathy and the dystrophin gene. Neuromusc Dis 1999; 9: 339-46.
41. Franz W-M, Müller M, Müller OJ, Herrmann R, Rothman T, Cremer M, Cohn RD, Voit T, Katus HA. Association of nonsense mutation of dystrophin gene with disruption of sarcoglycan complex in X-linked dilated cardiomyopathy. Lancet 2000; 355: 1781-5.
42. Bione S, D'Adamo P, Maestrini E, Gedeon AK, Bolhuis PA, Toniolo D. A novel X-linked gene, G4.5 is responsible for Barth syndrome. Nat Genet 1996; 12: 385-9.
43. D'Adamo P, Fassone L, Gedeon A, Janssen EAM, Bione S, Bolhuis PA, Barth PG, Wilson M, Haan E, Orstavik KH, Patton MA, Green AJ, Zammarchi E, Donati M, Toniolo D. The X-linked gene G4.5 is responsible for different infantile dilated cardiomyopathies. Am J Hum Genet 1997; 61: 862-7.
44. Bione S, Maestrini E, Rivella S, Manchini M, Regis S, Romei G, Toniolo D. Identification of a novel X-linked gene responsible for Emery-Dreifuss muscular dystrophy. Nat Genet 1994; 8: 323-7.
45. Wehnert M, Muntoni F. 60th ENMC International Workshop: non X-linked Emery-Dreifuss muscular dystrophy, 5-7 june 1998. Neuromusc disord 1999; 9: 115-20.

14. IDIOPATHIC VENTRICULAR FIBRILLATION

A.A. Wilde

Introduction

Ventricular fibrillation (VF) in the absence of structural heart disease is classified as 'idiopathic ventricular fibrillation' or 'primary electrical disease'. In those cases the arrhythmogenic substrate should in principle be looked for in the excitation and conduction properties of the heart. However, some minimal abnormalities are considered compatible with idiopathic VF (table 1) [1]. Moreover, it should be realized that even with all currently available highly sophisticated diagnostic techniques discrete structural abnormalities might be overlooked. Careful follow-up might indeed unmask structural heart disease in these patients.

On the other hand true primary electrical disease is now well recognized. Indeed, VF and/or polymorphic ventricular tachycardias (VT) might occur in structurally normal hearts (table 2). The differential diagnosis should include the congenital long QT syndrome (LQTS; chapter 15), the right bundle branch block-right precordial ST-segment elevation syndrome (Brugada syndrome; see below), exercise-induced polymophic (PM)VT (see below) and short-coupled Torsades de Pointes (see below). Occasionally, familial bradyarrhythmias, among others based on familial isolated conduction disease, may lead to sudden cardiac death.

A careful (family) history is pivotal for the correct diagnosis. Nocturnal sudden death in males is suggestive for Brugada syndrome, sudden death immediately upon arousal (with or without an acoustic stimulus) is suggestive for LQTS2 [2] and exercise-related events for LQTS1 [3] or exercise-induced PMVT (table 2). Resting ECGs and exercise recordings will disclose the diagnosis in most cases. Occasionally Holter recordings are useful, particularly if the onset of arrhythmias has been recorded (table 2).

Brugada syndrome

A clinical entity, recognized in (aborted) sudden cardiac death victims, electrocardiographically consisting of apparent right bundle branch block (RBBB) and right precordial ST-segment elevation was first recognized in 1953 [4], later elucidated

PA Doevendans and AA Wilde (eds.), Cardiovascular genetics, 169-176.

upon in 1988 [5] but first considered a functional disorder distinct from LQTS in 1992 by Pedro Brugada and Josep Brugada [6].

Table 1. Minimal abnormalities compatible with IVF [1]

- Mitral valve prolapse (lack of regurgitation, redundant valves, QT or ST-T wave abnormalities)
- Modest regional dyskinesia
- Thickening of septum or left ventricular wall (<10%)
- Paroxysmal atrial fibrillation
- Chronic atrial fibrillation
- AV block (first- or second-degree)
- Bundle-branch block
- Age > 60
- Hypertension (no hypertrophy)
- Nonspecific abnormalities at myocardial biopsy

Table 2. Differential diagnosis of Polymorphic Ventricular Tachycardia in structurally normal hearts (PMVT)

Disease [ref.]	**Age of onset**	**Gender (f/m)**	**Fam Hx**	**ECG**	**Typical symptom related trigger**	**Mode of onset**
LQTS1 [3]	>4	+/+	+++	QT↑	Exercise, swimming	Tachycardia
LQTS2 [2,3]	>10	++/+	+++	QT↑	Arousal, acoustic stimulus, emotion	pause
Cath. PMVT [21]	<10	+/++	++	Normal bradycardia	Exercise, stress	Tachycardia
Short-coupled TdP [28]	35 ± 10 (mean + SD)	+/+	++	Normal	No	Short-coupled
1q42 [26]	21 ± 10 (mean)	+/++	+++	Normal	Exercise, stress	AS
Brugada syndrome [7]	± 40 (mean)	+/+++	++	"RBBB, ST↑"	Nocturnal	Short-coupled
Idiopathic VF	± 36 (mean)	+/++	+	Normal	No	AS
ARVC2 [23,24,27]	>10	+/+	+++	Normal	Exercise, stress	AS

LQTS: long QT syndrome; Cath. PMVT: catecholamine induced polymorphic ventricular tachycardia; TdP: Torsade de Pointes; 1q42: primary arrhythmia syndrome linked to chromosome 1q42; VF: ventricular fibrillation; ARVC: arrhythmogenic right ventricular cardiomyopathy AS: no special initiation trigger.

The ECG characteristics (see figure 1), which may be variably present from day to day, are unrelated to structural heart disease, myocardial ischemia or electrolyte disturbances. The syndrome, now generally referred to as Brugada syndrome, may display a familial occurrence, affects symptomatically more males, seems to be associated with a high mortality rate, and is increasingly recognized [7]. The prevalence of this syndrome among patients with idiopathic VF critically depends on the criteria used [6].

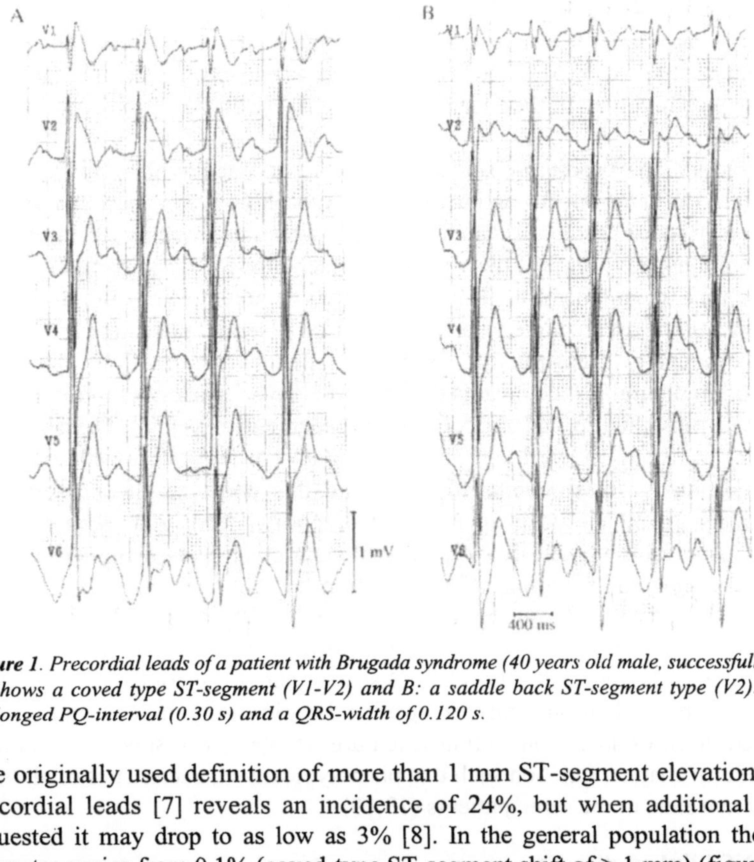

***Figure 1**. Precordial leads of a patient with Brugada syndrome (40 years old male, successfully resuscitated). A: shows a coved type ST-segment (V1-V2) and B: a saddle back ST-segment type (V2). Note also the prolonged PQ-interval (0.30 s) and a QRS-width of 0.120 s.*

The originally used definition of more than 1 mm ST-segment elevation in the right precordial leads [7] reveals an incidence of 24%, but when additional features are requested it may drop to as low as 3% [8]. In the general population the prevalence estimates varies from 0.1% (coved-type ST-segment shift of > 1 mm) (figure 1A) to 6% (saddle-back, figure 1B) in France to 0.7% (> 1 mm ST-segment shift, general male population) in Japan [9]. In Thailand (and probably other Southeast Asian countries) sudden unexplained death syndrome is the second most prevalent cause of death in young males. The 'endemic' nature of the disease in these countries is reflected by their local names like Lai-Tai (Thailand), Bangungut (Philippines) and Pokkuri (Japan).

The familial nature presumes the presence of causally related genes. Indeed, mutations in SCN5A, the gene encoding the alpha-subunit of the cardiac fast sodium channel were shown to co-segregate as an autosomal dominant trait in small families in which a high incidence of sudden cardiac death was present [11]. Similarly, in affected individuals, mutations in the SCN5A gene have been found [12]. Such genetic aberrations are generally not found in electrocardiographically unaffected family members nor in unrelated control individuals. When expressed in heterologous expression systems, functional alterations in sodium characteristics of the mutated sodium channels, could be demonstrated. Based on these genetic and electrophysiological observations a causal relationship is generally assumed [13].

SCN5A is not the only gene involved in Brugada syndrome. In fact, it is only found in 10-15% of patients, although a 33% 'hit' has also been observed [14]. Genetic heterogeneity has been demonstrated because SCN5A could be excluded as the causally related gene in a large family. The second disease-related gene is, however, located in the close vicinity of SCN5A (15). Theoretically, all genes encoding proteins responsible for the ion currents involved in the morphology of phase 1 of the action potential are candidate genes.

The causal relationship of sodium channel mutants is explained by the impact altered sodium currents do have on the action potential morphology, in particular in the epicardial layers. Reduced sodium channel amplitude, a common finding for all mutants studied, leads to a negative shift of the voltage at which phase 1 repolarization begins. This impacts on the magnitude of the L-type calcium current which may fail to activate properly. The resulting attenuation or loss of the action potential plateau phase creates electrical heterogeneity transmurally, with consequent current flow from the endocardial and midmural layers towards the epicardial layer. Electrodes located above these areas will pick this up and reflect it as ST-segment elevation. The abundant presence of the transient outward current in the right ventricular free wall creates a favorable condition for these events to occur and this underlies the predominant presence of ST-segment elevation in the right precordial leads. The dispersion in refractoriness, as a result of exclusive loss of right ventricular epicardial plateau phase creates an arrhythmogenic condition with arrhythmias resulting from phase 2 reentry [7].

Mutations in SCN5A may also cause Long QT syndrome (LQT3) [16] or Progressive Cardiac Conduction Defects (PCCD) [17]. Disease-related mutations are identified throughout the gene without any disease-specific location [12]. Indeed, these three SCN5A-linked diseases share some clinical features (table 3) and specific mutations may affect sodium channel function such that phenotypically characteristics of all three diseases may manifest in the same patients (18,19).

Table 3. *SCN5A* linked diseases

	LQT_3	BS	PCCD
Prolonged QT interval	+++	+	-
Conduction abnormalities	+	++	+++
Sudden death during sleep	++	+++	?
ST-segment elevation ($V_{1\text{-}3}$)	-	+++	?
ST-segment elevation (drugs)	++	+++	?

Electrocardiographic and clinical characteristics of arrhythmia syndromes linked to the cardiac sodium channel gene SCN5A. BS: Brugada syndrome, PCCD: Progressive cardiac conduction defects.

Exercise-induced polymorphic ventricular tachycardia

In 1978, Coumel described four paediatric patients with stress or emotion-induced syncope related to polymorphic VT [20]. A larger group of patients was described in 1995 [21]. A family history of sudden death was reported for 30% of patients. The typical patient has no structural heart disease and experiences polymorphic ventricular extrasystoles upon reaching a certain heart rate (usually between 100 and 120 bpm), culminating into bidirectional and polymorphic ventricular tachycardias eventually leading to syncope. Mean age of first syncope was 7.8 years (3-16.5). ß-Blocker treatment is usually effective. In 1999, Swan et al. described a similar phenotype in a large Finnish family [22]. Age of onset was significantly later, however. Genetic linkage to the long arm of chromosome 1 was demonstrated (1q42) [22]. This region harbours, among others, the gene encoding the cardiac ryanodine receptor gene (humanRyR2). Linkage to the same region was observed in an Italian family with exercise-induced polymorphic ventricular tachycardia in the presence of clinical evidence (including patho-anatomical observations) for arrhythmogenic right ventricular cardiomyopathy (ARVC) [23,24]. Very recently Priori et al. Identified mutations in this gene in 4 individuals with the typical phenotype [25]. Three patients carried a de novo mutation and in 1 case segregation of a genetic aberration with the phenotype was demonstrated in a small family [25]. Furthermore, also Laitinen et al. identified mutations in conserved regions of the hRyR2 gene [26]. Finally, Tisu et al. identified in the Italian families with an ARVC-like phenotype (ARVC2) aberrations in the hRyR2 gene [27].The phenotypes described thus represent allelic disorders based on mutations in the ryanodine receptor gene. Functional studies of these aberrant ryanodine receptors are not yet available, but some state of cellular calcium overload is anticipated.

Short coupled Torsades de Pointes

Torsades de Pointes is a polymorphic VT usually associated with prolongation of the QT-interval. The arrhythmia is characterized by a typical initiation sequence with a long coupling interval of the first extrasystole (from the terminal end of the T-wave) which follows a relative pause in the rhythm (short-long-short sequence). In contrast the initiating beat of the short coupled variant of Torsades de Pointes has, as the name implies, a short coupling interval [28]. The coupling interval is in fact extremely short and a preceding pause is not mandatory (figure 2; table 2). Typically, the initiating extrasystole has a left bundle branch block pattern and a left axis deviation. In the majority of cases the Torsade deteriorated into ventricular fibrillation and in 4 out of 14 cases a familial history of sudden death was present [28]. Mean age of occurrence is ± 35 years with an equal distribution between sexes [28]. Currently, no clue to the genetic basis is known.

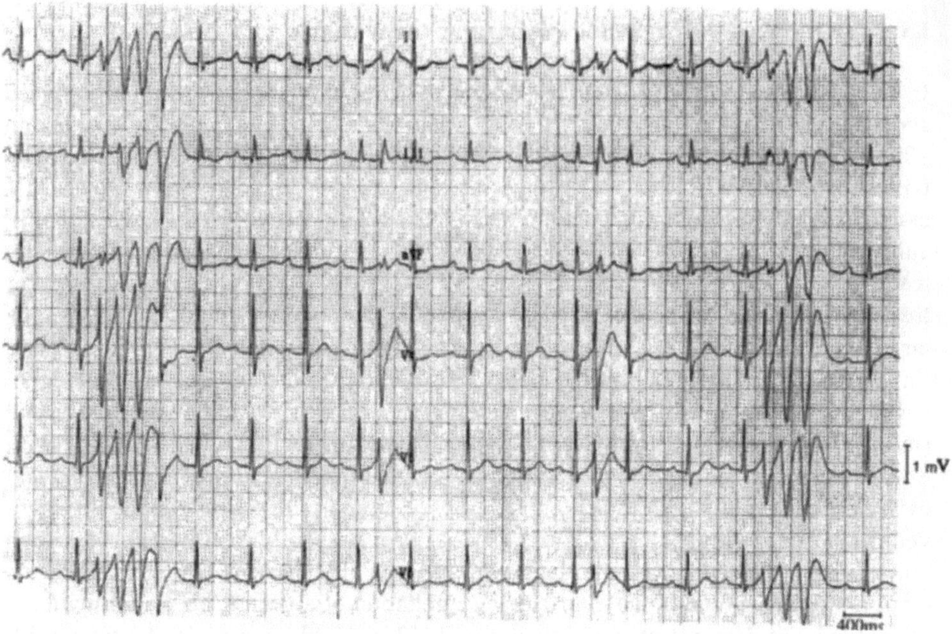

Figure 2: *6-Lead ECG (leads I, II, AVF, V_4-V_6) of a patient with short-coupled Torsades de Pointes. Note the very short coupling interval of the isolated extrasystoles and the initiating extrasystoles of the short runs of Torsade de Pointes. The QT-interval is normal.*

Table 4: Disease, chromosome, gene and category

Disease	Chromosome	Gene	Category
LQTS$_1$	11.15.5	KCNQ$_1$	A
LQTS$_2$	7.q35-36	K	A
Brugada syndrome	3.p21-23	SCN5A	B
Idiopathic VF	?	?	F
Cath-PMVT	1q42	hRyR2	B
ARVD2	1q42	hRyR2	B
Short-coupled TdP	?	?	F

For abbreviations see table 2.

Conclusion

Life-threatening ventricular arrhythmias in patients with structurally normal hearts is frequently associated with a positive family history for sudden cardiac death (at young age). The hitherto implied genetic basis is rapidly being uncovered. Currently the impact of genotyping is as follows:
Brugada Syndrome: diagnostics available. Molecular diagnosis does not alter treatment (Table 4, category B). Exercise-induced PMVT: diagnostics available. Molecular diagnosis does not alter treatment. Short-coupled TdP: No locus or gene is known.

References

1. Survivors of out-of-hospital cardiac arrest with apparently normal heart. Need for Definition and standardized clinical evaluation. Consensus Statement of the Joint Steering Committees of the Unexplained Cardiac Arrest Registry of Europe and of the Idiopathic Ventricular Fibrillation Registry in the United States. Circulation 1997; 95:265-72.
2. Wilde AAM, Jongbloed RJE, Doevendans PA, et al. Auditory stimuli as a trigger for arrhythmic events differentiate HERG-related ($LQTS_2$) patients from $KVLQT_1$-related patients ($LQTS_1$). J Am Coll Cardiol 1999; 33:327-32.
3. Schwartz PJ, Priori SG, Spazzolini C, et al. Genotype-phenotype correlation in the long-QT syndrome. Gene-specific triggers for life-threatening arrhythmias. Circulation 2001; 103:89-96.
4. Osher H.L., Wolff L.: Electrocardiographic pattern simulating acute myocardial injury. Am J Med Sci 1953; 226:541-45.
5. Martini B, Nava A, Thiene G, et al. Ventricular fibrillation without apparent heart disease: description of 6 cases. Am Heart J 1989; 118:1203-9.
6. Brugada P, Brugada J. Right bundle branch block, persistent ST segment elevation and sudden cardiac death: a distinct clinical and electrocardiographic syndrome. J Am Coll Cardiol 1992; 20:1391-6.
7. Alings M, Wilde A. "Brugada" Syndrome. Clinical data and suggested pathophysiological mechanism. Circulation 1999; 99:666-73.
8. Remme CA, Wever EFD, Wilde AAM et al. Diagnosis and long-term follow-up of the Brugada syndrome in patiënts with idiopathic ventricular fibrillation. Eur. Heart J. 2001; 22: 400-409.
9. Hermida JS, Lemoine JL, Bou Aoun F, et al. Prevalence of the Brugada syndrome in a apparently healthy population. Am J Cardiol 2000; 86:91-4.
10. Miyasaka Y, Yamada K, Sugiura T, et al. Prevalence and mortality of right bundle branch block and right precordial ST-segment elevation (Brugada type ECG) in a general population. Circulation 2000; 102 Supp II:676A.
11. Chen Q, Kirsch GE, Zhang D, et al. Genetic basis and molecular mechanism for idiopathic ventricular fibrillation. Nature 1998; 392:293-6.
12. Bezzina CR, Rook MB, Wilde AAM. The cardiac sodium channel and inherited arrhythmia syndromes. Cardiovasc Res 2001; 49:257-271.
13. Wilde AAM, Veldkamp MW. What we can learn from individual resuscitated patients. Cardiovasc Res 2000; 46:14-6.
14. Gasparini M, Priori SG, Mantica M, et al. Provocative test in the Brugada Syndrome: do we have the right tools? Circulation 2000; 102 Supp II:677A.
15. London B, Barmada M, Nguyen T, et al. Identifying a second Brugada Syndrome locus on chromosome 3. Circulation 2000; 102 Supp II:280A.
16. Way Q, Shen J, Splawski I, et al. SCN5A mutations associated with an inherited cardiac arrhythmia, long QT syndrome. Cell 1995; 80:805-11.
17. Schott JJ, Alshinawi C, Kyndt F, et al. Cardiac conduction defects associate with mutations in SCN5A. Nature Genet 1999; 23:20-1.
18. Bezzina C, Veldkamp MW, van den Berg MP, et al. A single Na^+ channel mutation causing both long-QT and Brugada syndromes. Circ Res 1999; 1206-13.
19. Veldkamp MW, Viswanathan PC, Bezzina C, et al. Two distinct congenital arrhythmias evoked by a multidysfunctional Na^+ channel. Circ Res 2000; 86:91-9.
20. Coumel P, Fidelle J, Lucet V, et al. Catecholamine-induced severe ventricular arrhythmias with Adam-Stokes syndrome in children: report of four cases. Br Heart J 1978; 40 suppl:28-37.
21. Leenhardt A, Lucet V, Denjoy I, et al. Catecholaminergic polymorphic ventricular tachycardia in children. A 7-year follow-up of 21 patients. Circulation 1995; 91:1512-9.

22. Swan H, Piipo K, Viitasalo M, et al. Arrhythmic disorder mapped to chromosome 1q42-q43 causes malignant polymorphic ventricular tachycardia in structurally normal hearts. J Am Coll Cardiol 1999; 34:2035-42.
23. Rampazzo A, Nava A, Erne P, et al. A new locus for arrhythmogenic right ventricular cardiomyopathy (ARVD2) maps to chromosome 1q42-q43. Hum Mol Genet 1995; 4:2151-54.
24. Nava A, Canciani B, Daliento L, et al. Juvenile sudden death and effort ventricular tachycardias in a family with right ventricular cardiomyopathy. Int J Cardiol 1988; 21:111-25.
25. Priori SG, Napolitano C, Tiso N, et al. Mutations in the cardiac ryanodine receptor gene (hRyR2) underlie catecholaminergic polymorphic ventricular tachycardia. Circulation 2000; 102:r49-53.
26. Laitinen PJ, Brown KM, Piippo K, et al. Mutations of the cardiac ryanodine receptor (RyR2) gene in familial polymorphic ventricular tachycardia. Circulation 2001; 103:485-90.
27. Tiso N, Stephan DA, Nava A, et al. Identification of mutations in the cardiac ryanodinge receptor gene in families affected with arrhythmogenic right ventricular cardiomyopathy type 2 (ARVD2). Hum Mol Genet 2001; 10:189-94.
28. Leenhardt A, Glaser E, Burguera M, et al. Short-coupled variant of Torsades de Pointes. A new electrocardiographic entity in the spectrum of idiopathic ventricular arrhythmias. Circulation 1994; 89:206-15.

15. DIAGNOSIS AND TREATMENT OF THE CONGENITAL LONG QT SYNDROME

X.H.T. Wehrens, M.A. Vos, A.A. Wilde

Introduction

Over the past decade, the congenital long QT syndrome (LQTS) has contributed significantly to our understanding of ventricular arrhythmias. Congenital LQTS is an inherited disease characterized by prolonged ventricular repolarization and a propensity for life-threatening ventricular tachyarrhythmias resulting in syncope and sudden death [1]. Two forms of inherited long QT syndrome are known: (1) the more common Romano-Ward syndrome (RWS), with an autosomal dominant inheritance, and (2) the Jervell and Lange-Nielssen syndrome (JLN), which is usually autosomal recessive long QT syndrome associated with inherited sensorineuronal deafness. Long QT syndrome, occurring secondary to heart failure, hypertrophy or drug-therapy, is called acquired LQTS [2].

An abrupt and important turn in the understanding of the congenital LQTS has resulted from the discovery that mutations in genes encoding ion channels are responsible for the manifestation of this disease [3]. As a consequence, it became clear that what has been going under the unifying name of the LQTS, actually represents a variety of different diseases caused by ion channel mutations, all producing alterations in ionic currents, leading to the same end result: prolonged ventricular repolarization [4]. In the past five years, this understanding has paved the way to a deeper level of comprehension of the syndrome, and as a result of that, a potentially genotype-specific treatment of LQTS mutation carriers (Category A disorder). In addition, several mutations and polymorphisms have been identified that predispose people to drug-provoked QT-interval prolongation (Category D disorder).

Genetics of the LQTS

LQTS is the first recognized inherited myocardial ion-channel disease. Genetic linkage mapping of the autosomal-dominant form of LQTS (Romano-Ward syndrome) has identified loci on six different chromosomes thus far (*LQT1-LQT6*) [5]. The autosomal

PA Doevendans and AA Wilde (eds.), Cardiovascular genetics, 177-190.

recessive variant of the LQTS (JLN) arises in individuals who inherit abnormal *KCNQ1(= KvLQT1)* or *KCNE1 (= minK)* alleles from both parents (*LQT1*, *LQT5*). The abnormal gene can be the same (usually in consanguineous families) or different (so-called compound heterozygosity) [6]. Parents of subjects with JLN are heterozygous for LQTS mutations, but are usually (but not always) asymptomatic (table 1) [7].

Most LQTS genes encode potassium channels, although the *LQT3 (SCN5A)* gene encodes the cardiac sodium channel (current indicated by I_{Na}) [8]. Two genes encode the slowly activating delayed rectifier potassium channel I_{Ks}, the α-subunit is encoded by *KCNQ1* and the β-subunit by *KCNE1*. Finally, the *LQT2 (KCNH2 = HERG)* and *LQT6 (KCNE2 = MiRP1)* genes encode the α- and β-subunit of the rapidly activating delayed rectifier potassium channel I_{Kr}, respectively [5]. Mutant channels result in repolarization abnormalities, that underlie clinical and ECG findings. The LQT genes *KCNQ1* (42%) and *KCNH2* (45%) account for most of the identified mutations so far, *SCN5A* (8%), *KCNE1* (3%), and *KNCE2* (2%) account for the remaining 13% (see Table 1). Missense mutations are most common (>70%), followed by frameshift mutations (10%), in-frame deletions, and nonsense and splice-site mutations (5-7% each) [5].

Table 1. Clinical characteristics in common forms of LQTS

	LQT1	LQT2	LQT3
Gene mutated	*KCNQ1* (=*KvLQT1*)	*KCNH2* (=*HERG*)	*SCN5A*
Current affected	I_{Ks}	I_{Kr}	I_{Na}
Estimated prevalence (%)	45	40	10
% events occurring with exercise or emotional stress	97	51	39
Exercise related trigger	+++	+	+
Other triggers	Swimming	Loud noise	
% with events to age 10	40	16	2
% with events to age 40	63	46	18
Median age 1st event	9	12	16
Mean QTc	490 ± 43	495 ± 43	510 ± 48
QT shortening with exercise	< normal	normal	> normal
Efficacy β-blockade to prevent events	+++	++	+?
Efficacy mexilletine to shorten QT	-	+	+++
Classification	Cat A disease	Cat A disease	Cat A disease

Adapted from: Wilde AAM, Roden DM. Circulation 2000; 102:2796-98 [48].

Functional consequences of LQTS mutations

The ventricular action potential is generated by the summation of individual currents moving through multiple ion channel proteins (figure 1). The rapidly activating and inactivating Na^+ current is primarily responsible for the initial upstroke of the action potential. The characteristic plateau phase of the human cardiac action potential is maintained by a fine balance of small inward and outward currents flowing through pumps, exchangers, and voltage-gated channels with unique voltage-dependent properties and kinetics. Because the plateau period is one of *very high input impedance*, small changes in any ionic component can cause pronounced effects on the duration and wave form of the action potential plateau [9]. Outward plateau current gradually increases over the time course of the plateau. The process of repolarization begins when net outward current exceeds inward current. The three major repolarizing currents are the rapidly activating delayed rectifier potassium current I_{Kr}, [10], the slowly activating delayed rectifier current I_{Ks} [11], and the inward rectifier current I_{K1} (figure 1).
Mutations in the cardiac Na^+ channels linked to LQT3 generally promote additional sodium channel activity during the plateau phase of the action potential leading to an extra component of inward current [12]. This additional inward current would be expected to prolong repolarization, and hence underlie the phenotype in carriers of these *SCN5A* mutations [13]. Mutations in the genes encoding the I_{Ks} and I_{Kr} potassium currents generally lead to a 'loss of function' of repolarizing current [14]. Hence, a reduction in repolarizing potassium current underlies the prolongation of the action potential duration (figure 1).

Clinical presentation and management of LQTS patients

Sudden death or a history of unexplained syncope in a child or young adult can bring a patient or family members under the clinician's attention. However, some of them are asymptomatic, despite the fact that they display the electrocardiographic characteristics of LQTS. Another group consists of patients that have been identified as LQTS mutation carriers without symptoms or any electrocardiographic feature related to LQTS. Finally, there is a group of patients that carries ion channel mutations or polymorphisms, that predispose them to drug-induced LQTS [15]. The diagnostic approach and guidelines for management of these categories of patients will be discussed in the following paragraphs.

Patients with symptoms of congenital LQTS

Symptoms
Recurrent syncopal attacks or cardiac arrest in a child or young adult should raise suspicion for the LQTS. Unexplained sudden cardiac death < 40 years among immediate family members or family members with definite LQTS can provide additional clues. The combination of syncope, epilepsy or cardiac arrest with congenital deafness should also alert the clinician.
The clinical course of LQTS is dependent on the genotype present in the mutation

carriers. Zareba et al. [16] found that cardiac events appear earlier in life in LQT1 compared to LQT3 patients. By the age of 15, more than 60% of LQT1 patients have had a cardiac event (syncope, cardiac arrest, or sudden cardiac death), compared to less than 10% in LQT3 patients [16,17]. The number of cardiac events that occurred till the age of 40 years was also higher among subjects with mutations at the LQT1 locus (63%) or LQT2 locus (46%) than among subjects with mutations at the LQT3 locus (18%). In contrast, the likelihood of death *during* a cardiac event was much higher among LQT3 mutation carriers (20%) compared to LQT1 and LQT2 (4%) [16]. Due to the low number of patients, no data are available yet for LQT5 and LQT6 patients.

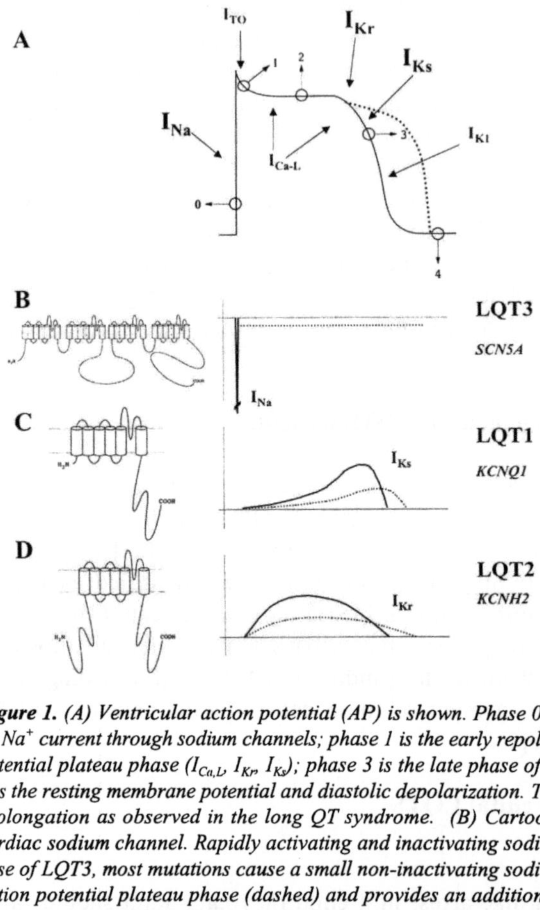

Figure 1. (A) Ventricular action potential (AP) is shown. Phase 0 is the action potential upstroke, initiated by Na^+ *current through sodium channels; phase 1 is the early repolarization phase* (I_{TO})*; phase 2 is the action potential plateau phase* ($I_{Ca,L}$, I_{Kr}, I_{Ks})*; phase 3 is the late phase of rapid repolarization* (I_{Ks}, I_{K1})*; and phase 4 is the resting membrane potential and diastolic depolarization. The dashed line represents action potential prolongation as observed in the long QT syndrome. (B) Cartoon of the gene* SCN5A, *that encodes the cardiac sodium channel. Rapidly activating and inactivating sodium current initiates phase 0 of the AP. In case of LQT3, most mutations cause a small non-inactivating sodium current that remains active during the action potential plateau phase (dashed) and provides an additional depolarizang current, which prolongs repolarization. (C) Cartoon of the* KCQN1 *gene, that encodes the cardiac potassium channel conducting* I_{Ks}. I_{Ks} *is the slowly activating delayed rectifier current that importantly contributes to repolarization. In case of LQT1, reduced* I_{Ks} *activity leads to action potential prolongation. (D) Cartoon of the* KCNH2 *gene, that encodes the potassium channel which conducts the rapidly activating delayed rectifier current* I_{Kr}. *In LQT2, a reduction of* I_{Kr} *causes prolongation of the repolarization phase (dashed line).*

Triggers of cardiac events

Triggers for arrhythmic episodes and syncope are also depending on the specific LQTS gene affected. In I_{Ks}-related LQTS (LQT1), exercise- and stress-related events dominate the clinical picture [17,18]. Diving and swimming, as triggers, are almost exclusive for LQT1 patients [17,19]. In contrast, patients with LQT3-associated Na^+ channel mutations are at particularly high risk, at rest or asleep, because their QT interval is excessively prolonged at slow heart rates. LQT2 patients have an intermediate pattern, and tend to display events both at rest and during exercise. However, events provoked by auditory stimuli such as an alarm clock or telephone ringing particularly occur in LQT2 patients [17,19]. No data are available yet for LQT5 and LQT6 patients.

Beta-blocker therapy for symptomatic patients

Among untreated *symptomatic* patients, mortality is high, being 20% in the first year after the initial syncope, and approximately 50% within 10 years [20]. The 10-year mortality rate dropped below 5% after LQTS patients were routinely put on adrenergic receptor blocking therapy [21]. In a large retrospective study in 869 LQTS patients (581 probands and 288 affected family members), the effectiveness and limitations of -blockers were evaluated [22] by comparing matched periods before and after starting β-blocker therapy. After initiation of β-blockers, there was a significant reduction in the rate of cardiac events in both probands and affected family members. Patients (> 10 years of age) who had cardiac symptoms before β-blocker therapy had, however, a high likelihood of experiencing recurrent cardiac events (32% within 5 years) despite the assumed usage of β-blockers. However, the risk of experiencing aborted cardiac arrest or sudden death in patients with only syncope before β-blocker therapy was <1.7% in 5 years. In patients with aborted cardiac arrest before β-blocker therapy, the probability to die was 6.6% and to experience another cardiac arrest or die was 14% [22]. In patients with recurrent cardiac symptoms or aborted cardiac arrest, β-blocker therapy might not be completely effective in preventing sudden cardiac death, and ICD therapy may be warranted for these high-risk patients.

Towards a genotype-specific therapy of symptomatic LQTS patients

As most LQT1 patients experience syncopal events during exercise, competitive sports should be avoided. Diving and swimming without supervision, identified as a common trigger for LQT1 patients, should also be avoided [19]. The high risk associated with auditory stimuli in LQT2 patients warrants the removal of telephones and alarm clocks from patients bedrooms.

Patients with LQT1 and LQT2 genotypes may benefit from β-blocker therapy as cardiac events rates were reduced [17,22]. Because the amplitude of I_{Kr} increased when extracellular potassium concentrations are increased, attempts have been undertaken to increase K^+ levels in LQT2 patients. Indeed, QT intervals have been shown to shorten significantly in response to K^+ in LQT2 patients [23]. Potassium supplementation is, however, hindered by difficulties in achieving high K^+ concentrations with chronic oral therapy [24].

A beneficial effect of β-blocker therapy has not been demonstrated for LQT3 patients [17,22]. LQT3 patients are at higher risk at slow heart rates, and therefore may benefit from pacemaker therapy. Several experimental and clinical studies suggest a beneficial effect of Na^+ channel blockers such as mexillitine [25] or flecainide [26] in LQT3 patients, although long-term follow-up data are not yet available. It should be noted, however, that flecainide causes a Brugada-like ECG (see chapter 14) in a significant number of LQT3 patients [27]. The impact of these changes which suggest the introduction of a different arrhythmogenic substrate is currently unknown. A further therapeutic differentiation on the basis of the specific mutation in the affected gene can be expected in the near future.

Patients without symptoms but with ECG characteristics suggestive of LQTS

ECG characteristics of the long QT syndrome

Some patients are not identified on the basis of their symptoms, but because of typical electrocardiographic features suggestive of LQTS. The principal diagnostic hallmark of LQTS is abnormal prolongation of ventricular repolarization, measured as lengthening of the QT interval on the 12-lead ECG. This is most easily identified in leads II or V1, V3, or V5, but all 12 leads should be examined to identify the longest QT interval [28]. Bazett' correction formula ($QTc = QT / \sqrt{RR}$) is often used to correct QT interval for heart rate.

The diagnosis 'LQTS' is easily confirmed when the QTc is markedly increased (eg. ≥ 500 ms), but often the QTc values are more modestly prolonged [29]. When QTc ≥ 460 ms is used, the positive predictive accuracy for LQTS is 96% in women and 91% in men; negative predictive accuracy of almost 100% is present with a QTc ≤ 410 ms in males and ≤ 440 ms in females [29]. When the QTc ≥ 480, positive predictive accuracy for LQTS is 100%. In any case of doubt, genetic studies are recommended.

The second electrocardiographic characteristic of the LQTS is QT interval dispersion, which can be measured as a lead-to-lead variability in QT intervals. In normal individuals, the difference between maximum and minimal QT intervals measured on the standard resting ECG has been reported to be 54 ± 27 [30] and 48 ± 18 msec [28]. In patients with the congenital LQTS, however, regional dispersion of ventricular repolarization times have been reported to vary from 109 to 185 msec [30,31].

In LQTS patients, not only the duration of repolarization is altered (QT interval), but also its morphology. The most typical presentation of the T wave may be biphasic or notched, and these findings are most prominent in the precordial leads [32].The appearance of notched T wave during the recovery phase of exercise occurs significantly more frequently in LQTS patients than in control patients (85% vs 3%). In addition, T wave alternans is an infrequently recorded highly arrhythmogenic electrocardiographic finding with transient beat-to-beat changes in amplitude, shape, and polarity of the T wave during sinus rhythm without concomitant QRS changes. T wave alternans is encountered in about 2.5% of all patients [33].

Signs of sinus node dysfunction, consisting of sinus bradycardia, sinus pauses, and a lower than expected heart rate during exercise have been reported in patients with the LQTS [34]. Slow heart rates are particularly striking in younger children. During submaximal exercise testing, many LQTS patients reach a lower maximal heart rate level than that achieved by healthy controls matched by sex and age [35].

Genotype-specific ECG finding

The different time- and voltage-dependence of the ionic currents involved in LQTS are probably responsible for distinct ECG-phenotypes that have been reported for the different genotypes. Initial studies by Moss et al. [36] reported an association of certain T-wave patterns with LQT1, LQT2, and LQT3. Recenty, Zhang et al. [37] recognized 10 typical ST-T wave patterns that are genotype specific (4 LQT1, 4 LQT2, and 2 LQT3) (see figure 2). Prolonged broad-based T waves and widened bifid T-waves, mostly low in amplitude, are characteristic for LQT1 and LQT2. Most notable for LQT3 is the long isoelectric segment followed by a normal T-wave duration with a relatively sharp deflection [37]. These ECG characteristics cannot be used to diagnose LQTS, but are rather useful to stratify molecular genetic studies.

In a recent study by Swan et al. [35], a reduced maximum heart rate during exercise was found for LQT1 patients, whereas this was normal for LQT2 patients, compared to controls. During recovery from exercise, LQT1 patients showed an exaggeration of the QT interval prolongation and steeper QT/heart rate slopes compared to LQT2 and in controls [35]. Finally, Schwartz et al. reported that LQT3 patients display a higher degree of QT interval shortening in response to increase in heart rate than LQT2 patients [25] (see table 1).

Treatment of asymptomatic patients with ECG characteristics of LQTS

Treatment of asymptomatic patients is still controversial, because the majority of LQTS patients will never experience symptoms, and sudden death during the first syncopal episode is unlikely to occur [16]. While waiting for more definitive data, Schwartz recommended to begin treatment for asymptomatic patients only under the following six conditions: in those with congenital deafness; in neonates and for the first year of life because of the enhanced risk during the first months in life; in siblings of children who have already died suddenly; in patients with documented evidence of T wave alternans; when the QTc exceeds 600 ms; and whenever there is manifest anxiety or explicit request for treatment [38].

Mutation carriers without symptoms or ECG characteristics of LQTS

It is estimated that approximately 10% of all patients that carry a LQTS ion channel mutation have a normal QTc $\leq$ 440 ms [37]. However, only 2% of all LQTS mutation carriers have a normal ST-T wave pattern with a normal QT interval. Priori et al. [39] showed that in some families penetrance can be as low as 25%. This implies that family members considered normal on clinical grounds could be silent gene carriers, and thus would be unexpectedly at risk of generating affected offspring and perhaps also of developing torsade de pointes arrhythmias if exposed to either cardiac or noncardiac drugs that block potassium channels [15,40]. It is therefore recommended to perform molecular screening in all family members of genotyped patients [39]. On the other hand, few LQTS patients present with sudden death as their first symptom. Conservative management of silent gene carriers seems advisable, as the value of -blocker therapy is still unknown.

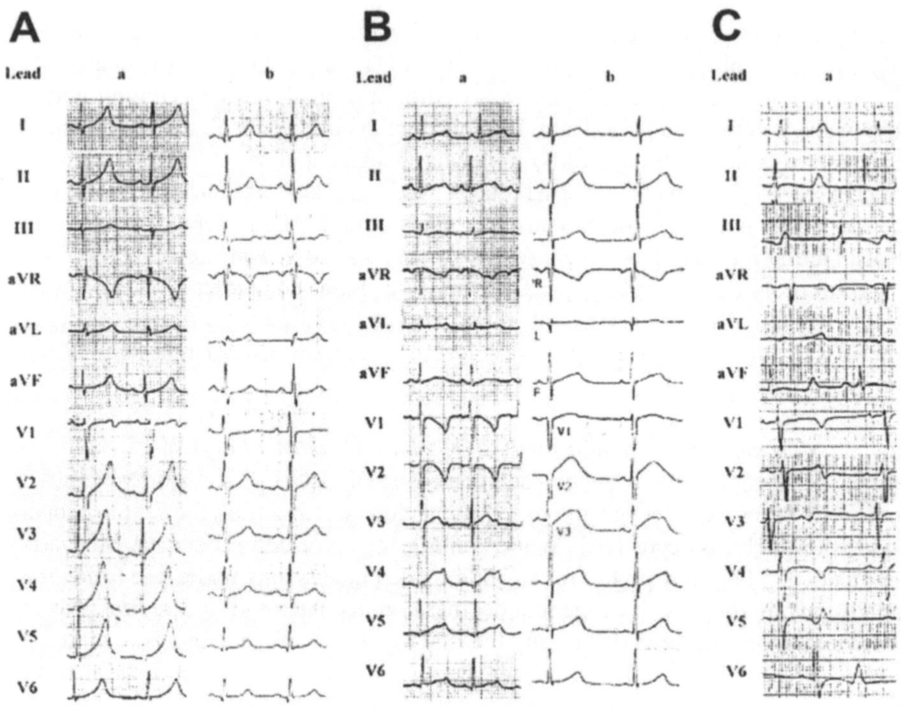

Figure 2. (A). The two most common LQT1 ECG patterns: (a) Broad-based T-wave pattern, (b) normal-appearing T-wave pattern. (B). The two most frequently encountered LQT2 ECG manifestations: (a) Obvious bifid T-waves, (b) Subtle bifid T-wave with a second component on top of the T-wave in limb and left precordial leads (or alternatively the second component on the downslope of T-wave; not shown). (C). Most typical LQT3 ECG pattern: (a) Late-onset peaked/biphasic T-wave. From: Zhang et al. Circulation 2000;102:2849-55 [37]

Patients carrying polymorphisms associated with drug-induced LQTS

Some patients carry a predisposition for drug-induced torsade de pointes arrhythmias on the basis of congenital LQTS, hypertrophy, heart failure, conduction defects, or hypokalemia [2]. Acquired LQTS can also be a side effect of treatment with commonly used medications, including some antiarrhythmic, antihistamine, antibiotic, psychoactive, and gastrointestinal prokinetic agents [41] (see table 2). A minority of patients with drug-provoked LQTS has a *genetic* predisposition to torsade de pointes because of mutations in the *KCNE2* subunit of their I_{Kr} potassium channel [42,43] or a mutation in the *KCNQ1* subunit of their I_{Ks} channel [40]. In addition, a polymorphism in the *KCNE1* gene [44], as well as two relatively common polymorphisms in *KCNE2* (allelic frequency in both cases around 1.6%) have been associated with quinidine- and erythromycin-induced LQTS [15,42]. However, in most patients with acquired LQTS, no ion channel mutations have been identified thus far.

In patients without ion channel mutations, it is believed that pro-arrhythmia is induced by block of the potassium current I_{Kr} [45]. Recent studies have shed some light on the fact why so many structurally diverse compounds block *KCNH2* channels but not other potassium channels. Because the *KCNH2* channel has a unique group of amino acids in the S6 domain which are not present in other voltage-gated K^+ channels (Kv1-Kv4), many commonly used drugs preferentially block *KCNH2* channels [15], placing patients at risk for cardiac arrhythmias.

There are no data to support genetic diagnostic approaches in these patients, unless they participate in a study. The relevance of the polymorphisms is not yet clear, and there is no well defined set of genes that have to be analyzed. A pragmatic approach is to provide a list of compounds that should not be used in the future and should be known to both mutation carriers and patients with LQTS (see table 2).

Table 2. List of drugs associated with acquired long QT syndrome

Cardiovascular

Antianginal
Bepridil

Antiarrhythmic
Amiodarone, Disopyramide, Dofetilide, Flecainide, Ibutilide, Procainamide, Quinidine, Sotalol

Antihypertensive agent
Isradipine, Moexipril, Nicardipine,

Diuretic
Indapamide

Lipid lowering drugs
Probucol

Central nervous system

Anesthetic
Droperidol

Anticonvulsant
Felbamate, Fosphenytoin

Antidepressant
Amitriptyline, Desipramine, Doxepin, Fluoxetine, Imipramine, Venlafaxinee

Antimigraine
Naratriptan, Sumatryptan, Zolmitriptan

Antipsychotics
Chlorpromazine, Haloperidol, Meroidazine, Quetiapine, Pimozide, Risperidone, Thioridazine

Muscle relaxant
Tizanidine

Opiate agonist
Levomethadyl

Gastrointestinal

Antidiarrhea
Octreotide

Prokinetic agent
*Cizapride, Clemastine

Microbiological

Antibiotics
Clarithromycin, Erythromycin, Gatifloxacin, *Grepafloxacin, Levofloxacin, Moxifloxacin
Pentamidine, Sparfloxacin, Trimethoprim, Sulfamethoxazole

Antifungal
Fluconazole, Itraconazole, Ketoconazole

Antiviral
Foscarnet

Antimalarial
Halofantrine

Other

Anti cancer
Arsenic trioxide, Tamoxifen

Antihistamine
*Astemizole, Azelastine, *Terfenadine

Immunosuppressant
Tracolimus

Sympathicomimetic
Salmeterol

* *Removed from the market. For regularly updated information concerning drugs that prolong the QT interval and/or induce Torsade de Pointes, see the website **www.QTdrugs.org** by Dr R.L. Woosley.*

Conclusion

In approximately 60-70% of all patients with clinical signs of LQTS, a mutation has been identified despite thorough screening of all known LQTS loci. It is therefore expected that possibly new genes encoding cardiac ion channel or associated regulatory proteins will be related with LQTS. The same accounts for drug-provoked LQTS, where ion channel mutations and polymorphisms seem to predispose certain patients to drug-induced arrhythmias. Future identification of more mutations, polymorphisms, and novel LQTS genes will enable the prospective identification of groups of patients that are at risk for drug-induced LQTS.

Recent and ongoing studies into the mechanisms that relate the molecular defects to the clinical manifestation of the long QT syndrome contribute to the development of a gene- and even mutation-specific therapy for the congenital LQTS. This is most apparent for LQT3, where carriers of certain mutations respond well to mexiletine therapy [25], whereas patients with a different mutation seem to benefit more from flecainide therapy [25,46]. It is to be expected that also for *KCNH2*-related LQTS a mutation-specific therapeutic strategy might develop, as it is reasonable to assume that mutations leading to intracellular trafficking defects require a different intervention strategy compared to mutations that exert a dominant-negative effect on healthy channel subunits [47,48]. The therapeutic strategies in relation to the genetic diagnosis that are available for physicians dealing with LQTS patients at this moment have been listed.

References

1. Schwartz PJ. Idiopathic long QT syndrome: progress and questions. Am Heart J. 1985; 109:399-411.
2. Roden DM. Mechanisms and management of proarrhythmia. Am J Cardiol. 1998; 82:49-57I.
3. Wang Q, Shen J, Splawski I, et al. SCN5A mutations associated with an inherited cardiac arrhythmia, long QT syndrome. Cell. 1995; 80:805-11.
4. Kass RS. Genetically induced reduction in small currents has major impact. Circulation. 1997; 96:1720-21.
5. Splawski I, Shen J, Timothy KW, et al. Spectrum of mutations in long-QT syndrome genes. KVLQT1, HERG, SCN5A, KCNE1, and KCNE2. Circulation. 2000; 102:1178-85.
6. Schulze-Bahr E, Wang Q, Wedekind H, et al. KCNE1 mutations cause Jervell and Lange-Nielsen syndrome. Nat Genet. 1997; 17:267-68.
7. Priori SG, Schwartz PJ, Napolitano C, et al. A recessive variant of the Romano-Ward long-QT syndrome? Circulation. 1998; 97:2420-25.
8. Geelen JL, Doevendans PA, Jongbloed RJ, et al. Molecular genetics of inherited long QT syndromes. Eur Heart J. 1998; 19:1427-33.
9. Kass RS, Davies MP. The roles of ion channels in an inherited heart disease: molecular genetics of the long QT syndrome. Cardiovasc Res. 1996; 32:443-54.
10. Sanguinetti MC, Jurkiewicz NK. Lanthanum blocks a specific component of I_K and screens membrane surface change in cardiac cells. Am J Physiol. 1990; 259:H1881-89.
11. Sanguinetti MC, Jurkiewicz NK. Delayed rectifier outward K^+ current is composed of two currents in guinea pig atrial cells. Am J Physiol. 1991; 260:H393-99.
12. Bennett PB, Yazawa K, Makita N, et al. Molecular mechanism for an inherited cardiac arrhythmia. Nature. 1995;376: 683-85.
13. Clancy CE, Rudy Y. Linking a genetic defect to its cellular phenotype in a cardiac arrhythmia. Nature. 1999; 400:566-69.
14. Sanguinetti MC, Curran ME, Spector PS, et al. Spectrum of HERG K^+-channel dysfunction in an inherited cardiac arrhythmia. Proc Natl Acad Sci U S A. 1996; 93:2208-12.
15. Sesti F, Abbott GW, Wei J, et al. A common polymorphism associated with antibiotic-induced cardiac arrhythmia. Proc Natl Acad Sci U S A. 2000; 97:10613-18.
16. Zareba W, Moss AJ, Schwartz PJ, et al. Influence of genotype on the clinical course of the long-QT syndrome. International Long-QT Syndrome Registry Research Group. N Engl J Med. 1998; 339:960-65.
17. Schwartz PJ, Priori SG, Spazzolini C, et al. Genotype-phenotype correlation in the long-QT syndrome : gene-specific triggers for life-threatening arrhythmias. Circulation. 2001; 103:89-95.
18. Wilde AA, Jongbloed RJ, Doevendans PA, et al. Auditory stimuli as a trigger for arrhythmic events differentiate HERG-related (LQTS2) patients from KVLQT1-related patients (LQTS1). J Am Coll Cardiol. 1999; 33:327-32.
19. Moss AJ, Robinson JL, Gessman L, et al. Comparison of clinical and genetic variables of cardiac events associated with loud noise versus swimming among subjects with the long QT syndrome. Am J Cardiol. 1999; 84:876-79.
20. Schwartz PJ, Periti M, Malliani A. The long Q-T syndrome. Am Heart J. 1975;89:378-90.
21. Moss AJ, Schwartz PJ, Crampton RS, et al. The long QT syndrome: a prospective international study. Circulation. 1985; 71:17-21.
22. Moss AJ, Zareba W, Hall WJ, et al. Effectiveness and limitations of beta-blocker therapy in congenital long-QT syndrome. Circulation. 2000; 101:616-23.
23. Compton SJ, Lux RL, Ramsey MR, et al. Genetically defined therapy of inherited long-QT syndrome. Correction of abnormal repolarization by potassium. Circulation. 1996;

94:1018-22.
24. Tan HL, Alings M, Van Olden RW, et al. Long-term (subacute) potassium treatment in congenital HERG-related long QT syndrome (LQTS2). J Cardiovasc Electrophysiol. 1999; 10:229-33.
25. Schwartz PJ, Priori SG, Napolitano C, et al. Long QT syndrome patients with mutations of the SCN5A and HERG genes have differential responses to Na^+ channel blockade and to increases in heart rate. Implications for gene-specific therapy. Circulation. 1995; 92:3381-86.
26. Benhorin J, Taub R, Goldsmit M, et al. Effects of flecainide in patients with new SCN5A mutation: mutation-specific therapy for long-QT syndrome? Circulation. 2000; 101:1698-706.
27. Priori SG, Napolitano C, Schwartz PJ, et al. The elusive link between LQT3 and Brugada syndrome : the role of flecainide challenge. Circulation. 2000; 102:945-947.
28. Cowan JC, et al. Importance of lead selection in QT interval measurement. Am J Cardiol. 1988; 61:83-87.
29. Vincent GM, Timothy KW, Leppert M, et al. The spectrum of symptoms and QT intervals in carriers of the gene for the long-QT syndrome. N Engl J Med. 1992; 327:846-52.
30. Sylven JC, Horacek BM, Spencer CA, et al. QT interval variability on the body surface. J Electrocardiol. 1984; 17:179-88.
31. Linker NJ, Colonna P, Kelwick CA, et al. Assessment of QT dispersion in symptomatic patients with congenital long QT syndromes. Am J Cardiol. 1992; 69:634-38.
32. Malfatto G, Beria G, Sala S, et al. Quantitative analysis of T wave abnormalities and their prognostic implications in the idiopathic long QT syndrome. J Am Coll Cardiol. 1994; 23:296-301.
33. Schwartz PJ, Malliani A. Electrical alternation of the T-wave: clinical and experimental evidence of its relationship with the sympathetic nervous system and with the long Q-T syndrome. Am Heart J. 1975; 89:45-50.
34. Moss AJ, Schwartz PJ, Crampton RS, et al. The long QT syndrome. Prospective longitudinal study of 328 families. Circulation. 1991; 84:1136-44.
35. Swan H, Viitasalo M, Piippo K, et al. Sinus node function and ventricular repolarization during exercise stress test in long QT syndrome patients with KvLQT1 and HERG potassium channel defects. J Am Coll Cardiol. 1999; 34:823-29.
36. Moss AJ, Zareba W, Benhorin J, et al. ECG T-wave patterns in genetically distinct forms of the hereditary long QT syndrome. Circulation. 1995; 92:2929-34.
37. Zhang L, Timothy KW, Vincent GM, et al. Spectrum of ST-T-wave patterns and repolarization parameters in congenital long-QT syndrome : ECG findings identify genotypes. Circulation. 2000; 102:2849-55.
38. Schwartz PJ. The long QT syndrome. Armonk,NY: Futura Publishing Company,Inc.; 1997.
39. Priori SG, Napolitano C, Schwartz PJ.Low penetrance in the long-QT syndrome: clinical impact. Circulation. 1999; 99:529-33.
40. Napolitano C, Schwartz PJ, Brown AM, et al. Evidence for a cardiac ion channel mutation underlying drug-induced QT prolongation and life-threatening arrhythmias. J Cardiovasc Electrophysiol. 2000; 11:691-96.
41. Roden DM. Acquired long QT syndromes and the risk of proarrhythmia. J Cardiovasc Electrophysiol. 2000; 11:938-40.
42. Abbott GW, Sesti F, Splawski I, et al. MiRP1 forms I_{Kr} potassium channels with HERG and is associated with cardiac arrhythmia. Cell. 1999; 97:175-87.
43. Wei J, Abbott GW, Sesti F, et al. Prevalence of KCNE2 (MiRP1) mutations in acquired long QT syndrome [Abstract]. Circulation. 1999; 100:I495.
44. Wei J, Yang ICH, Tapper AR, et al. KCNE1 polymorphism confers risk of drug-induced long QT syndrome by altering kinetic properties to Iks potassium channels [Abstract]. Circulation. 1999; 100:I495.

45. Roden DM, Lazzara R, Rosen M, et al. Multiple mechanisms in the long-QT syndrome. Current knowledge, gaps, and future directions. The SADS Foundation Task Force on LQTS. Circulation. 1996; 94:1996-2012.
46. Abriel H, Wehrens XHT, Benhorin J, et al. Molecular pharmacology of the sodium channel mutation D1790G linked to the long-QT syndrome. Circulation. 2000; 102:921-25.
47. Zhou Z, Gong Q, January CT. Correction of defective protein trafficking of a mutant HERG potassium channel in human long QT syndrome. Pharmacological and temperature effects. J Biol Chem. 1999; 274:31123-26.
48. Wilde AA, Roden DM. Predicting the long-QT genotype from clinical data : from sense to science. Circulation. 2000; 102:2796-98.

16. ATRIAL FIBRILLATION

R. Brugada, R. Roberts

Introduction

Few trials in Cardiology have been so ascertaining of our limited knowledge of cardiac physiology as the Cardiac Arrhythmia Suppression Trial, CAST. That trial made us aware of the complexity of the interaction between antiarrhythmic drugs and factors that control cardiac contractility and rhythm. A balance between structural and ionic components is required for the electromechanical impulse to propagate orderly across the myocardial cells. When structural heart disease or genetic or iatrogenic factors modify this interaction, the result can be the formation of a chaotic electrical activity or fibrillation which can affect either chamber of the heart, atria or ventricles. The atrial chaos or atrial fibrillation (AF) is defined as an erratic activation of the atria, causing an irregular heart rhythm at the ventricular level. AF remains the Achilles' heel of cardiac rhythmology. Despite the overall advance in the treatment of the cardiac dysrhythmias with the introduction of radiofrequency ablation, therapeutic options in AF have remained largely unchanged and aimed at controlling the heart rate and anticoagulation. New surgical and ablation techniques are being developed, while promising they are still extremely laborious and available only to a handful of patients. The limited success in the therapy of AF is in part due to our poor understanding of its molecular pathophysiology. Advances in genetics and molecular biology will likely give new insights into the development of the disease. Molecular research of AF has focused on two main fields, identification of the genes that play a role in the initiation of the disease and altered gene expression during the disease state. These studies are aimed at identifying not only the triggering factors in the acute form but also those that perpetuate the arrhythmia and convert it into a chronic form.

Clinical Background

AF is the most common sustained arrhythmia encountered in clinical practice. It affects over 3 million Americans and its prevalence increases with age to about 6% in people over the age of 65 [1]. The disease doubles the mortality and it accounts for over one third of all cardioembolic episodes [2]. In addition, AF is usually associated with

PA Doevendans and AA Wilde (eds.), Cardiovascular genetics, 191-198.

disease, or atherosclerotic cardiovascular disease [3].
AF can be transient (paroxysmal) or persistent. Paroxysmal AF accounts for 35-40% of all cases of AF seen by physicians and is not a benign entity in individuals with underlying cardiac pathology [4]. The disease carries a high mortality and high incidence of stroke, and despite being a self-terminating arrhythmia, there is a 30-50% chance of converting to a chronic state depending on the underlying pathology. In some instances, especially in the young, the disease has no apparent etiology, and is called "lone" AF. Lone AF accounts for 2-16 % of all cases [5,6] and in the absence of risk factors like hypertension, diabetes or previous stroke, has a low risk of embolism and does not require the use of anticoagulation before the age of 65 [7]. Among the "lone" AF group falls the familial forms of the disease, in which a genetic basis and no cardiac pathology are the main characteristics. Limited studies have shown that the familial form has also a higher risk of embolism after the age of 65, data that supports the use of anticoagulation in these individuals [8].
There are three main goals in the therapy of AF: control of heart rate, prevention of thromboembolism and restoration of sinus rhythm. The first two are successfully achieved in the majority of cases with the use of medications. The latter remains a challenge. While the pharmacological approach to restore sinus rhythm can be helpful in some cases, it carries a high recurrence rate and a potential proarrhythmic effect, especially in individuals with underlying cardiac pathology. Surgery and ablation have emerged in the last decade as promising techniques to terminate the arrhythmia, but to date they are very time consuming and therefore, only few patients can benefit from these procedures.

Genetic background

Several elements are needed for a coordinated cardiac activity. Among them, ion currents, ion channels, structural proteins and gap junctions, which are responsible for the transmission of the electrical and mechanical impulse across the cardiac myocites. The complexity of this process continues to be a tremendous limitation to our understanding of arrhythmogenesis. With the incorporation of molecular biology in cardiology, we are able to resolve some of the challenges. The discovery of the structure of the ion channels, their function and pathophysiology have helped unravel in part the role played by the different ionic currents in both the electrical activity and electromechanical coupling. While basic mechanisms of arrhythmia have been provided by the functional analysis of the ion channels involved in the generation of the cardiac action potential, it has not been until the development of genetics and the discovery of mutations causing familial diseases that we have been able to jump from the most basic level to the clinical arena. Cardiac arrhythmias predisposing to sudden death, like Long QT and Brugada syndrome, have benefited tremendously from the advances in genetics and molecular biology. Most importantly, these discoveries have provided the possibility for genetic diagnosis. These familial diseases due to a single gene, despite being rather uncommon, allow the study of a pure form of a disease, in which a single abnormal protein is the trigger responsible for the arrhythmogenecity. However, our knowledge from genetics is not limited to the inherited forms of the disease. They have also opened new insights into how the abnormal and ultimately the normal gene interact with the damaged heart muscle, drugs, or environment and trigger the arrhythmia in the acquired forms. The simple subdivision of familial and acquired is no longer applicable as genetic modifiers are being identified. It is clear that each disease depends on the interaction between the genetic background and environmental factors to ultimately determine which individuals will be at higher risk to develop disease.

In the human, research efforts to elucidate the molecular basis of AF are focused into three main areas: genetic defects that cause the familial forms of the disease, genetic backgrounds that predispose to the disease and alterations in the gene expression of ion channels currents involved in the formation of the atrial action potential. The latter will mainly provide some understanding on the molecular changes triggered by the disease and may explain some of the mechanisms that perpetuate the arrhythmia into a chronic form. However, it will be very difficult to prove whether the molecular changes that occur in the atria are the etiology of the disease or one of its consequences. This hypothesis could be in part clarified by the identification of the genetic defects that cause the familial form of the disease. In this case, the genetic defect triggers the development of the pathology, and provides definitive insight into the etiology of the disease.

Atrial Fibrillation as a monogenic disease

We have known for a long time that certain arrhythmias are inherited. There are multiple publications of families with many of its members affected by the same arrhythmia. It is not generally appreciated that AF may be familial. This was evident from a search in the literature, which showed only a few publications referring to the familial form of the disease. It was first reported as a familial form in 1943 [9], and while it is probably very uncommon, there has been no systematic study to determine the overall prevalence of the disease. One report in the Spanish Journal of Cardiology helped identify five families in Catalonia, Spain [8] (figure 1) with AF inherited with an autosomal dominant pattern. In these families there were a total of 103 individuals. Forty-two of them presented with AF The age of diagnosis of the arrhythmia was from 1 to 45 years. The penetrance of the disease was very high; in latter generations three individuals were diagnosed in their first month of life. The elderly generations were diagnosed at a later age although the age of presentation of the disease is unknown, mainly due to the lack of symptoms and lack of routine examinations until recently.

The echocardiograms were within the normal range when the patients were diagnosed. Some of them have subsequently developed dilatation of the left atrium on follow-up. Two patients have mild left ventricular dysfunction, one of them probably related to her advanced age and the other possibly due to tachycardiomyopathy secondary to poorly controlled heart rate. In six patients electrical cardioversion was unsuccessful despite a structurally normal heart. The majority of the individuals in these five families are asymptomatic, and only six patients presently suffer from palpitations, but otherwise continue a normal life. The disease is chronic in all but two individuals.

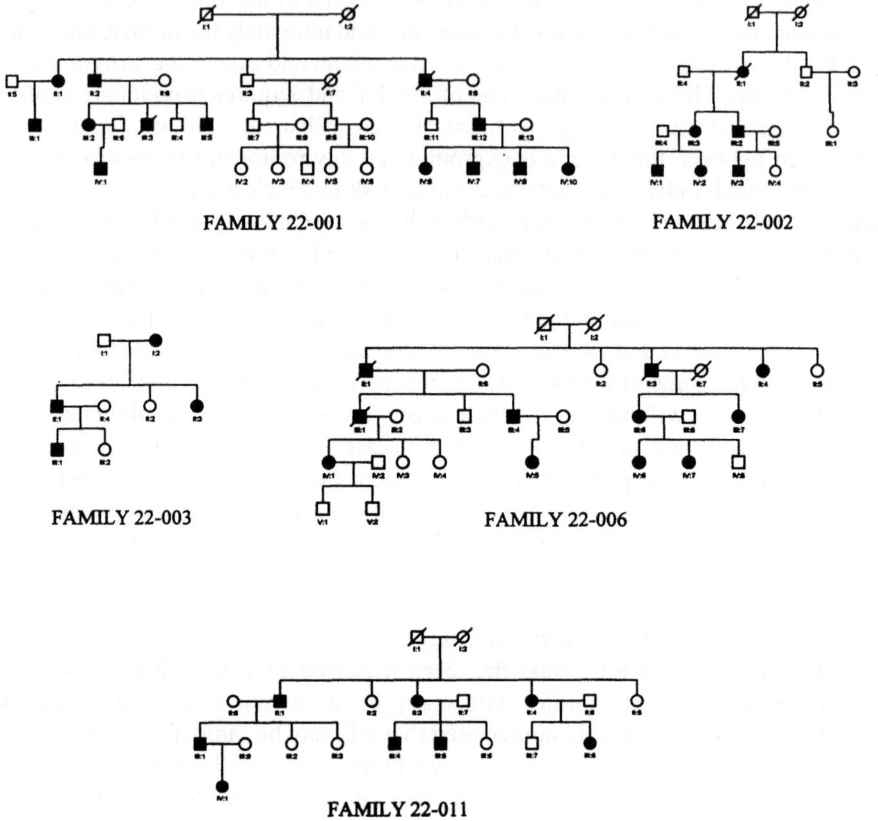

***Figure 1**. Pedigree of the families collected in Catalonia, Spain with common locus on chromosome 10, segregating with familial atrial fibrillation.*

One of these two patients died suddenly, while being treated with antiarrhythmic drugs. With techniques of linkage analysis in family 22-001 (figure 1) we were able to identify an area of 28 cM in chromosome 10q22, which was segregating with the affected individuals [10]. The LOD score of 3.6 indicated to us that the association was not due to chance. Analysis of the additional families from the same geographical area confirmed linkage with a LOD score of 17 and provided us the opportunity to narrow the region to 0.5 cM, around 500.000 base pairs which has enabled us to undertake positional cloning to identify the gene and the underlying mutation. At this point eight genes have been identified in the area and are presently being characterized.

Since the beginning of the project, we have collected more than 100 probands with familial AF and we have finished the phenotypic characterization in 32 families. The analysis of these families has shown that AF is a heterogeneous disease, caused by more than one gene [11]. The continuous identification of families indicate that this is more common than previously suspected, and that it is particularly important to screen family members of individuals presenting with lone AF because otherwise since it is relative benign, it will go undetected. Thus far familial AF is considered a category E genetic disease (table 1).

Atrial fibrillation concomitant with other monogenic diseases

AF has been described in other cardiac monogenic diseases as a concomitant disease. It has been identified in families with hypertrophic cardiomyopathy [12-13], skeletal myopathies [14-15], familial amyloidosis [16] and in monogenic diseases predisposing to atrial abnormalities [17]. In these cases, the disease is probably related to morphological changes in the atria caused by the underlying cardiac pathology.

Genetic predisposition to acquired atrial fibrillation

The familial form of AF is uncommon. The majority of the cases are acquired and related to structural abnormalities. Though, it is still important to remember that not all individuals with the same cardiac pathology develop AF, and probably, among other, there are genetic factors that predispose for the development of the arrhythmia. Few centers have been trying to unravel some of these genetic backgrounds, but the results have been disappointing to date. One report from Japan [18] tested the hypothesis that genetic factors that increase cardiac fibrosis would be a determinant for the development of lone AF. These investigators analyzed a polymorphism in the ACE gene, an enzyme that interacts with angiotensin II and affects cardiac remodeling. ACE gene can be inherited with an intronic deletion, which has been linked to higher circulating levels of enzyme and higher degree of hypertrophy and myocardial fibrosis [19]. While this cardiac fibrosis has been described at the ventricular level, they hypothesized that it would also affect the atria and cause the arrhythmia. They compared the genotypes of 77 patients with lone AF to 83 controls. They did not find any difference in the distribution of the ACE genotypes between the affected individuals and controls. There was no correlation with the type of AF, namely, paroxysmal or chronic and the genotype.

Table 1: Genes and loci in atrial fibrillation

Disease	Phenotype	*Loci*	Gene	Cat
Fam AF	Lone AF	10q22-24	?	E
Isolated AF	Lone AF	16	ACE	D

Alterations in ion channels currents involved in the formation of the atrial action potential

Heterogeneity in action potential is considered to play an important role in the development of reentrant arrhythmias and previous studies have proven that defects in ion channels involved in the action potential are responsible for some of the familial ventricular arrhythmias [20,21]. Animal models have shown that there is heterogeneity in the action potential within and among different atrial regions [22]. This variability correlates in part with the ionic currents, a higher density of L_{Ca} in the areas with the longest action potential duration, and smaller I_{to} density in the areas with smaller phase 1 amplitude. There is electrophysiological adaptation to AF consisting of a decrease in effective refractory period, shortening of the atrial action potential and increased dispersion of refractoriness [23]. Therefore it is tempting to speculate that abnormalities in ion channels will be responsible for the development of the chaotic reentry in the atrial tissue. Channels that control repolarization and the refractory period (potassium and calcium channels) are excellent candidates for the triggering and sustaining of AF. This electrophysiological variability together with the structural remodeling of the atrial tissue caused by the arrhythmia can be responsible for its maintenance and conversion to a chronic form. Van Wagoner et al. investigated this hypothesis in the human subject [24]. Contrary to the beliefs that there should be an increase in the outward potassium currents to shorten the action potential, he showed a decrease in the outward potassium currents I_{to} and I_{Ksus} and an increase in the inward rectifier K current I_{K1} in patients with chronic AF. The decrease in the outward current was similar in both the left and right atrium, while the increase in I_{K1} was more pronounced in the left atrium than the right. The changes in outward currents were similar in the different myocytes according to size and in those isolated from the dilated left atrium when compared to the normal right atrium, indicating that these changes were not related to myocyte size or chamber dilation. Likewise, Grammer et al. [25] described a reduction in I_{to} current due to transcriptional down-regulation of Kv4.3, but no change in Kv1.4, Kv1.5 or the current densities of I_{sus}. Lai et al. [26] measured the mRNA amounts of KVLQT1, Mink, HERG and KV1.5. He found an up-regulation of Mink, while the other potassium currents were down-regulated. All these results can in part be explained probably by the different arrhythmia etiology, duration or underlying pathology of the patient population. Goette et al. [27] analyzed the tissue expression of angiotensin receptor subtypes. He found that in both chronic and paroxysmal AF, AT(1)-R was down-regulated, while AT (2)-r was up-regulated. Grammer et al. [28] described decreased expression of the alpha 1c subunit and beta b/beta c-subunits of L-typeCa^{2+} channels with resulting decreased availability. From all this information, what seems clear, is that, once AF is initiated, many changes appear in the atrial electrical activity and gene expression which can contribute to the perpetuation of the arrhythmia and development of the chronic form.

Conclusion

Molecular biology and genetics are giving and will continue to give new insights into the development of cardiac diseases. Arrhythmias like AF will undoubtedly benefit from the discovery of the genes that cause the familial forms of the disease and from the understanding of the altered gene expression as a consequence of it. The interaction of all these genes with the structural cardiac abnormalities will probably shed light not only on the factors that induce the first episode but on the determinants that prolong this episode into a chronic form.

References

1. Feinberg WM, Blackshear JL, Laupacis A, Kronmal R, Hart RG. Prevalence, age distribution, and gender of patients with atrial fibrillation: analysis and implications. Arch Intern Med 1995; 155:469-73.
2. Wolf PA, Abbot RD, Kannel WB. Atrial Fibrillation: a major contributor to stroke in the elderly: the Framingham Study. Arch Intern Med 1987; 147:1561-4.
3. Lok NS, Lau CP. Presentation and management of patients admitted with atrial fibrillation: A review of 291 cases in a regional hospital. Int J Cardiol 1995; 48:271-278.
4. The Boston Area Anticoagulation Trial for Atrial Fibrillation Investigators: The effect of low-dose warfarin on the risk of stroke in patients with nonrheumatic atrial fibrillation. N Engl J Med 1990; 323 :1505-1511.
5. Kopecky SL, Gersh BJ, McGoon MD, Whisnant JP, Holmes DR Jr, Ilstrup DM, Frye RL. The natural history of lone atrial fibrillation. A population-based study over three decades. N Engl J Med 1987; 317:669-674.
6. Brand FN, Abbott RD, Kannel W, Wolf PA: Characteristics and prognosis of lone atrial fibrillation. 30-year follow-up in the Framingham study. JAMA 1985; 254:3449-3453
7. Atrial fibrillation Investigators: risk factors for stroke and efficacy of antithrombotic therapy in atrial fibrillation: Analysis of pooled data from five randomized controlled trials. Arch Intern Med 1994; 154:1449-1457.
8. Girona J, Domingo A, Albert D, Casaldàliga J, Mont L, Brugada J, Brugada R. Fibrilacion auricular familiar. Rev. Esp. Cardiol 1997; 50:548-551.
9. Wolff, L. Familial auricular fibrillation. New Engl J Med 1943; 229:396.
10. Brugada R, Tapscott T, Czernuszewicz GZ, Marian AJ, Iglesias A, Mont L, Brugada J, Girona J, Domingo A, Bachinski LL, Roberts R. Identification of a genetic locus for familial atrial fibrillation. N Engl J Med 1997; 336:905-911.
11. Brugada R, Bachinski L, Hill R, Roberts R. Familial atrial fibrillation is a genetically heterogeneous disease. JACC, 1998; 31:349A.
12. Gruver EJ, Fatkin D, Dodds GA, Kisslo J, Maron BJ, Seidman JG, Seidman CE. Familial hypertrophic cardiomyopathy and atrial fibrillation caused by Arg663His beta-cardiac myosin heavy chain mutation.Am J Cardiol. 1999; 83:13H-18H.
13. Richard P, Charron P, Leclercq C, Ledeuil C, Carrier L, Dubourg O, Desnos M, Bouhour JB, Schwartz K, Daubert JC, Komajda M, Hainque B. Homozygotes for a R869G mutation in the beta -myosin heavy chain gene have a severe form of familial hypertrophic cardiomyopathy. J Mol Cell Cardiol. 2000; 32:1575-83.
14. Ohkubo R, Nakagawa M, Higuchi I, Utatsu Y, Miyazato H, Atsuchi Y, Osame M. Familial skeletal myopathy with atrioventricular block. Intern Med. 1999; 38:856-60.
15. Ruchardt A, Eisenlohr H, Lydtin H. Myocardial involvement in carrier states for Duchenne muscular dystrophy. A rare cause of supraventricular arrhythmia. Dtsch Med Wochenschr. 1998; 123:930-5.
16. Gillmore JD, Booth DR, Pepys MB, Hawkins PN. Hereditary cardiac amyloidosis associated with the transthyretin Ile122 mutation in a white man. Heart 1999; 82:e2.
17. Stephan E, Ashoush R, Megarbane A, Kassab R, Salem N, Loiselet J, Bouvagnet P. Autosomal dominant Mendelian midline complex. Secundum atrial septal defect associated with cardiac and facial-thoracic defects. A familial case. Arch Mal Coeur Vaiss. 2000; 93:641-7.
18. Yamashita T, Hayami N, Ajiki K, Oikawa N, Sezaki K, Inoue M, Omata M, Murakawa Y. Is ACE gene polymorphism associated with lone atrial fibrillation? Jpn Heart J 1997; 38:637-41.

19. Nakai K, Itoh C, Miura Y, Hotta K, Musha T, Itoh T, Miyakawa T, Iwasaki R, Hiramori K. Deletion polymorphism of the angiotensin I-converting enzyme gene is associated with serum ACE concentration and increased risk for CAD in the Japanese. Circulation 1994; 90:2199-202.
20. Roden DM, Lazzara R, Rosen M, Schwartz PJ, Towbin J, Vincent M. Multiple mechanisms in the long-QT syndrome. Current knowledge, gaps and future directions. Circulation. 1996; 94:1996-2012.
21. Chen Q, Kirsch GE, Zhang D, Brugada R, Brugada J, Brugada P, Potenza D, Moya A, Borggrefe M, Breithardt G, Ortiz-Lopez R, Wang Z, Antzelevitch C, O'Brien RE, Schulze-Bahr E, Keating MT, Towbin JA, Wang Q. Genetic basis and molecular mechanisms for idiopathic ventricular fibrillation. Nature, 1998; 392:293-296.
22. Feng J, Yue L, Wang Z, Nattel S. Ionic mechanisms of regional action potential heterogeneity in the canine right atrium.Circ Res 1998; 83:541-51.
23. Morillo CA, Klein GJ, Jones DL, Guiraudon CM. Chronic rapid atrial pacing. Structural, functional, and electrophysiological characteristics of a new model of sustained atrial fibrillation. Circulation 1995; 91:1588-95.
24. Van Wagoner DR, Pond AL, McCarthy PM, Trimmer JS, Nerbonne JM. Outward K+ current densities and Kv1.5 expression are reduced in chronic human atrial fibrillation. Circ. Res. 1997; 80:772-81.
25. Grammer JB, Bosch RF, Kuhlkamp V, Seipel L. Molecular remodeling of Kv4.3 potassium channels in human atrial fibrillation. J Cardiovasc Electrophysiol. 2000; 11:626-33.
26. Lai LP, Su MJ, Lin JL, Lin FY, Tsai CH, Chen YS, Tseng YZ, Lien WP, Huang SK. Changes in the mRNA levels of delayed rectifier potassium channels in human atrial fibrillation. Cardiology. 1999; 92:248-55.
27. Goette A, Arndt M, Rocken C, Spiess A, Staack T, Geller JC, Huth C, Ansorge S, Klein HU, Lendeckel U. Regulation of angiotensin II receptor subtypes during atrial fibrillation in humans. Circulation 2000; 101:2678-81.
28. Grammer JB, Bosch RF, Kuhlkamp V, Seipel L. Molecular and electrophysiological evidence for "remodeling" of the L-type Ca2+ channel in *persistent atrial fibrillation in humans. Z Kardiol. 2000; 89:IV23-9.*

17. GENETICS OF ARRHYTHMOGENIC RIGHT VENTRICULAR CARDIOMYOPATHY

A. Rampazzo, G. Thiene, C. Basso, A. Nava, G.A. Danieli

Introduction

Arrhythmogenic right ventricular cardiomyopathy is a morbid entity characterized by myocardial electrical instability with increased risk of sudden death [1-3]. The acronym ARVD (Arrhythmogenic Right Ventricular Dysplasia) pointed to the peculiar morphology of the heart in the affected subjects, showing an altered composition of the right ventricular free wall. More recently, the acronym was changed into ARVC (Arrhythmogenic Right Ventricular Cardiomyopathy), since a segmental or diffuse myocardial dystrophy of the right ventricle free wall, with massive fibro-fatty infiltration, was typically observed in this disease (figure 1) [4]. This degenerative pattern seems to be more frequent in adult cases, manifesting cardiac symptoms and arrhythmias, than in younger subjects, thus providing indirect evidence that the disease is progressive [5]. Often, myocardial degeneration may extend to the left ventricle [5-8], less frequently to the interventricular septum [5]. Therefore, ARVD/C should no longer be regarded as cardiomyopathy confined to the right ventricle, as suggested by early observations. Patchy acute myocarditis patterns with myocyte death and focal round cell inflammatory infiltrates (mostly lymphocytes) [9] are present in two-third of the cases [5]. On the other hand, a role for apoptosis in the progressive death of cardiomyocytes has been postulated [10]. Thirthy to 50% of ARVD/C cases which come to the attention of the Cardiologist, show a familial history for the disease [11]. Often one or more cases of sudden death are reported in the family. In general, the disease is inherited as an autosomal dominant trait with incomplete penetrance [12]. An autosomal recessive pattern has been reported only in a peculiar form of ARVD/C, associated with palmoplantar keratosis and woolly hair, called "Naxos disease" [13].

The problem of the origin of the disease in isolated cases is still a matter of debate. An isolated case may be a phenocopy, which mimics the affected phenotype of genetic origin; it may be the result of a novel mutation or, more simply, it may appear "isolated" because the pathogenic trait was not fully penetrant in the parent.

PA Doevendans and AA Wilde (eds.), Cardiovascular genetics, 199-210

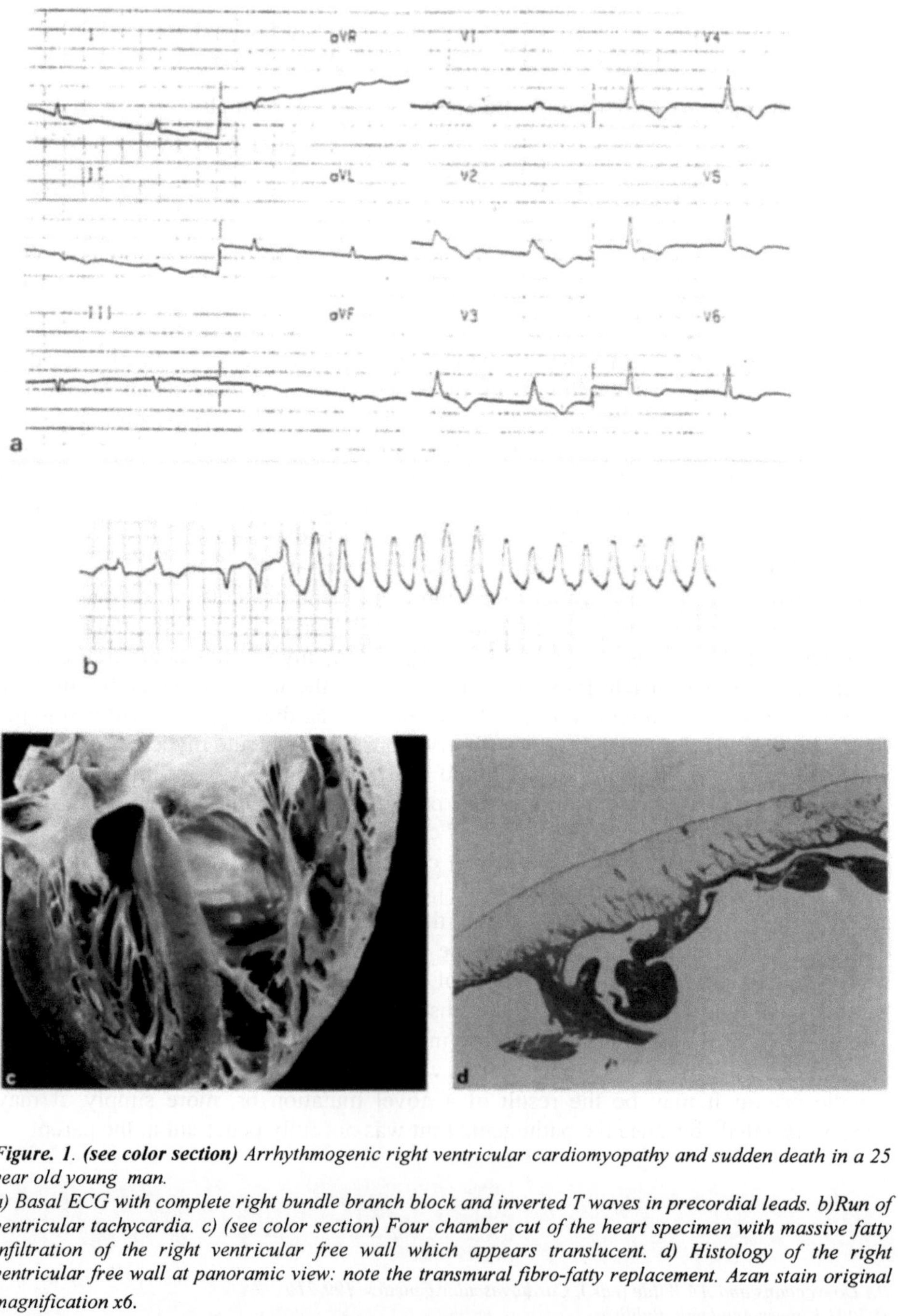

***Figure. 1*. (see color section)** *Arrhythmogenic right ventricular cardiomyopathy and sudden death in a 25 year old young man.*
a) Basal ECG with complete right bundle branch block and inverted T waves in precordial leads. b)Run of ventricular tachycardia. c) (see color section) Four chamber cut of the heart specimen with massive fatty infiltration of the right ventricular free wall which appears translucent. d) Histology of the right ventricular free wall at panoramic view: note the transmural fibro-fatty replacement. Azan stain original magnification x6.

The incidence and prevalence of ARVD/C in the general population are still unknown. Preliminary observations concerning Venetia (North-East Italy) indicated that the prevalence for all the forms of ARVD/C could be 1 in 5000 [14]. This value was possibly underestimated, since patients with a clinical diagnosis of ARVD/C (based on symptoms, right precordial ECG changes, RV arrhythmias, and structural and functional RV abnormalities) are only the extreme of the disease spectrum. A number of cases may run asymptomatic until the first presentation, which may coincide with sudden death. In general, isolated and asymptomatic cases are very difficult to diagnose by conventional non-invasive methods [15,16].

Diagnostic criteria

Few years ago, ARVD/C was listed for the first time among the cardiomyopathies in the WHO classification [17].

Diagnosis of ARVD/C is based on the clinical demonstration of structural, functional, and electrocardiographic abnormalities caused by the underlying histological changes [18]. The clinical presentation of ARVD/C usually consist of arrhythmias of right ventricular (RV) origin ranging from isolated premature ventricular beats to sustained ventricular tachycardia or ventricular fibrillation leading to sudden death [19]. Other clinical manifestations of the disease include global and/or regional dysfunction and structural alterations of the right ventricle, ECG depolarization/repolarization changes characteristically in right precordial leads, and evolution to right or biventricular heart failure mimicking dilated cardiomyopathy [20]. The pattern of VT with LBBB morphology may be considered almost pathognomonic of this cardiomyopathy [16,19,21-23].

Diagnostic criteria are based on the identification of structural abnormalities, fatty or fibro-fatty replacement of the RV myocardium, electrocardiographic changes, arrhythmias of RV origin and familial disease [18]. The diagnosis of ARVD/C is established by the presence of 2 major criteria or 1 major criteria plus 2 minor criteria or 0 major criteria and 4 minor criteria (Table 1). The major criteria include: 1) the presence of structural abnormalities in the right ventricle, 2) abnormal myocardial tissue in the right ventricle with fatty infiltration, 3) repolarization abnormalities on the electrocardiogram with T wave inversion in leads V1 to V3 or beyond, 4) conduction abnormalities on the electrocardiogram such as a QRS duration >= 100 msec in V1, V2, or V3 or an epsilon wave, and 5) a family history of ARVD/C confirmed by autopsy results. The minor criteria for ARVD/C include: 1) mild to moderate structural abnormalities of the right ventricle, 2) ECG abnormalities such as T wave inversion in V2 and V3 or late potentials on a signal averaged ECG, 3) ventricular arrhythmias such as sustained or nonsustained ventricular tachycardia with a left bundle morphology or more than 1000 PVCs per 24 hour, and 4) a family history of premature sudden cardiac death or ARVD/C.

Usually, after the diagnosis of one subject affected with ARVD/C, the clinical evaluation of all family members leads to early identification of additional ARVD/C cases, characterized by a broad clinical spectrum with a favourable outcome. In the setting of positive family history, even minor ECG and echocardiographic abnormalities may help in raising the suspicion of the presence of ARVD/C [24].

Table 1. Criteria for diagnosis of arrhythmogenic right ventricular cardiomyopathy [17].

I. Global and/or Regional Dysfunction and Structural Alterations detected by echocardiography, angiography, magnetic imaging, or radionuclide scintigraphy.

MAJOR:

Severe dilatation and reduction of right ventricular ejection fraction with no (or only mild) LV impairment.

Localized right ventricular aneurysms (akinetic or dyskinetic areas with diastolic bulging.)

Severe segmental dilatation of the right ventricle.

MINOR:

Mild global right ventricular dilatation and/or ejection fraction reduction with normal left ventricle.

Mild segmental dilatation of the right ventricle.

Regional right ventricular hypokinesia.

II. Tissue Characterization of Walls

MAJOR:

Fibrofatty replacement of myocardium on endomyocardial biopsy.

III. Repolarisation Abnormalities

MINOR:

Inverted T waves in right precordial leads (V2 and V3) (people aged>12 years, in absence of right bundle branch block.)

IV. Depolarisation/Conduction Abnormalities

MAJOR:

Epsilon waves or localised prolongation (>110ms) of the QRS complex in right precordial leads (V1-V3.)

MINOR:

Late potentials (signal averaged ECG.)

V. Arrhythmias

MINOR:

Left bundle branch block type ventricular tachycardia (sustained and nonsustained) ECG, Holter, exercise testing.

Frequent ventricular extrasystoles (>1000/24 hours) (Holter.)

VI. Family History

MAJOR:

Familial disease confirmed at necropsy or surgery.

MINOR:

Familial history of premature sudden death (<35 years) due to suspected right ventricular dysplasia.

Familial history (clinical diagnosis based on present criteria)

Clinical heterogeneity

Clinical and pathologic data suggest a wide life span, from adolescence to adulthood, during which the disease may become symptomatic and fatal [25]. Study of the natural history allowed to distinguish (a) a covert phase in apparently normal subjects who have risk of abrupt electrical instability and sudden death, (b) an overt arrhythmic phase with palpitations and impending cardiac arrest, (c) congestive heart failure with pump depression, sometimes so severe as to require heart transplantation [15, 26]. The clinical phenotype often shows inter- and intra-familial variability.
The clinical findings may differ in the distinct form of ARVD/C. Two ARVD/C types are characterized by peculiar clinical phenotypes.
Naxos disease was first described in 1986 by Protonotarios et al, [13] by the study of the population of the Greek island of Naxos. This disease is characterized by ARVC, diffuse non-epidermolytic palmoplantar keratoderma and woolly hair. All three aspects of the disease appear to be expressed in affected individuals; its stereotyped expression in all affected subjects means that early or mild disease can be readily recognized, making the diagnosis more accurate [27,28]. Clinical genetic assessment revealed high penetrance and expression. It appears in families descending from the Hellenic island of Naxos showing an autosomal recessive inheritance.
Arrhythmogenic right ventricular cardiomyopathy type 2 (ARVD2) is clinically different from the other forms of ARVD/C because of the presence of peculiar polymorphic effort-induced ventricular arrhythmias, by its high penetrance and by a 1:1 male:female ratio among the affected subjects (see also chapter 13) [29]. In ARVD2 cases the standard electrocardiograms do not show the typical features of ARVD/C, such as incomplete right bundle branch block or negative T-waves in the right precordial leads [29]; polymorphic ventricular tachycardia is characterized by premature ventricular beats with left and right bundle branch block morphology and different axis deviation, that appear in response to vigorous exercise [30]. In the autopsy cases, myocardial fibro-fatty replacement is segmental and mostly involving the right ventricular apex. Correct and early identification of this disease is crucial, taking into account the poor prognosis of patients with this arrhythmia, due to the high risk of sudden death, and the good results obtained with β-blocker therapy [29].

Genetic heterogeneity of ARVD/C

Linkage analyses in large pedigrees showing autosomal dominant ARVD/C inheritance demonstrated high genetic heterogeneity in ARVD/C. Analysis of highly informative polymorphic DNA microsatellites showed that at least six different genomic loci are independently involved in the inheritance of ARVD/C disease (table 2). Our group mapped the first ARVD/C locus (ARVD1) in a large multiple generation pedigree to human chromosome 14q23-q24 [14]. In spite of the long-standing effort toward the positional cloning of the ARVD1 gene, the primary defect is still unidentified. Several genes mapped to the critical region, including a novel intronless gene predominantly expressed in the heart tissue [31], were unsuccessfully screened for mutations. On the contrary, the gene involved in ARVD2, which was mapped by our group to chromosome 1q42-q43 [32], was recently identified in our laboratory [33].

Table 2. Chromosomal localization of ARVD/C loci

ARVD/ C TYPE	CHROMOSOMAL LOCATION	FLANKING MARKERS	GENE	CAT
ARVD1	14q23-24	D14S42, D14S254, D14S279	?	E
ARVD2	1q42-q43	D1S163, D1S2680, D1S184	RyR2	A
ARVD3	14q12-q22	D14S257, D14S70, D14S252	?	E
ARVD4	2q32.1-32.3	D2S152, D2S103, D2S389	?	E
ARVD5	3p23	D33610, D3S3613, D3S3659	?	E
ARVD6	10p12-p14	D10S1707, D10S1664, D10S191	?	E
Naxos	17q21	D17S800, D17S1299, D17S1789	Plakoglobin	A

An independent study, performed on three small families in a different Italian laboratory, provided significant positive lod scores for markers located in the region 14q12-q22, suggesting the existence of a third ARVD/C locus (ARVD3) [34]. Evidence in favour of a fourth ARVD/C locus (ARVD4) was obtained in 1997 in our laboratory [35]. In a North-American three-generation family, the haplotype defined by seven polymorphic DNA markers of the chromosome 2 long arm (2q32.1-q32.3) was found to be invariably transmitted in association with the disease. The linkage was confirmed in two additional unrelated families. In these families, the clinical features of ARVD/C are typical of the disease, however, the left ventricle always appears partially affected, thus supporting the hypothesis that a different gene is involved. [35]

Genetic linkage analysis of a large North-American kindred performed by Ahmad et coll. [36] indicated that a gene responsible for ARVD/C (ARVD5) is located on the short arm of chromosome 3 (3p23). Recently, a sixth ARVD/C locus (ARVD6) was identified at 10p12-p14, in a North–American family, characterized by having a high incidence of sudden death, early disease onset, and high penetrance [37]. The human protein tyrosine phosphatase-like gene was selected as a candidate gene possibly responsible for ARVD6 in this family [38]. DNA analysis of the family detected a sequence variation that was present in all affected but also present in the general population, so it is a benign polymorphism rather than a disease causing mutation.

Up to now, 28 families were analysed by our group with the sets of markers associated with the different ARVD/C loci [24]. Six of them had the disease locus mapped to chromosome 14q23-q24. Four families were linked to ARVD2 locus on chromosome 1q42-q43 and four families had the disease locus mapped to chromosome 2q32.1-q32.3. Four large families did not show linkage with any of the ARVD/C known loci, providing evidence of further genetic heterogeneity. The remaining 10 families were uninformative, due to their small size.

Both the identification of ARVD/C loci and the availability of several DNA polymorphic markers in their close proximity, open the way to pre-symptomatic detection of ARVD/C carriers by DNA analysis. This opportunity will greatly facilitate early prophylaxis of life-threatening complications in the at-risk subjects in the affected families. However, the real focus of the problem in molecular genetics of ARVD/C is the identification and cloning of the involved genes. Identification of the responsible gene(s) will be crucial for future genetic screening and will significantly improve diagnostic accuracy for this disorder.

Identification of ARVD/C genes

So far, two ARVD/C genes have been identified, one involved in the Naxos disease [39] and one in the arrhythmogenic right ventricular cardiomyopathy type 2 (ARVD2) [33].

In 1998, the Naxos disease locus was mapped to chromosome 17q21 [39], where the gene coding for plakoglobin is located. A homozygous 2 base pair deletion (Pk2157del2) in the plakoglobin gene was identified in the 19 affected subjects; 29 clinically unaffected family members were found heterozygous for the mutation. This deletion caused a frameshift and premature termination of the protein [40]. Plakoglobin is a key component of desmosomes and adherens junctions, and is important for the tight adhesion of many cell types, including those in the heart [41] and skin [42]. The finding of a deletion in plakoglobin in Naxos disease suggests that the proteins involved in cell-cell adhesion play an important role in maintaining myocyte integrity, and when junctions are disrupted, cell death and fibro-fatty replacement occur. Interestingly, the plakoglobin-null mouse model mirrors cardiac and skin features seen in patients with Naxos disease [43,44].

The ARVD2 disease locus was mapped to chromosome 1q42-q43 [32]; three ARVD2 candidate genes were mapped to the ARVD2 critical region: α-actinin (ACTN2), nidogen (NID) and the cardiac ryanodine receptor gene (RYR2). The investigation on ACTN2 and NID failed to detect ARVD2 causative mutations. On the contrary, four RyR2 mutations (R176Q, L433P, N2386I and T2504M) were shown to be invariably transmitted from patient to patient along generations in four independent Italian families and were never detected among their healthy relatives or among the control population [33]. These four RyR2 mutations occurred in two highly conserved regions, strictly matching those where mutations causing malignant hyperthermia or central core disease are clustered in the RYR1 gene, the corresponding skeletal muscle ryanodine receptor [45]. Ryanodine receptor function is fundamental for intracellular calcium homeostasis and for excitation-contraction coupling [46]. In myocardial cells, the RyR2 protein, activated by calcium, induces the release of calcium from the sarcoplasmic reticulum (SR) into the cytosol. The current research hypothesis is that RyR2 missense mutations might alter the ability of the calcium channel to remain closed. Thus, on physical perturbation (i.e. membrane depolarisation or mechanical stress), the defect would allow calcium to leak from the channel and promote a massive SR calcium release. This situation might be viewed as a gain of function, in agreement with the dominant inheritance.

The detection of RyR2 mutations causing ARVD2 opens the way to pre-symptomatic detection of carriers of the disease. In families in which a single ARVD2 case was diagnosed, DNA tests could reveal which infants are carriers, thus enabling early

monitoring and treatment. Moreover, the discovery that RyR2 is involved in ARVD2 might possibly lead to a specific and effective pharmacological treatment.
Two different studies [47,48] showed that mutations of the RyR2 gene might cause inherited polymorphic tachycardia. In the first study [47], four single-nucleotide substitutions leading to missense mutations (S2246L, R2474S, N4104K and R4497C) were identified among twelve patients presenting with typical catecholaminergic polymorphic ventricular tachycardia. These patients didn't show overt structural heart abnormalities. Genetic analysis of the asymptomatic parents revealed that 3 cases carried de-novo mutations, whereas the fourth mutation was identified in the proband and in 4 clinically affected family members. Recently, in 3 large families with polymorphic ventricular tachycardia, but in the absence of any evident structural myocardial disease, 3 different RyR2 mutations (P2328S, Q4201R and V4653F) were detected. They were shown to fully cosegregate with the characteristic arrhythmic phenotype [48].
The finding of RyR2 mutations in ARVD2, in cathecolaminergic ventricular tachycardias and in familial polymorphic ventricular tachycardia, raises the question of the possible allelism of these diseases, thus probably forming another group of ryanodine receptor syndromes in addition to that composed of malignant hyperthermia and central core disease and showing subtle phenotypic variations that originate from similar molecular defects

Conclusion

The progress of molecular genetics studies enabled us to resolve genetic heterogeneity of ARVD/C. The definition of linkage groups and the usage of flanking polymorphic DNA markers made it possible to follow the segregation of the "affected" haplotypes even in those families the small seize of which would prevent standard linkage analysis. Therefore, the genetic approach may be conveniently used for a preliminary identification of "at-risk" subjects in families with recurrence of ARVD/C cases.
On the other hand, this kind of "genetic" diagnosis may be faulty in some cases, due to short-distance recombination. Therefore, the optimal situation in perspective would be the detection of the causative mutation in the index case. Presently this is possible in Naxos disease, where all patients described so far share the same mutation, and in ARVD2, where, on the contrary, heterogeneity of mutations seems to be the rule. Once a causative mutation is detected in an affected subject, the identification of the same mutation in other members of the same family should be indicative of a potential affection. However, for the time being, the equation mutation=affection cannot be held, since data on genotype-phenotype correlations are still too limited, while ARVD/C trait often shows incomplete penetrance.
The identification of genes involved in different ARVD/Cs is very promising for the development of specific treatments. However, even in the present situation, definition of the linkage group in a given family might be very helpful, since retrospective analysis of trial data might reveal common trends in families belonging to the same clinical-genetic entity.

Acknowledgments

This work was financially supported by Telethon-Italy (Grant no.1288 to A. Nava), by MURST (Grant 1998 to G.A. Danieli) and by Fondazione Cassa di Risparmio di Padova e Rovigo.

References

1. Nava A, Rossi L, Thiene G. Arrhythmogenic right ventricular cardiomyopathy. 1997, Elsevier Science B.V., Amsterdam.
2. Thiene G, Nava A, Corrado D, Rossi L, Pennelli N. Right ventricular cardiomyopathy and sudden death in young people. N Engl J Med 1988; 318:129-33.
3. Corrado D, Thiene G, Nava A, Rossi L, Pennelli N. Sudden death in young competitive athletes: clinicopathologic correlations in 22 cases. Am J Med 1990; 89:588-96.
4. Thiene G, Basso C, Danieli GA, Rampazzo A, Corrado D, Nava A. Arrhythmogenic right ventricular cardiomyopathy. A still underrecognized clinical entity. Trends Cardiovasc Med 1997; 7:84-90.
5. Basso C, Thiene G, Corrado D, Angelini A, Nava A, Valente M Arrhythmogenic right ventricular cardiomyopathy. Dysplasia, dystrophy, or myocarditis? Circulation 1996; 94:983-91.
6. Manyari DE, Klein GJ, Gulamhusein S, Boughner D, Guiraudon GM, Wyse G, Mitchell LB, Kostuk WJ. Arrhythmogenic right ventricular dysplasia: a generalized cardiomyopathy? Circulation 1983; 68:251-57.
7. Pinamonti B, Sinagra G, Salvi A, Di Lenarda A, Morgera T, Silvestri F, Bussani R, Camerini F. Left ventricular involvement in right ventricular dyspalsia. Am Heart J 1992; 123:711-24.
8. Gallo P, D'Amati G, Pelliccia F. Pathologic evidence of extensive left ventricular involvement in arrhythmogenic right ventricular cardiomyopathy. Hum Pathol 1992; 23:948-52.
9. Thiene G, Corrado D, Nava A, Rossi L, Poletti A, Boffa GM, Daliento L, Pennelli N. Right ventricular cardiomyopathy: is there evidence of an inflammatory aetiology? Eur Heart J 1991; 12:22-25.
10. Valente M, Calabrese F, Thiene G, Angelini A, Basso C, Nava A, Rossi L. In vivo evidence of apoptosis in arrhythmogenic right ventricular cardiomyopathy. Am J Pathol 1998; 152:479-84.
11. Nava A, Rampazzo A, Villanova C, Muriago M, Buja G. Familiar occurrence of arrhythmogenic right ventricular cardiomyopathy. In Nava A, Rossi L, Thiene G, eds: Arrhythmogenic right ventricular cardiomyopathy/dysplasia, 1997, Elsevier Science B.V., p. 159-65.
12. Nava A, Thiene G, Canciani B, Scognamiglio R, Daliento L, Buja G, Martini B, Stritoni P, Fasoli G. Familial occurrence of right ventricular dysplasia: a study involving nine families. J Am Coll Cardiol 1988; 12:1222-28.
13. Protonotarios N, Tsatsopoulou A, Patsourakos P, Alexopoulos D, Gezerlis P, Simitsis S, Scampardonis G. Cardiac abnormalities in familial palmoplantar keratosis. Br Heart J 1986; 56:321-26.
14. Rampazzo A, Nava A, Danieli GA, Buja G, Daliento L, Fasoli G, Scognamiglio R, Corrado D, Thiene G. The gene for arrhythmogenic right ventricular cardiomyopathy maps to chromosome 14q23-q24. Hum Mol Genet 1994; 3:959-62.
15. Corrado D, Basso C, Thiene G, McKenna WJ, Davies MJ, Fontaliran F, Nava A, Silvestri F, Blomstrom-Lundqvist C, Wlodarska EK, Fontaine G, Camerini F. Spectrum of clinicopathologic manifestations of arrhythmogenic right ventricular cardiomyopathy/dysplasia: a multicenter study. J Am Coll Cardiol 1997; 30:1512-20.
16. Nava A, Thiene G, Canciani B, Martini B, Daliento L, Buja G, Fasoli G. Clinical profile of concealed form of arrhythmogenic right ventricular cardiomyopathy presenting with apparently idiopathic ventricular arrhythmias. Int J Cardiol 1992; 35:195-206.
17. Richardson P, McKenna W, Bristow M, Maisch B, Mautner B, O'Connell J, Olsen E, Thiene G, Goodwin J, Gyarfas I, Martin I, Nordet P. Report of the 1995 World Health Organization/International Society and Federation of Cardiology Task Force on the Definition and Classification of cardiomyopathies. Circulation 1996; 93:841-42.

18. McKenna WJ, Thiene G, Nava A, Fontaliran F. Blomstrom-Lundqvist C, Fontaine G, Camerini on behalf of the Working Group Myocardial and Pericardial Disease of the European Society of Cardiology and of the Scientific Council on Cardiomyopathies of the International Society and Federation of Cardiology. Diagnosis of Arrhythmogenic Right Ventricular Dysplasia/cardiomyopathy. Br Heart J 1994; 71:215-218.
19. Marcus FI, Fontaine GH, Guiraudon G, Frank R, Laurenceau JL, Malergue C, Grosgogeat Y. Right ventricular dysplasia: a report of 24 adult cases. Circulation 1982; 65:384-98.
20. Rowland E, McKenna WJ, Sugrue D, Barclay R, Foale RA, Krikler DM. Ventricular tachycardia of left bundle branch block configuration in patients with isolated right ventricular dilatation. Clinical and electrophysiological features. Br Heart J 1984; 51:15-24.
21. Fontaine G, Frank R, Tonet JL, Guiraudon G, Cabrol C, Chomette G, Grosgogeat Y. Arrhythmogenic right ventricular dysplasia: a clinical model for the study of chronic ventricular tachycardia. Jpn Circ J 1984; 48:515-38.
22. Fontaine G, Frank R, Fontaliran F, Lascault G, Tonet J. Right ventricular tachycardias. In Parmely WW, Chatteryce K, eds. Cardiology. New York, JB Lippincott Company, p. 1-17.
23. Martini B, Nava A, Thiene G, Buja GF, Canciani B, Miraglia G, Scognamiglio R, Boffa GM, Daliento L. Accelerated idioventricular rhythm of infundibular origin in patients with a concealed form of arrhythmogenic right ventricular dysplasia. Br Heart J 1988; 59:564-71.
24. Nava A, Bauce B, Basso C, Muriago M, Rampazzo A, Villanova C, Daliento L, Buja G, Corrado D, Danieli GA, Thiene G. Clinical profile and long-term follow-up of 37 families with arrhythmogenic right ventricular cardiomyopathy. J Am Coll Cardiol 2000; 36:2226-33.
25. Daliento L, Turrini P, Nava A, Rizzoli G, Angelini A, Buja G, Scognamiglio R, Thiene G. Arrhythmogenic right ventricular cardiomyopathy in young versus adult patients: similarities and differences. J Am Coll Cardiol 1995; 25:655-64.
26. Thiene G, Nava A, Angelini A, Daliento L, Scognamiglio R, Corrado D. Anatomoclinical aspects of arrhythmogenic right ventricular cardiomyopathy. In Camerini F, Gavazzi A, DeMaria R, (Eds.) (1998) Advances in cardiomyopthies. Berlin, Springer Verlag, 1997; p. 397-408.
27. Protonotarios N, Tsatsopoulou A. The Naxos disease. In Nava A, Rossi L, Thiene G, eds: Arrhythmogenic right ventricular cardiomyopathy/dysplasia, 1997, Elsevier Science B.V., 1997p. 454-62.
28. Fontaine G, Fontaliran F, Frank R. Arrhythmogenic ventricular cardiomyopathies: clinical forms and main differential diagnoses. Circulation 1998; 97:1532-35.
29. Bauce B, Nava A, Rampazzo A, Daliento L, Muriago M, Basso C, Thiene G, Danieli GA. Familial effort polymorphic ventricular arrhythmias in arrhythmogenic right ventricular cardiomyopathy map to chromosome 1q42-43. Am J Cardiol 2000; 85:573-79.
30. Reid DS, Tynan M, Braidwood L, Fitzgerald GR. Bidirectional tachycardia in a child. A study using His bundle electrography. Br Heart J 1975; 37:339-44.
31. Rampazzo A, Pivotto F, Occhi G, Tiso N, Bortoluzzi S, Rowen L, Hood L, Nava A, Danieli GA. Characterization of C14orf4, a novel intronless human gene containing a polyglutamine repeat, mapped to the ARVD1 critical region. Biochem Biophys Res Commun 2000; 278:766-74.
32. Rampazzo A, Nava A, Erne P, Eberhard M, Vian E, Slomp P, Tiso N, Thiene G, Danieli GA. A new locus for arrhythmogenic right ventricular cardiomyopathy (ARVD2) maps to chromosome 1q42-q43. Hum Mol Genet 1995; 4:2151-54.
33. Tiso N, Stephan DA, Nava A, Bagattin A, Devaney JM, Stanchi F, Larderet G, Brahmbhatt B, Brown K, Bauce B, Muriago M, Basso C, Thiene G, Danieli GA, Rampazzo A. Identification of mutations in the cardiac ryanodine receptor gene in families affected with arrhythmogenic right ventricular cardiomyopathy type 2 (ARVD2). Hum Mol Genet 2001; 10:189-94.
34. Severini GM, Krajinovic M, Pinamonti B, Sinagra G, Fioretti P, Brunazzi MC, Falaschi A, Camerini F, Giacca M, Mestroni L. A new locus for arrhythmogenic right ventricular dysplasia on the long arm of chromosome 14. Genomics 1996; 31:193-200.

35. Rampazzo A, Nava A, Miorin M, Fonderico P, Pope B, Tiso N, Livolsi B, Zimbello R, Thiene G, Danieli GA. ARVD4, a new locus for arrhythmogenic right ventricular cardiomyopathy, maps to chromosome 2 long arm. Genomics 1997; 45:259-63.
36. Ahmad F, Li D, Karibe A, Gonzalez O, Tapscott T, Hill R, Weilbaecher D, Blackie P, Furey M, Gardner M, Bachinski LL, Roberts R. Localization of a gene responsible for arrhythmogenic right ventricular dysplasia to chromosome 3p23. Circulation 1998; 98:2791-95.
37. Li D, Ahmad F, Gardner MJ, Weilbaecher D, Hill R, Karibe A, Gonzalez O, Tapscott T, Sharratt GP, Bachinski LL, Roberts R. The locus of a novel gene responsible for arrhythmogenic right-ventricular dysplasia characterized by early onset and high penetrance maps to chromosome 10p12-p14. Am J Hum Genet 2000; 66:148-56.
38. Li D, Gonzalez O, Bachinski LL, Roberts R. Human protein tyrosine phosphatase-like gene: expression profile, genomic structure, and mutation analysis in families with ARVD. Gene 2000; 256:237-43.
39. Coonar AS, Protonotarios N, Tsatsopoulou A, Needham EW, Houlston RS, Cliff S, Otter MI, Murday VA, Mattu RK, McKenna WJ. Gene for arrhythmogenic right ventricular cardiomyopathy with diffuse nonepidermolytic palmoplantar keratoderma and woolly hair (Naxos disease) maps to 17q21. Circulation 1998; 97:2049-58.
40. McKoy G, Protonotarios N, Crosby A, Tsatsopoulou A, Anastasakis A, Coonar A, Norman M, Baboonian C, Jeffery S, McKenna WJ. Identification of a deletion in plakoglobin in arrhythmogenic right ventricular cardiomyopathy with palmoplantar keratoderma and woolly hair (Naxos disease). Lancet 2000; 355:2119-24.
41. Hertig CM, Butz S, Koch S, Eppenberger-Eberhardt M, Kemler R, Eppenberger HM. N-cadherin in adult rat cardiomyocytes in culture II. Spatio-temporal appearance of proteins involved in cell-cell contact and communication. Formation of two distinct N-cadherin/catenin complexes. J Cell Sci 1996; 109:11-20.
42. Haftek M, Hansen MU, Kaiser HW, Kreysel HW, Schmitt D. Interkeratinocyte adherens junctions: immunocytochemical visualization of cell-cell junctional structures, distinct from desmosomes, in human epidermis. J Invest Dermatol 1996; 106:498-504.
43. Ruiz P, Brinkmann V, Ledermann B, et al. Targeted mutation of plakoglobin in mice reveals essential functions of desmosomes in the embryonic heart. J Cell Biol 1996; 135:215-25.
44. Bierkamp C, Mclaughlin KJ, Schwarz H, Huber O, Kemler R. Embryonic heart and skin defects in mice lacking plakoglobin. Dev Biol 1996; 180:780-85.
45. McCarthy TV, Quane KA, Lynch PJ. Ryanodine receptor mutations in malignant hyperthermia and central core disease. Hum Mutat 2000; 15:410-17.
46. Brillantes AB, Ondrias K, Scott A, Kobrinsky E, Ondriasova E, Moschella MC, Jayaraman T, Landers M, Ehrlich BE, Marks AR. Stabilization of calcium release channel (ryanodine receptor) function by FK506-binding protein. Cell 1994; 77:513-23.
47. Priori SG, Napolitano C, Tiso N, Memmi M, Vignati G, Bloise R, Sorrentino VV, Danieli GA. Mutations in the Cardiac Ryanodine Receptor Gene (hRyR2) Underlie Catecholaminergic Polymorphic Ventricular Tachycardia. Circulation 2001; 103:196-200.
48. Laitinen PJ, Brown KM, Piippo K, Swan H, Devaney JM, Brahmbhatt B, Donarum EA, Marino M, Tiso N, Viitasalo M, Toivonen L, Stephan DA, Kontula K. Mutations of the cardiac ryanodine receptor (RyR2) gene in familial polymorphic ventricular tachycardia. Circulation 2001; 103:485-90.

18. GENOME RESEARCH AND FUTURE HEALTHCARE

G.B. van Ommen

Introduction

The last decade has seen many great successes of linkage analysis and positional cloning, now scaled up in the Human Genome Project. Paradigm changes in medical genetics have brought major progress in unraveling the etiology of most of the major genetic diseases (e.g. Duchenne, cystic fibrosis, Huntington disease, myotonic dystrophy, X-linked mental retardation) and hereditary cancer syndromes (e.g. retinoblastoma, neurofibromatosis, colon, skin and breast cancer). The genome project has enormously stimulated the development of advanced technology to characterize DNA and study genes. Consequently a spectacular rise has occurred in the identification of causes of genetic disease. Nearly all important, frequent diseases (about 100-150), and a large number of rarer diseases have been traced back to their causally defective gene. In most cases (in total for ca. 1500-2000 genes) also the underlying mutations have been identified. The first, highly valuable spin-off has been the development of specific and reliable diagnostics, thus relieving insecurity and long and burdening diagnostic odysseys. A welcome development first and foremost for patients and their relatives, but also for their medical caretakers.

While often reviled as boring routine by the classical cell- and molecular biologist favoring detailed functional study, in reality the tale of the isolation of major disease genes has been one of original strategies and resourceful tinkering, of large-scale collaboration and competition, rewarded by the finding of entirely novel disease mechanisms and inheritance modes. The study of human genetic disease and animal model systems has highlighted the existence of several novel genetic mechanisms, the impact of which could never have been conceived otherwise, like genetic imprinting, germline mosaicism, trinucleotide repeat expansion and anticipation. In turn, the study of these processes has greatly deepened our fundamental insights in genetics. These worldwide advances have yielded a better understanding of the chain of events connecting the molecular defects in genes, via the functional disturbances in cells and organs, to the clinical effects on the organism as a whole. This so-called 'Genotype-Phenotype correlation' is of paramount importance, not only in optimal patient and family counseling, but also to define proper groups for the

PA Doevendans and AA Wilde (eds.), Cardiovascular genetics, 211-216

evaluation of strategie for therapy and prevention, especially when more experimental, pharmacological and gene therapies will come within reach. Unfortunately, many of the processes determining the genotype-phenotype correlation are still elusive, as they depend on more complex interactions between multiple genes, different variant alleles of these genes and, last but not least, between genes, gene variants and the environment.

Functional genomics

The combination of genomic information with large-scale miniaturization and automation, will bring great advances in insights. Even today, the increasing power of bioinformatics (databases, image processing and Internet use), nanotechnology (the DNA-chip) and automation (laboratory robotics) is putting us on the eve of a quantum leap in understanding of functional networks in living organisms, via an unprecedented scaling-up of information gathering, processing and interpretation. The systematic description of the data in genome projects of man and other organisms, is just the first essential step on a long way. The descriptive stages of the genome project are currently being complemented by high-throughput technology to discover the functions and interactions of the newly found genes. The combined results of cross-comparison of the data between different genes of one organism and between the genes and genomes of different organisms, the development of targeted animal models for human disease and the large-scale parallel analysis of gene-expression profiles of tissues in normal versus diseased state and during growth and development, will fundamentally improve our capacities at complex pattern recognition. In scientific research, this is the ever-recurrent basis for new, verifiable hypotheses. Predictably therefore, the quest for the biological functions and interactions of our genes and the subsequent development of medical interventions, be it via gene therapy, or probably more often through pharmacological routes, uncovered by our improved understanding, will undergo an unparalleled blossoming time. This will apply equally to 'classical' genetic diseases and to common, multifactorial disorders like cardiovascular disease, cancer, hypertension, rheumatic arthritis, migraine, Parkinson and Alzheimer and even to infectious diseases and injury hazards.

Pharmacogenomics

The aim of the human genome diversity (HGD) project, a population-based offspring of the genome project, is the elucidation of the individual variation of genes. Recently, a section of this variation has attracted major attention of the biotech/pharma industry. The study of genetic factors governing drug response, a field dubbed 'pharmacogenetics', is widely expected to hold tremendous promise for better targeted pharmacological treatment. Currently ill-understood differences in efficacy and side-effects of medicine between different persons are most likely based on genetic differences in drug uptake and metabolism. It is easy to see how the elucidation of these differences could unlock major possibilities for more effective, individually-tailored medical treatments. This promises to greatly reduce health care cost due to ineffective or even disadvantageous drug treatments.

HUGO

Early in the genome research era, scientists worldwide recognized that a free international competition, while healthy as a mechanism to stimulate rapid progress, could potentially cause important wasting of abilities and resources. In contrast, a basic level of coordination and international collaboration, when properly monitored, was envisaged to greatly increase efficiency and assist in generating resources and defining problem areas requiring special attention. To stimulate this coordination, the Human Genome Organization (HUGO) was conceived in 1988 and founded in 1989. In line with the state of research, the major emphasis of HUGO has initially been on guiding the mapping, which previously had proceeded under an even looser, self-imposed scientific regime, the Human Gene Mapping (HGM) workshops, organized biannually by the gene mapping community. HUGO monitors and assists the genome mapping process on one hand by organizing annual Human Genome Mapping Meetings, and on the other hand by a program of smaller meetings and workshops on specific topics, including, for example, the program of single-chromosome workshops of the past five years, supported by the European Community and National Institute of Health (NIH) and Department of Energy (DOE) in America.

Mapping, sequencing or both?

Until recently, the emphasis of genome mapping has been on the detailed mapping of genes on a chromosome-by-chromosome basis. However, with the current methodological advances, novel whole-genome mapping methods have been established both for genomic DNA and genes. By these methods, currently about 30.000 human expressed genes have been ordered on refined subchromosomal maps, based on the location of short sequences of tissue-specific cDNAs (Expressed Sequence Tags, EST). The coordination of this mapping stage, in cDNA/EST Full mapping meetings, initiated by the Wellcome Trust in 1994, was subsequently organized by HUGO, with funding from many government and industry parties. For the current stage of whole genome sequencing, the debate is still ongoing on whether refined regional or chromosome-by-chromosome maps are still required to generate reliably-mapped raw material 'sequence-ready contigs'), or alternatively, if sequence-based techniques have become cheap and non-redundant enough to abolish the need for scrupulous mapping altogether. The demise and subsequent resurrection of the genome database GDB, established in 1989 and until now the world's mapping database par excellence, may precipitate at short term a decision in favor of sequence-based data acquisition and storage. However, the reactions in the gene mapping and clinical fields following GDB's problems underscore that the existence of a well-curated, comprehensive mapping database, providing not only gene maps but also a resource of unique, internationally agreed, freely accessible mapping and application data for genetic and physical markers, is an indispensable condition for the fruitful translation of genome knowledge into practical applications. This is both true for the mapping of major common diseases and for direct clinical applications in (differential) diagnosis. Indeed, to secure optimal societal value from the advances in the genome project - one of the prime rationales for the entire endeavor - funding agencies worldwide should seriously consider investing, jointly if necessary, into a "meaner and leaner" successor of GDB.

Intellectual property

In the wake of the rapid advances in discovering new genes, a fierce debate has emerged on public-versus-private aspects of our genome heritage. Especially in the field of the analysis of human cDNA/gene sequences and their comparison with other species to unravel function, major issues are still unresolved on how to strike the balance between, on one hand, maximal scientific progress and public benefit - typically served by immediate public access of newly generated data - and proper patent protection of intellectual property of inventions on the other hand, required to safeguard the staggering investments to develop therapies. The existence of an independent international organization like HUGO, which does not report directly to specific governments, industries or funding bodies, is an important asset to an unbiased international discussion. In 1992, 1996, 1997 and 2000. HUGO has generated policy papers on public access, patenting and related intellectual property issues including SNPs and the effect of the European Directive on patenting biologicals.

Genetic services and education

On the side of caution, major points have yet to be addressed to convert the new opportunities of genetic services into beneficial healthcare: First, the provision of requested information, which may be very burdensome to the applicant, needs to be properly embedded in expert clinical-genetic healthcare and preceded as well as guided by well-designed, understandable information. This requires additional research into the impact of genetic information and expansion of the professional field, to deal with increased possibilities and demand. The future implementation of screening programs for major genetic diseases, to widen the access of the public to voluntary preventive and therapeutic options, including life-style choices, increases the need to politically address the level of professional care provision. Furthermore, also the public needs to be better educated into the value, impact and limitations of genetics, especially adolescents as consumers of these services in the immediate future.

Global ethics

An entirely different, but equally important question is whether our society is ready to assimilate these profound changes. One should not overestimate the adaptive capacity of societies. Not even regionally, let alone worldwide. Nationally, and more in general in Western societies, the threat looms of privacy infringements, unequal access to health care and selective in- or exclusion from insurances or labor. Clearly, it would defeat the purpose of genetics research, when exactly those who should benefit most from the developments are put in jeopardy by them. The threat of social inequity also exists on a global scale: There is a great diversity in cultures, social priorities and economic strength between Europe, Asia and America. Even greater health and wealth differences exist between the North and the South. Thus, the establishment of ethically and morally acceptable standards has to be approached with great caution, involving many more parties than only the western scientists, industry and policy makers. This is yet another field where an independent, worldwide organization of knowledgeable professionals with genomics and genetics background has an invaluable contribution, next to regional genetics societies like the American, European and Australian Societies for Human Genetics and other world agencies like UNESCO. In 1996, the HUGO Ethics committee has published a 'Statement on the Principled Conduct of Genetics Research', which has been widely acclaimed. This is the basis of further refinements applicable to specific situations. The first specific issue has been addressed in the statement "DNA Samples: Control and Access", which has been published in march 1998, at HUGO's HGM98 Meeting in Turin. This statement seeks to carefully balance privacy issues versus the value of coded maintenance of sample identity, with a view on future validation of epidemiological and specific studies. In march 1999, at the Brisbane HUGO Meeting HGM99 the HUGO Ethics Statement on Cloning was issued, placing this contentious issue in the current framework of human genetics. I April 2000 at the HAM 2000 meeting in Vancouver, a new statement was released, addressing the complex matter of benefit sharing in genetic research. These statements are typically prepared by the HUGO Ethics committee after thoroughly reviewing 60-80 statements and documents from national and international bodies, private and governmental, and are intended to assist national and supranational policy determination and standardization of ethical review.

Economics and funding

As witnessed by the ongoing fierce debate on public versus private issues, commercial development in different western regions and increased attention for less privileged populations, an international dialogue is in order on how to reap the profits of our insights on a balanced, worldwide scale and how to prevent just another increase of the technological gap. Indeed, most European nations could easily end up on the 'wrong' side of this gap. The increasing hi-tech nature of advanced biomedical research and the recent enormous funding increase in biomedical research in the US and Japan, combined with the comparatively limited investments in fundamental biomedical research in Europe, are about to put a heavy mortgage on the role which Europe may still play in areas of decisive impact on health care and economy in the 21st century. In order to reap major benefits for human health care in diagnostic, therapeutic and preventive medicine and to realize the vast array of business opportunities, a more active stimulation of genome research should be considered a priority task by national ministries of health, education and economy, supranational bodies such as the European Union and funding agencies in healthcare such as the Wellcome Trust, where possible assisted by the biotech and pharmaceutical industrial field.

Literature

www.gene.ucl.ac.uk
www.hugo-international.org/hugo
www.gdb.org
www.onfobiogen.fr
www.geneclinics.com
www.ebi.ac.uk
www.ncbi.nlm.nih.gov/dbEST
www.celera.come
www.ncbi.nlm.nih.gov/entrez
www.ornl.gov/hgmis/

COLOR SECTION

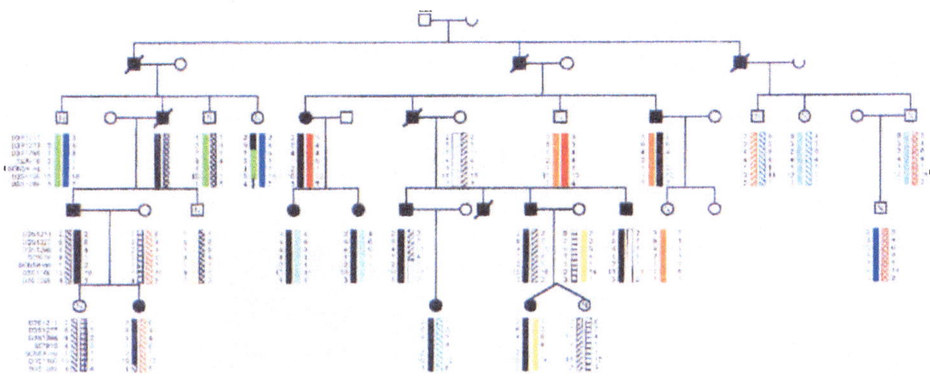

Figure 1. *(see Chapter 1, p. 2) Linkage analyses in a familypresenting with "Brugada" syndrome and LQT3. The haplotype indicated with a black bar segregates with the disease. Affected persons are indicated with filled symbols. N = not affected. Deceased persons are indicated with a crossed line. Alleles are numbered for each marker on chromosome 3.*

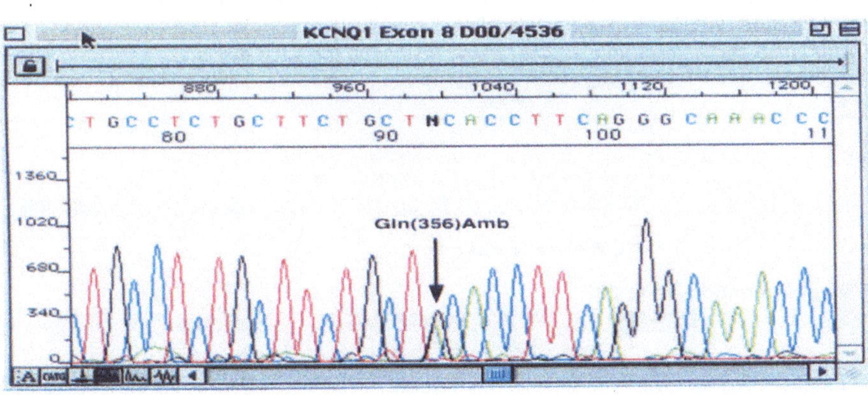

Figure 3. *(see Chapter 1, p. 8) Sequence analysis. A DNA mutation was found leading to a change from aminoacid glutamine to a full stop at position 356. The result is an incomplete non-functional ion channel protein (KCNQ1) that causes the long QT syndrome type 1 (Romano-Ward syndrome) in this patient.*

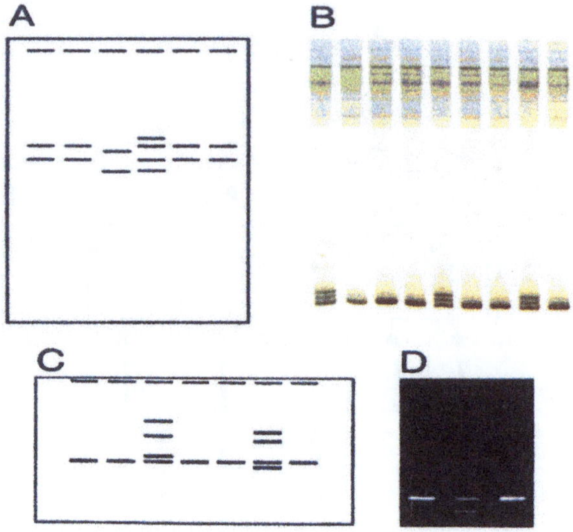

Figure 4. (see Chapter 1, p. 9) *SSCP-analysis. The theoretical change in mobility is shown (figure 4a). Normally 2 bands are visible, the sense and the antisense strand of the DNA (controls in lanes 1,2,5 and 6). If a DNA fragment is homzygously mutated, theoretically 2 new bands might appear since both sense and antisense DNA changes for both alleles (lane 3). In case of a heterozygote (one normal and one mutated gene, lane 4), a total of four bands can be seen. Figure 4b shows a base deletion at position 754 in the HERG gene of a Long-QT2 patient. Affected family members are shown in lanes 1, 5 and 8. Figure 4c shows a theoretical DGGE analysis. Mutants are seen in lanes 3 and 6, revealing homo and heteroduplexes. Figure 4d shows a N543H heterozygous mutation in the LDL receptor gene (lane 2) causing familial hypercholesterolemia compared to control DNA (lane 1 and 3). The aberrant homo and heteroduplexes are clearly visible on this DGGE gel.*

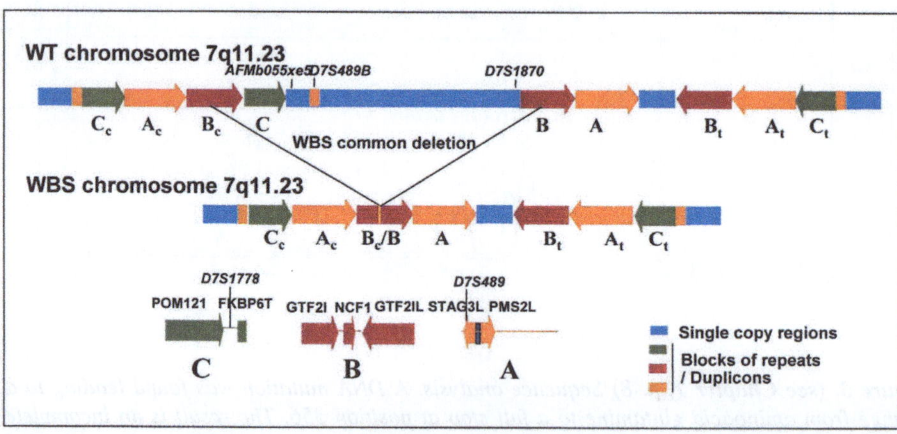

Figure 2 (see Chapter 10, p. 116) *Schematic representation of the 7q11.23 genomic region. The single copy region that is commonly deleted in WBS patients (blue square from AFMb055xe5 to D7S1870 in the upper panel) contains 25-30 genes and is flanked by a complex arrangement of blocks of chromosome 7-specific low copy repeats or duplicons*

(called A, B and C) [47]. The arrow orientation from centromere to telomere of the middle duplicons is arbitrarily depicted as a reference for the relative orientation of the centromeric (A_c, B_c, C_c) and telomeric (A_t, B_t, C_t) blocks.The location of single copy polymorphic markers that internally limit the deleted interval (AFMb055xe5 and D7S1870) and two multiple copy polymorphic loci (D7S489 and D7S1778) within the duplicons are indicated. Most WBS chromosomes (middle panel) arise as a consequence of unequal recombination between the centromeric B_c and middle B duplicons. The lower panel shows the gene/pseudogene composition of each putatively ancestral duplicon. Block A contains sequences related to the PMS2 mismatch repair gene (PMS2L) and the stromal antigen 3 gene (STAG3L) that are also present in other chromosome 7 locations. Block B contains the GTF2I, NCF1 genes, and another gene related to GTF2I (GTF2IL). Block C comprises the POM121 gene and the four first exons of FKBP6.

Next page:

Figure 1 (see Chapter 17, p. 200) *Arrhythmogenic right ventricular cardiomyopathy and sudden death in a 25 year old young man.*
a) Basal ECG with complete right bundle branch block and inverted T waves in precordial leads. b) Run of ventricular tachycardia. c) Four chamber cut of the heart specimen with massive fatty infiltration of the right ventricular free wall which appears translucent.
d) Histology of the right ventricular free wall at panoramic view: note the transmural fibro-fatty replacement. Azan stain original magnification x6.

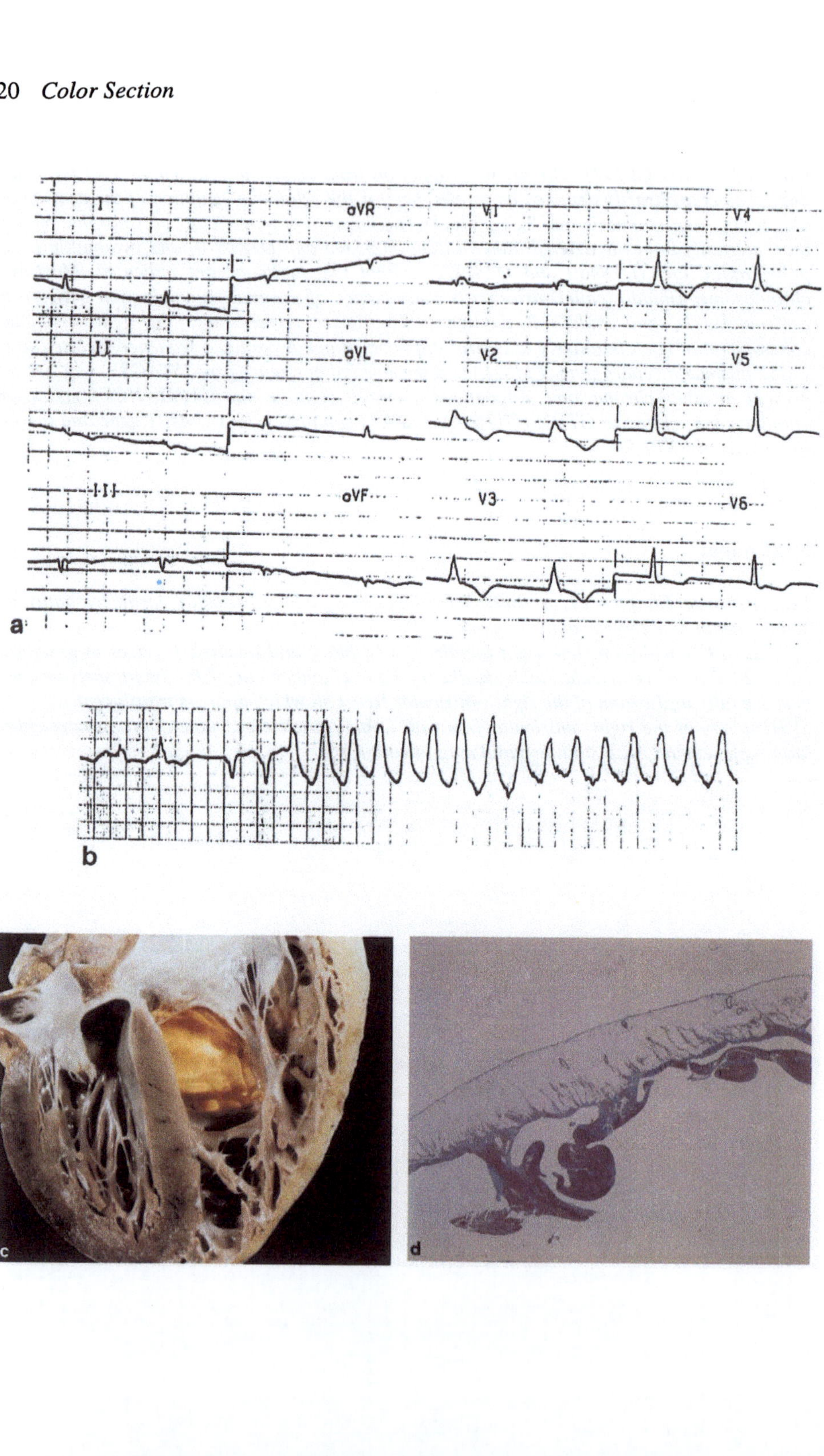
I
aVR
V1
V4
II
aVL
V2
V5
III
aVF
V3
V6
a
b
c
d

INDEX

INDEX

Developments in Cardiovascular Medicine

138. A.-M. Salmasi and A.S. Iskandrian (eds.): *Cardiac Output and Regional Flow in Health and Disease.* 1993 ISBN 0-7923-1911-7
139. J.H. Kingma, N.M. van Hemel and K.I. Lie (eds.): *Atrial Fibrillation, a Treatable Disease?* 1992 ISBN 0-7923-2008-5
140. B. Ostadel and N.S. Dhalla (eds.): *Heart Function in Health and Disease.* Proceedings of the Cardiovascular Program (Prague, Czechoslovakia, 1991). 1992 ISBN 0-7923-2052-2
141. D. Noble and Y.E. Earm (eds.): *Ionic Channels and Effect of Taurine on the Heart.* Proceedings of an International Symposium (Seoul, Korea, 1992). 1993 ISBN 0-7923-2199-5
142. H.M. Piper and C.J. Preusse (eds.): *Ischemia-reperfusion in Cardiac Surgery.* 1993 ISBN 0-7923-2241-X
143. J. Roelandt, E.J. Gussenhoven and N. Bom (eds.): *Intravascular Ultrasound.* 1993 ISBN 0-7923-2301-7
144. M.E. Safar and M.F. O'Rourke (eds.): *The Arterial System in Hypertension.* 1993 ISBN 0-7923-2343-2
145. P.W. Serruys, D.P. Foley and P.J. de Feyter (eds.): *Quantitative Coronary Angio- graphy in Clinical Practice.* With a Foreword by Spencer B. King III. 1994 ISBN 0-7923-2368-8
146. J. Candell-Riera and D. Ortega-Alcalde (eds.): *Nuclear Cardiology in Everyday Practice.* 1994 ISBN 0-7923-2374-2
147. P. Cummins (ed.): *Growth Factors and the Cardiovascular System.* 1993 ISBN 0-7923-2401-3
148. K. Przyklenk, R.A. Kloner and D.M. Yellon (eds.): *Ischemic Preconditioning: The Concept of Endogenous Cardioprotection.* 1993 ISBN 0-7923-2410-2
149. T.H. Marwick: *Stress Echocardiography.* Its Role in the Diagnosis and Evaluation of Coronary Artery Disease. 1994 ISBN 0-7923-2579-6
150. W.H. van Gilst and K.I. Lie (eds.): *Neurohumoral Regulation of Coronary Flow.* Role of the Endothelium. 1993 ISBN 0-7923-2588-5
151. N. Sperelakis (ed.): *Physiology and Pathophysiology of the Heart.* 3rd rev. ed. 1994 ISBN 0-7923-2612-1
152. J.C. Kaski (ed.): *Angina Pectoris with Normal Coronary Arteries: Syndrome X.* 1994 ISBN 0-7923-2651-2
153. D.R. Gross: *Animal Models in Cardiovascular Research.* 2nd rev. ed. 1994 ISBN 0-7923-2712-8
154. A.S. Iskandrian and E.E. van der Wall (eds.): *Myocardial Viability.* Detection and Clinical Relevance. 1994 ISBN 0-7923-2813-2
155. J.H.C. Reiber and P.W. Serruys (eds.): *Progress in Quantitative Coronary Arteriography.* 1994 ISBN 0-7923-2814-0
156. U. Goldbourt, U. de Faire and K. Berg (eds.): *Genetic Factors in Coronary Heart Disease.* 1994 ISBN 0-7923-2752-7
157. G. Leonetti and C. Cuspidi (eds.): *Hypertension in the Elderly.* 1994 ISBN 0-7923-2852-3
158. D. Ardissino, S. Savonitto and L.H. Opie (eds.): *Drug Evaluation in Angina Pectoris.* 1994 ISBN 0-7923-2897-3
159. G. Bkaily (ed.): *Membrane Physiopathology.* 1994 ISBN 0-7923-3062-5
160. R.C. Becker (ed.): *The Modern Era of Coronary Thrombolysis.* 1994 ISBN 0-7923-3063-3
161. P.J. Walter (ed.): *Coronary Bypass Surgery in the Elderly.* Ethical, Economical and Quality of Life Aspects. With a foreword by N.K. Wenger. 1995 ISBN 0-7923-3188-5
162. J.W. de Jong and R. Ferrari (eds.), *The Carnitine System.* A New Therapeutical Approach to Cardiovascular Diseases. 1995 ISBN 0-7923-3318-7
163. C.A. Neill and E.B. Clark: *The Developing Heart: A "History' of Pediatric Cardiology.* 1995 ISBN 0-7923-3375-6
164. N. Sperelakis: *Electrogenesis of Biopotentials in the Cardiovascular System.* 1995 ISBN 0-7923-3398-5
165. M. Schwaiger (ed.): *Cardiac Positron Emission Tomography.* 1995 ISBN 0-7923-3417-5
166. E.E. van der Wall, P.K. Blanksma, M.G. Niemeyer and A.M.J. Paans (eds.): *Cardiac Positron Emission Tomography.* Viability, Perfusion, Receptors and Cardiomyopathy. 1995 ISBN 0-7923-3472-8
167. P.K. Singal, I.M.C. Dixon, R.E. Beamish and N.S. Dhalla (eds.): *Mechanism of Heart Failure.* 1995 ISBN 0-7923-3490-6
168. N.S. Dhalla, P.K. Singal, N. Takeda and R.E. Beamish (eds.): *Pathophysiology of Heart Failure.* 1995 ISBN 0-7923-3571-6
169. N.S. Dhalla, G.N. Pierce, V. Panagia and R.E. Beamish (eds.): *Heart Hypertrophy and Failure.* 1995 ISBN 0-7923-3572-4

Developments in Cardiovascular Medicine

170. S.N. Willich and J.E. Muller (eds.): *Triggering of Acute Coronary Syndromes.* Implications for Prevention. 1995 ISBN 0-7923-3605-4
171. E.E. van der Wall, T.H. Marwick and J.H.C. Reiber (eds.): *Advances in Imaging Techniques in Ischemic Heart Disease.* 1995 ISBN 0-7923-3620-8
172. B. Swynghedauw: *Molecular Cardiology for the Cardiologist.* 1995 ISBN 0-7923-3622-4
173. C.A. Nienaber and U. Sechtem (eds.): *Imaging and Intervention in Cardiology.* 1996 ISBN 0-7923-3649-6
174. G. Assmann (ed.): *HDL Deficiency and Atherosclerosis.* 1995 ISBN 0-7923-8888-7
175. N.M. van Hemel, F.H.M. Wittkampf and H. Ector (eds.): *The Pacemaker Clinic of the 90's.* Essentials in Brady-Pacing. 1995 ISBN 0-7923-3688-7
176. N. Wilke (ed.): *Advanced Cardiovascular MRI of the Heart and Great Vessels.* Forthcoming. ISBN 0-7923-3720-4
177. M. LeWinter, H. Suga and M.W. Watkins (eds.): *Cardiac Energetics: From Emax to Pressure-volume Area.* 1995 ISBN 0-7923-3721-2
178. R.J. Siegel (ed.): *Ultrasound Angioplasty.* 1995 ISBN 0-7923-3722-0
179. D.M. Yellon and G.J. Gross (eds.): *Myocardial Protection and the K_{ATP} Channel.* 1995 ISBN 0-7923-3791-3
180. A.V.G. Bruschke, J.H.C. Reiber, K.I. Lie and H.J.J. Wellens (eds.): *Lipid Lowering Therapy and Progression of Coronary Atherosclerosis.* 1996 ISBN 0-7923-3807-3
181. A.-S.A. Abd-Eyattah and A.S. Wechsler (eds.): *Purines and Myocardial Protection.* 1995 ISBN 0-7923-3831-6
182. M. Morad, S. Ebashi, W. Trautwein and Y. Kurachi (eds.): *Molecular Physiology and Pharmacology of Cardiac Ion Channels and Transporters.* 1996 ISBN 0-7923-3913-4
183. M.A. Oto (ed.): *Practice and Progress in Cardiac Pacing and Electrophysiology.* 1996 ISBN 0-7923-3950-9
184. W.H. Birkenhäger (ed.): *Practical Management of Hypertension.* Second Edition. 1996 ISBN 0-7923-3952-5
185. J.C. Chatham, J.R. Forder and J.H. McNeill (eds.): *The Heart in Diabetes.* 1996 ISBN 0-7923-4052-3
186. J.H.C. Reiber and E.E. van der Wall (eds.): *Cardiovascular Imaging.* 1996 ISBN 0-7923-4109-0
187. A-M. Salmasi and A. Strano (eds.): *Angiology in Practice.* 1996 ISBN 0-7923-4143-0
188. M.W. Kroll and M.H. Lehmann (eds.): *Implantable Cardioverter Defibrillator Therapy: The Engineering – Clinical Interface.* 1996 ISBN 0-7923-4300-X
189. K.L. March (ed.): *Gene Transfer in the Cardiovascular System.* Experimental Approaches and Therapeutic Implications. 1996 ISBN 0-7923-9859-9
190. L. Klein (ed.): *Coronary Stenosis Morphology: Analysis and Implication.* 1997 ISBN 0-7923-9867-X
191. J.E. Pérez and R.M. Lang (eds.): *Echocardiography and Cardiovascular Function: Tools for the Next Decade.* 1997 ISBN 0-7923-9884-X
192. A.A. Knowlton (ed.): *Heat Shock Proteins and the Cardiovascular System.* 1997 ISBN 0-7923-9910-2
193. R.C. Becker (ed.): *The Textbook of Coronary Thrombosis and Thrombolysis.* 1997 ISBN 0-7923-9923-4
194. R.M. Mentzer, Jr., M. Kitakaze, J.M. Downey and M. Hori (eds.): *Adenosine, Cardioprotection and Its Clinical Application.* 1997 ISBN 0-7923-9954-4
195. N.H.J. Pijls and B. De Bruyne: *Coronary Pressure.* 1997 ISBN 0-7923-4672-6
196. I. Graham, H. Refsum, I.H. Rosenberg and P.M. Ueland (eds.): *Homocysteine Metabolism: from Basic Science to Clinical Medicine.* 1997 ISBN 0-7923-9983-8
197. E.E. van der Wall, V. Manger Cats and J. Baan (eds.): *Vascular Medicine – From Endothelium to Myocardium.* 1997 ISBN 0-7923-4740-4
198. A. Lafont and E. Topol (eds.): *Arterial Remodeling.* A Critical Factor in Restenosis. 1997 ISBN 0-7923-8008-8
199. M. Mercury, D.D. McPherson, H. Bassiouny and S. Glagov (eds.): *Non-Invasive Imaging of Atherosclerosis* 1998 ISBN 0-7923-8036-3
200. W.C. De Mello and M.J. Janse (eds.): *Heart Cell Communication in Health and Disease.* 1997 ISBN 0-7923-8052-5

Developments in Cardiovascular Medicine

201. P.E. Vardas (ed.): *Cardiac Arrhythmias Pacing and Electrophysiology.* The Expert View. 1998 ISBN 0-7923-4908-3
202. E.E. van der Wall, P.K. Blanksma, M.G. Niemeyer, W. Vaalburg and H.J.G.M. Crijns (eds.): *Advanced Imaging in Coronary Artery Disease.* PET, SPECT, MRI, IVUS, EBCT. 1998 ISBN 0-7923-5083-9
203. R.L. Wilenski (ed.): *Unstable Coronary Artery Syndromes, Pathophysiology, Diagnosis and Treatment.* 1998 ISBN 0-7923-8201-3
204. J.H.C. Reiber and E.E. van der Wall (eds.): *What's New in Cardiovascular Imaging?* 1998 ISBN 0-7923-5121-5
205. J.C. Kaski and D.W. Holt (eds.): *Myocardial Damage.* Early Detection by Novel Biochemical Markers. 1998 ISBN 0-7923-5140-1
206. M. Malik (ed.): *Clinical Guide to Cardiac Autonomic Tests.* 1998 ISBN 0-7923-5178-9
207. G.F. Baxter and D.M. Yellon (eds.): *Delayed Preconditioning and Adaptive Cardioprotection.* 1998 ISBN 0-7923-5259-9
208. B. Swynghedauw: *Molecular Cardiology for the Cardiologist, Second Edition.* 1998 ISBN 0-7923-8323-0
209. G. Burnstock, J.G. Dobson, Jr., B.T. Liang, J. Linden (eds.): *Cardiovascular Biology of Purines.* 1998 ISBN 0-7923-8334-6
210. B.D. Hoit and R.A. Walsh (eds.): *Cardiovascular Physiology in the Genetically Engineered Mouse.* 1998 ISBN 0-7923-8356-7
211. P. Whittaker and G.S. Abela (eds.): *Direct Myocardial Revascularization: History, Methodology, Technology.* 1998 ISBN 0-7923-8398-2
212. C.A. Nienaber and R. Fattori (eds.): *Diagnosis and Treatment of Aortic Diseases.* 1999 ISBN 0-7923-5517-2
213. J.C. Kaski (ed.): *Chest Pain with Normal Coronary Angiograms: Pathogenesis, Diagnosis and Management.* 1999 ISBN 0-7923-8421-0
214. P.A. Doevendans, R.S. Reneman and M. van Bilsen (eds.): *Cardiovascular Specific Gene Expression.* 1999 ISBN 0-7923-5633-0
215. G. Pons-Lladó, F. Carreras, X. Borrás, M. Subirana and L.J. Jiménez-Borreguero (eds.): *Atlas of Practical Cardiac Applications of MRI.* 1999 ISBN 0-7923-5636-5
216. L.W. Klein and J.E. Calvin: *Resource Ultilization in Cardiac Disease.* 1999 ISBN 0-7923-8509-8
217. R. Gorlin, G. Dangas, P.K. Toutouzas and M.M. Konstadoulaks: *Contemporary Concepts in Cardiology, Pathophysiology and Clinical Management.* 1999 ISBN 0-7923-8514-4
218. S. Gupta and A.J. Camm: *Chronic Infection, Chlamydia and Coronary Heart Disease.* 1999 ISBN 0-7923-5797-3
219. M. Rajskina: *Ventricular Fibrillation in Sudden Cardiac Death.* 1999 ISBN 0-7923-8570-5
220. Z. Abedin and R. Conner: *Interpretation of Cardiac Arrhythmias: Self Assessment Approach.* 1999 ISBN 0-7923-8576-4
221. J.E. Lock, J.F. Keane and S.B. Perry (eds.): *Diagnostic and Interventional Catheterization in Congenital Heart Disease, second edition.* 1999 ISBN 0-7923-8597-7
222. J.S. Steinberg (ed.): *Atrial Fibrillation after Cardiac Surgery.* 1999 ISBN 0-7923-8655-8
223. E.E. van der Wall, A. van der Laarse, B.M. Pluim and A.V.G. Bruschke (eds.): *Left Ventricular Hypertrophy.* Physiology versus Pathology. 1999 ISBN 0-7923-6038-9
224. J.F. Keaney, Jr. (ed.): *Oxidative Stress and Vascular Disease.* 1999 ISBN 0-7923-8678-7
225. R.G. Masters (ed.): *Surgical Options for the Treatment of Heart Failure.* 2000 ISBN 0-7923-6130-X
226. A.E. Iskandrian and E.E. van der Wall: *Myocardial Viability. 2nd Completely Revised Edition.* 2000 ISBN 0-7923-6161-X
227. N.H.J. Pijls and B. De Bruyne: *Coronary Pressure.* Second Edition. 2000 ISBN 0-7923-6170-9
228. B.E. Jaski: *Basics of Heart Failure.* A Problem Solving Approach. 2000 ISBN 0-7923-7786-9
229. H.-H. Osterhues, V. Hombach and A.J. Moss (eds.): *Advances in Noninvasive Electrocardiographic Monitoring Techniques.* 2000 ISBN 0-7923-6214-4
230. K. Robinson (ed.): *Homocysteine and Vascular Disease.* 2000 ISBN 0-7923-6248-9
231. C.I. Berul and J.A. Towbin (eds.): *Molecular Genetics of Cardiac Electrophysiology.* 2000 ISBN 0-7923-7829-6

Developments in Cardiovascular Medicine

232. A. Bayés de Luna, F. Furlanello, B.J. Maron and D.P. Zipes (eds.): *Arrhythmias and Sudden Death in Athletes*. 2000 ISBN 0-7923-6337-X
233. J-C. Tardif and M.G. Bourassa (eds.): *Antioxidants and Cardiovascular Disease*. 2000 ISBN 0-7923-6564-X
234. J. Candell-Riera, J. Castell-Conesa and S. Aguandé-Bruix (eds.): *Myocardium at Risk and Viable Myocardium*. Evaluation by SPET. 2000 ISBN 0-7923-6724-3
235. M.H. Ellestad and E. Amsterdam (eds.): *Exercise Testing*. Current Concepts and Recent Advances. 2001 ISBN 0-7923-7378-2
236. D.L. Mann (eds.): *The Role of Inflammatory Mediators in the Failing Heart*. 2001 ISBN 0-7923-7381-2

Previous volumes are still available

KLUWER ACADEMIC PUBLISHERS – DORDRECHT / BOSTON / LONDON

MIX
Papier aus verantwortungsvollen Quellen
Paper from responsible sources
FSC® C105338

If you have any concerns about our products,
you can contact us on
ProductSafety@springernature.com

In case Publisher is established outside the EU,
the EU authorized representative is:
Springer Nature Customer Service Center GmbH
Europaplatz 3, 69115 Heidelberg, Germany

Printed by Libri Plureos GmbH
in Hamburg, Germany